The Road to Universal Health Coverage

Innovation, Equity, and the New Health Economy

EDITED BY

Jeffrey L. Sturchio

Ilona Kickbusch

Louis Galambos

WITH

Christian Franz

FOREWORD BY

Tedros Adhanom Ghebreyesus

Director-General, World Health Organization

JOHNS HOPKINS UNIVERSITY PRESS BALTIMORE

© 2018 Johns Hopkins University Press
All rights reserved. Published 2018
Printed in the United States of America on acid-free paper
9 8 7 6 5 4 3 2 1

Johns Hopkins University Press
2715 North Charles Street
Baltimore, Maryland 21218-4363
www.press.jhu.edu

Library of Congress Cataloging-in-Publication Data

Names: Sturchio, Jeffrey L. (Jeffrey Louis), 1952– editor. | Kickbusch, Ilona, 1948– editor. |
    Galambos, Louis, editor.
Title: The road to universal health coverage : innovation, equity, and the new health economy /
    edited by Jeffrey L. Sturchio, Ilona Kickbusch, and Louis Galambos with Christian Franz ;
    foreword by Tedros Adhanom Ghebreyesus.
Description: Baltimore : Johns Hopkins University Press, 2018. | Includes bibliographical
    references and index.
Identifiers: LCCN 2018041197 | ISBN 9781421429557 (pbk. : alk. paper) |
    ISBN 1421429551 (pbk. : alk. paper) | ISBN 9781421429564 (electronic) |
    ISBN 142142956X (electronic)
Subjects: | MESH: Universal Coverage | Insurance, Health—economics
Classification: LCC RA412.3 | NLM W 100 | DDC 368.38/2—dc23
LC record available at https://lccn.loc.gov/2018041197

A catalog record for this book is available from the British Library.

*Special discounts are available for bulk purchases of this book. For more information, please contact
Special Sales at 410-516-6936 or specialsales@press.jhu.edu.*

Johns Hopkins University Press uses environmentally friendly book materials, including
recycled text paper that is composed of at least 30 percent post-consumer waste, whenever
possible.

The Road to Universal Health Coverage

For Devi Sridhar:
fellow student of
global health.

J-L Shrchis
13.8.19

Contents

Foreword

All roads lead to universal health coverage—and this is our top priority at the World Health Organization (WHO). For me, the key question of universal health coverage is an ethical one. Do we want our fellow citizens to die because they are poor? Or millions of families to be impoverished by catastrophic health expenditures because they lack financial risk protection? Universal health coverage is a human right.[1]

There's no single path to universal health coverage, or UHC. All countries must find their own way, in the context of their own social, political, and economic circumstances. But the foundation everywhere must be a strong health system, based on primary care, with an emphasis on disease prevention and health promotion. Such health systems do not only provide the best health outcomes; they're also the best defense against outbreaks and other health emergencies. In that sense, UHC and health security are truly two sides of the same coin. There are many steps on the road to UHC. But the key is political commitment.[2]

To bring this commitment about and transform it into action, we need to convince more than health policy makers alone. Financing health systems in a sustainable way, building a motivated health workforce, and establishing efficient institutions are challenges that need to be tackled in several policy fields.

This book makes an important contribution in this regard. The health economy it conceptualizes aims at a comprehensive perspective on the contribution of health to stable economic prosperity. The work of the United Nations High-Level Commission on Health Employment and Economic Growth showed not only how urgently countries need to invest in the education and training of health workers; it also revealed how important health workers are for countries' economic growth.

This message is a vital one: Health cannot be left to health ministers alone. Ministers of finance and of the economy need to be involved, too. Their policies can have a profound impact on the health of the population and on how equitable health system reforms turn out to be.

In a similar way, the private sector has a crucial role. Research and development for new medicines and diagnostic tools is just one area where private sector investments are needed. While health financing is the role of the public sector in most countries, private sector actors can facilitate efficient supply chains, health service delivery, and infrastructure investments. However, strong public stewardship is necessary to harness this potential of the private sector. This book gives some evidence of how barriers to private sector involvement can be overcome.

From a health perspective, the idea of a broad health economy allows us to point to the importance of health in many (if not most) of the Sustainable Development Goals (SDGs) adopted by the 70th United Nations General Assembly in 2015.

The WHO's 13th General Programme of Work is based on the SDGs and is designed to help countries stay on track toward Goal 3 and the other health-related targets. Its three strategic priorities—universal health coverage, health security, and improved health and well-being—encapsulate this commitment. We at the WHO have also developed an impact framework to enable us to measure progress and remain focused on outcomes rather than outputs.[3]

Tedros Adhanom Ghebreyesus
Director-General, World Health Organization

REFERENCES

1. Tedros Adhanom Ghebreyesus, "All Roads Lead to Universal Health Coverage," http://www.who.int/news-room/commentaries/detail/all-roads-lead-to-universal-health-coverage. Originally published in *Lancet Global Health* 5, no. 9 (September 2017): e839–40.
2. Tedros Adhanom Ghebreyesus, address (UHC Roundtable, Abuja, Nigeria, April 12, 2018), http://www.who.int/dg/speeches/2018/uhc-roundtable/en/.
3. Tedros Adhanom Ghebreyesus, address (Launch of Sustainable Development Goals–themed issue of the *Bulletin of the World Health Organization*, Geneva, Switzerland, August 31, 2018), http://www.who.int/dg/speeches/2018/sustainable-development-goals-who-bulletin-launch/en/.

Preface

The road to universal health coverage (UHC) has become a central theme in global public health in recent years as countries large and small, rich and poor, contemplate how to extend healthcare to more of their citizens in a way that guards against the risk of catastrophic out-of-pocket expenditures, improves health outcomes equitably, and uses available resources efficiently. As United Nations member states contemplate the new agenda around the post-2015 Sustainable Development Goals, UHC has been adopted as a target to capture the degree to which different societies are realizing their ambition to provide "health for all."

Of course, countries will differ in the way they address UHC, based on a wide range of factors—political, economic, social, epidemiological, and technical. But the concept is here to stay, and multilateral organizations, their member states, civil society, and the private sector are engaged in lively and critical debates about the meaning of UHC and the mechanisms and resources required to achieve it by 2030.

With these thoughts in mind, the Global Health Centre at the Graduate Institute of International and Development Studies in Geneva, Switzerland; the Johns Hopkins Institute for Applied Economics, Global Health, and the Study of Business Enterprise in Baltimore, Maryland; and Rabin Martin, a global health strategy consultancy based in New York and London, embarked on a collaboration in 2014, together with a working group of advisors from academe, civil society, and the public and private sectors, to explore several critical dimensions of the transition to UHC. Our starting point was the insight that health and healthcare constitute a major economic force in most countries. This "health economy," estimated to account for roughly 10% of global gross domestic product, comprises all stakeholders concerned with and involved in issues related to efficiency, effectiveness, values, and behaviors in health and healthcare. The diverse actors who participate in the health economy shape the health of populations and the delivery of health services, while also ensuring linkages with the wider macroeconomic, social, and political context.

Our goal was to spark lively discussion of this dimension of complex health systems that could help countries bring new resources and new partners into their efforts to move toward UHC. How should policy makers think about the dynamism, the opportunities, and the risks of this new health economy? How could attention to the health economy drive innovation and improve equity in the supply of health services to all, beginning with a focus on primary healthcare? What capabilities and growth opportunities are private companies and private providers bringing to the challenges of expanding delivery of essential health services? This book explores these and related questions through a series of chapters that frame the debate, with accompanying case studies that illustrate the sometimes-controversial dimensions of the innovative roles the private sector can play in helping countries achieve UHC.

The editors acknowledge the helpful insights, generous assistance, and thoughtful engagement of many colleagues and friends in the course of our joint work on this project. We thank the speakers and audience members at a series of advisory meetings and workshops we organized at the Graduate Institute for International and Development Studies in Geneva in February 2014; at Johns Hopkins University in Baltimore, Maryland, in October 2014; at the World Health Summit in Berlin in October 2014, jointly with HANSHEP (Harnessing Non-State Actors for Better Health for the Poor), the German Healthcare Partnership (GHP), and the German Federal Ministry for Economic Cooperation and Development (BMZ); at the World Health Summit in Berlin in October 2015 (again jointly with the BMZ and GHP); and at the World Health Summit in Berlin in October 2016 (jointly with the GHP and the M8 Alliance). We are also grateful to the speakers and audiences at a series of panel discussions we organized in conjunction with the World Health Assembly in Geneva in May 2015; the United Nations General Assembly in New York in September 2015; the Corporate Council on Africa's 10th Biennial US-Africa Business Summit in Addis Ababa, Ethiopia, in February 2016; the World Health Assembly in Geneva in May 2016; and the World Health Assembly in Geneva in May 2018. These dialogues afforded us useful opportunities to test and sharpen our ideas on the private sector and UHC and to gain additional critical perspectives from an important cross section of key stakeholders. An authors' workshop in Geneva in January 2018 helped us to shape the book's final form.

Without the indefatigable support of colleagues closer to home, this project and publication would not have been possible. We thank Christian Franz of CPC Analytics in Berlin, Germany, for his collaboration throughout the project, particularly for his persistence in helping the authors and editors complete their work. Tanya Mounier, who was, at the time, head of Rabin Martin's Geneva office, played a central role in generating and sustaining momentum during the early stages. At the Geneva Graduate Institute, Michaela Told and Lyndsey Canham were indispensable, as were Martina Szabo, Tina Flores, Kathy Chase-Gaudreau, and Nina Grigoriev at Rabin Martin. Others who also contributed to a series of annotated bibliographies on UHC included Luke Allen, Thorsten Behrendt, Sahil Deo, Amanda Fales, Rebecca Hoppy, Isabelle Lindenmayer, and Ayjeren Rozyjumayeva. At Johns Hopkins, Jim Ashton provided astute and skillful editorial help in shaping the early drafts of the chapters. Robin Coleman and his colleagues at Johns Hopkins University Press, particularly Juliana McCarthy and Robert M. Brown, have been exemplary publishing partners. We also gratefully acknowledge the support of unrestricted educational grants from the International Federation of Pharmaceutical Manufacturers and Associations; Merck KGaA, Darmstadt, Germany; Novartis Pharmaceuticals; Pfizer Inc.; and Pharmaceutical Research and Manufacturers of America.

The Road to Universal Health Coverage

The Road to Universal Health Coverage

Progress, Prospects, and the Private Sector

Jeffrey L. Sturchio and Louis Galambos

In September 2015, the 70th United Nations General Assembly adopted the Sustainable Development Goals (SDGs), which provide a framework for promoting greater equity and prosperity around the world. This remarkable achievement, which entailed the 193 Member States agreeing to a set of 17 goals and 169 targets, was hard won.[1] Health for All is the objective of Goal 3—"ensure healthy lives and promote well-being for all at all ages"—a vision first articulated at Alma-Ata 40 years ago. For many in the global health community, the inclusion of universal health coverage (UHC) as target 3.8 in the health goal was particularly significant. The World Health Organization's (WHO) definition of UHC "means that all people and communities can use the promotive, preventive, curative, rehabilitative and palliative health services they need, of sufficient quality to be effective, while also ensuring that the use of these services does not expose the user to financial hardship."[2] Indeed, some would argue that UHC is at the heart of the SDGs, for it is the only way to ensure greater health quality and equity in all countries around the world. According to Dr. Tedros Adhanom Ghebreyesus, director-general of the WHO: "All roads lead to universal health coverage—and this is our top priority at WHO. For me, the key question of universal health coverage is an ethical one. Do we want our fellow citizens to die because they are poor? Or millions of families impoverished by catastrophic health expenditures because they lack financial risk protection? Universal health coverage is a human right." UHC, Dr. Tedros observes, "is ultimately a political choice. It is the responsibility of every country and national government to pursue it."[3]

Like many ambitious global goals, UHC remains an aspiration for many countries. Today, the WHO estimates that half the world's population continues to be without access to basic health services.[4] Moreover, this already staggering number masks inequities that continue to exist from country to country: gaps between rich and poor, men and women, young and old, and among people of different ethnic backgrounds. UHC promises to give people greater access to higher quality health services without the fear of financial hardship. But the task of turning this vision into a reality poses a significant challenge for countries, rich and poor alike.[5]

Each country will chart its own course to UHC, deciding which health services to cover, who will be covered, how to pay for those services, and how to ensure effective and efficient delivery.[6] Already, more than 100 countries have begun to make efforts toward this goal—some with more success than others.[7] Some will need help. As we know, many of the countries that are still striving to achieve modern economic development cannot do this alone. Weak health infrastructures, a lack of trained health workers, poor financing, fragile economies, and the high burdens of infectious diseases and chronic illness will continue to pose challenges, particularly in lower- and middle-income countries.

If we look at the experience of countries that have achieved some measure of universal health coverage, we can see several important lessons about successful implementation: top to bottom political commitment is needed; adequate sources of health system financing must be acquired and secured; the institutional capacity to expand services must be strengthened; and the nongovernmental sectors—nongovernmental organizations (NGOs) and private firms—will have to be engaged in planning and delivering on the promise of UHC. The vigorous support of NGOs and the sustained engagement of the private sector can give the movement to achieve UHC the political, economic, and social momentum it needs.[8] Some policy analysts and advocates are both skeptical and cautious in considering the prospects for engaging more extensively with the private sector on the path to UHC, wondering if the risks and costs of this path might hinder expansion of equitable access to all. In a provocative commentary on the "perils and possibilities of the private health sector," Richard Horton and Stephanie Clark argue:

Our collective goal should not be to arrive at some settled ideological position either for or against the private sector. Instead, we should keep the objective of universal health coverage firmly in mind, ensuring that whatever mix of public and private health provision exists in a particular setting meets that goal. What we do know is that the public and private sectors cannot be seen as mutually exclusive entities within a health system. Each depends upon the other, and the performance of one is often intimately linked to the performance of the other. Public and private sectors therefore should be viewed as entwined elements of a whole health system, and managed as such.[9]

With this sense of the importance of understanding how a mixed health system works in practice very much in mind, we probe these issues in the rest of this book. We begin with a brief historical review of the ideal of universal health coverage from its nineteenth-century origins through the vision of "health for all" at Alma-Ata in 1978, to the recent incorporation of UHC into the SDGs. While the goal remains elusive in many countries, there are certainly examples of success to emulate. We consider these successful ventures as well as the movement's major challenges.

The successes encourage us to look at the global health economy from a fresh perspective, one that stresses the many positive aspects of developments currently satisfying important demands by providing new goods and services. The health sector is highly innovative in some countries and has made effective use of digital modes of communication, storage of information, and control. All other things being equal, economies that invest in health and provide strong healthcare services and outcomes bolster their human capital and are more successful over the long run. In an age in which the importance of human capital has at last been fully recognized, the role of the health economy is of central importance. As World Bank President Jim Yong Kim has said, "when you invest in human beings, you're putting in place the capital you need to grow your economies. . . . Investing in people *is* investing in economic growth."[10]

The emerging health systems also provide a remarkable array of jobs, including important work for women in a distinctly labor-intensive sector. In some countries, these jobs frequently provide entry points for workers who are interested in improving their standing in the technologically advanced healthcare sector. In societies that lack adequate educational facilities, on-the-job training can help boost the capabilities of the workforce and promote economic growth.

Some of these employees will strengthen both the public and the private sectors. Our sweep through the UHC experience points directly to the current-day importance of private involvement in healthcare around the world. Given their established positions, resources, and medical capabilities, these private firms and professionals need to be brought into the UHC movement at the planning and the implementation stages. As our contributors point out, private sector actors are already experimenting with a wide range of initiatives that have yet to receive the attention they deserve. In many cases, dynamic health markets are leading to improvements in population health, and public-private partnerships have emerged as important contributors to the UHC movement.[11]

What are the conditions required for countries to begin to translate their successful experiences and policy promises into practical results for population health? We look to the political, economic, and social implications of moving from aspiration to implementation. Throughout, we attempt to be realistic about the public and the private sectors' resources and capabilities. What range of capabilities are private providers and companies already bringing to the challenges of expanding delivery of essential health services to all? Which of those capabilities blend best with existing public institutions and programs? How can these trends be encouraged while ensuring appropriate attention to questions of governance, stewardship, and equity in evolving health systems? There are many opportunities ahead as companies continue to work with governments and civil society partners to help achieve the goal of UHC.

UHC Is Not New

In the nineteenth century, as modern economic development and rapid urbanization transformed European societies, their political leaders began to consider various means of improving the well-being of their populations.[12] In the new national state of Germany, Imperial Chancellor Otto von Bismarck introduced policies that he hoped would further unify the country and also fend off his socialist opponents. One of the most important of those policies was his Social Health Insurance Law in 1883. Part of a series of innovative welfare programs, the new insurance measure established local health bureaus and provided workers with sickness insurance. Britain and France were slow to follow Germany's lead, but both developed somewhat similar programs in the early twentieth century.[13]

World War II and its immediate aftermath produced the next decisive move toward expanded health coverage.[14] The horrors of the war, the Holocaust, and the enormous number of persons displaced in the 1940s created a new political and social environment for healthcare policy. Seeking to create international institutions that would help the world avoid another such disaster, the victorious allies and other nations combined to develop the United Nations and its associated organizations, including the World Health Organization. The UN and the WHO set out a new global program aimed at closing the economic and healthcare gap between the developed and the developing nations. Initially, the gap in healthcare was actually growing as Britain, France, Germany, the Soviet Union, and the Scandinavian countries all developed national programs that provided vaccines and treatments for a range of conditions, eventually expanding coverage to more and more population groups and conditions as they built public health systems.

With the European and Soviet systems as models, the United Nations pushed forward with assistance to the developing countries in Africa, Asia, and Latin America that were able to muster their own political and economic support for expanded healthcare. In the context of the Cold War between democratic capitalism and communism, the WHO, a growing array of NGOs and private sector actors, and many of the world's countries made substantial progress in overcoming the financial, social, and political barriers to universal care. These efforts reached what appeared to be a climax in an epochal International Conference on Primary Health Care in Alma-Ata, Kazakhstan. The conference produced a declaration that called for "Health for All," a goal that would be echoed decades later as universal health coverage.[15]

During the 1980s and 1990s, however, the global public health movement would focus largely on specific vertical programs for improving access to care and treatment—especially the great campaigns for vaccines, family planning, child survival, and then HIV/AIDS rather than on primary healthcare. Those campaigns experienced outstanding successes, but the objective of Health for All would never be forgotten. It reemerged as an element of the SDGs in the present century in response to a growing awareness that vertical programs would not work effectively in the long run.

The United Nations responded to the significant gaps and disparities in extending life expectancy and to the rising global expectations for health with a new global plan (the Millennium Development Goals) in 2000. The objectives, which ranged from eradicating extreme poverty and hunger to achieving universal primary education, also focused on health-related issues. These issues included reducing child mortality and improving maternal health while combating specific infectious diseases, especially HIV/AIDS, tuberculosis, and malaria. The target date was 2015, and while the progress was uneven across nations and within nations, the results were encouraging enough to persuade the UN and its many supporting organizations and governments to advance a new set of SDGs.[16] In the long history of joint efforts to combat mortality and morbidity, the SDGs, which revived the Alma-Ata plan to achieve Health for All, represented substantial progress toward UHC, with a health goal (SDG 3) that addresses the need to establish and strengthen health systems and not work only on disease-specific programs—and an explicit commitment to "leave no one behind."[17]

What Needs to Be Done?

The basic elements of universal health coverage have been well defined and carefully considered in a number of public health forums. Those nations, regions, and local societies that have made the most progress toward UHC all have efficient health systems that include effective primary healthcare.[18] Their healthcare institutions are well-staffed with trained health workers. Their staffs of physicians, nurses, and other workers have access to a package of essential medicines, technologies, and services. The system at all levels has sufficient and relatively stable financing over the long term. There is, as well, adequate financial support for patients to avoid catastrophic expenses. The best of these systems balance equity and quality, while ensuring access by their entire populations with no discrimination on the basis of gender, class, or ethnic origins. These systems are resilient and have successfully worked through the challenges posed by pandemics and by major shifts in global and national economies. They have also developed institutional mechanisms to encourage the adoption and diffusion of innovations in training and educating health workers, from community clinics to tertiary care facilities; in novel medications, vaccines, diagnostics, and medical devices; in service delivery; and in patient engagement and shared decision making. In practice, the systems are highly varied, with differing levels of efficiency and different degrees of comfort in incorporating the private provision of health services and supply of health products. We are seeing, however, an increasing trend toward developing mixed health systems that make effective use of the complementary skills and resources of the private as well as the public sector.

How the Private Sector Contributes to UHC

For those countries that have achieved a measure of success with UHC, two factors stand out. The countries with mixed public-private systems have done a better job, on average, of providing universal access to a package of essential health services; they have done so while maintaining a higher measure of financial protection than those that have relied solely on the public sector.[19] The most successful systems have found a variety of ways to integrate the private sector more fully with public resources. Nations as different as the United Kingdom and Thailand, which many take as paradigms of public sector health systems, rely heavily on the private sector in providing many forms of care to their citizens.[20]

Several of the chapters in this volume describe in some detail how the private sector—including companies large and small, academic hospital centers, private for-profit providers and not-for-profit providers as well—has improved access to health around the world.[21] From implementing childhood immunization programs, to training health workers, the private sector has been an enabler of better health for millions of communities. Seen in the context of UHC, these private programs have balanced the national policies and planning efforts, exercising a stabilizing influence. The private entities and the services they provide vary by country, from hospitals, clinics, and laboratories to drugs, vaccines, diagnostics, and medical devices, to ancillary services like ambulances and health insurance. Their quality varies from state-of-the-art facilities that attract patients from around the world to unlicensed drug vendors. All, however, combine to produce the global healthcare system we have and hope now to understand, improve, and extend until we are providing Health for All.

That goal will not be achieved if we are not mindful of the many ways the private sector has contributed and can continue to contribute to UHC. The paths charted by the private sector are many, and the chapters that follow detail some of them. Research and development is currently important, as are programs to improve policy and governance. Advances in technology can be of decisive importance, as can human resources management and workforce development. Capacity building, logistics and supply-chain management deserve attention, along with innovations in communications, marketing, and the financial mechanisms employed to help advance health. Companies are engaged in multisectoral partnerships to support countries trying to strengthen their health systems by training more health workers, developing new finance models, and building the body of knowledge that will be crucial to realizing the vision of UHC.

A few salient examples will give a better idea of what is already being done:

- Merck for Mothers and the Bill & Melinda Gates Foundation partnered with IntraHealth International and the Senegalese Ministry of Health and Social Action to scale up an innovative supply-chain model linking private suppliers—skilled in forecasting, ordering, and delivery of supplies—with health facilities to help maintain adequate stocks of a range of contraceptive options.
- In India, Unilever organized a hand-washing campaign during an important Hindu festival by distributing the bread known as roti with hand-washing messages to 5 million people.
- In Uganda, Merck KGaA worked with the Ministry of Health to launch an SMS mobile messaging campaign to raise awareness about diabetes.
- In several countries, Johnson & Johnson supports efforts to strengthen frontline health workers, including nurses, midwives, community health workers, and pharmacists.[22]

Why is the private sector pursuing opportunities to contribute to universal health coverage? The main reason is both simple and compelling: strong health systems are good for much more than health. They are also good for business. Weak supply chains, lack of regulatory harmonization, and insufficient human health resources, for example, create issues that companies grapple with constantly in developed and developing markets. Corporate social responsibility in this case is different and the difference is important. Building the health infrastructure encourages economic development and helps countries become better equipped to provide all of the services, private and public, required for healthier populations. Companies large and small have a vested interest in UHC because healthy employees help their businesses flourish.

Let us suggest five areas where collaborative efforts will pay off in coming years.

First, *in low- and middle-income countries, addressing the burden of chronic disease, including cancer, cardiovascular disease, diabetes, and respiratory conditions.* Like UHC, noncommunicable diseases (NCDs) are a key focus of the post-2015 sustainable development agenda. They collectively comprise a significant proportion of the global disease burden, so ramping up our work on them is critical to achieving UHC. We know that reducing risk factors for disease is an effective means of prevention; it is also less expensive to prevent than to treat disease. UHC fosters a greater focus on primary and secondary prevention, early detection, and management of chronic illness through the life course. Ultimately, the combination of these strategies will lead to better health outcomes and lower healthcare costs for individuals and their families, not to mention for economies overall.[23]

Second, we cannot forget *the challenge of neglected tropical diseases (NTDs)* such as river blindness, blinding trachoma, schistosomiasis, lymphatic filariasis, Guinea Worm, and others, which continue to plague the world's poorest people. Nor can we ignore emerging health threats such as Ebola and MERS, which tax all health systems but especially those in countries with already fragile health infrastructures and struggling economies.[24]

Third, to increase access to quality health services, we will need *to work with partners to muster private as well as public resources or the job will not get done.* Such mixed health systems must be able to withstand shocks such as natural disasters, disease outbreaks, and global economic crises that can devastate developed and developing nations' essential health services, including the management of chronic illness. If the private sector is a full partner in planning processes, governments and international institutions will be better prepared to address such crises in the years ahead.[25]

Fourth: building robust health workforces. *The lack of adequate numbers of trained health workers is arguably one of the biggest barriers to UHC implementation.* An estimated one billion people never see a health worker in their lifetimes. We must continue to increase the density and number of health workers at all levels, particularly in underserved and hard-to-reach areas. Especially as UHC is targeted more and more to the growing burden of noncommunicable diseases, the human resource challenges will be magnified. We have several opportunities to fully exploit the potential of the training and management of a wide range of frontline health workers, including physicians' assistants and community health workers. This is particularly applicable to management of hypertension and diabetes. Mobile devices and apps now provide health workers with new means of integrating their work into a national or regional system. But first, we need to be certain the health workers will be there to sustain care.[26]

Finally, to address the health system challenges in achieving UHC, *we should work to foster a new range of multisectoral partnerships to mobilize and share the knowledge, creativity, and resources of the public sector, private sector, and civil society alike.* Partnerships matter, particularly when they are embedded within national UHC plans. They help societies develop the dialogue and engagement necessary to establish trust and to find common ground on which to build innovative solutions. Ideally, those solutions will reach beyond the health sector. Policies and practices in the environment, transportation, information and communications, and education sectors, to note just a few obvious examples, have long-term implications for health and well-being. Without partnerships, we will not achieve UHC. With partnerships, particularly "partnerships for public purpose," we should be able to achieve the sustainable solutions that can make universal health coverage possible.[27]

The following chapters explore these issues in depth and provide guidelines to the new health economy, an economy full of promise as well as challenges. By focusing on the present and potential private sector contributions to UHC, we hope to broaden the global discussion and deepen our understanding of what needs to be done to achieve the global goal to "ensure healthy lives and promote well-being for all at all ages." That goal is simply stated and compelling, but the path to its attainment will be complex and deeply contested. In this book, readers will find critical perspectives and constructive suggestions that help to illuminate these issues. Good practices, cooperative behavior, and multisectoral partnerships will, we believe, enable societies to meet those challenges and realize the full promise of universal health coverage by 2030.

NOTES

1. "Transforming our world: the 2030 Agenda for Sustainable Development," resolution adopted by the UN General Assembly, September 25, 2015, A/Res/70/1 (New York: United Nations, 2015); http://www.un.org/ga/search/view_doc.asp?symbol=A/RES/70/1&Lang=E.

2. http://www.who.int/health_financing/universal_coverage_definition/en/; accessed July 3, 2018. The WHO definition of UHC embraces certain aspects of population-level coverage (clean air, for instance) that will be entirely in the public sector. Because we are focusing on specific ways to bring the private sector into the UHC movement, we have emphasized a somewhat narrower definition of the goal that focuses on health services. On Alma-Ata, see *Declaration of Alma-Ata: international conference on primary health care, Alma-Ata, USSR, 6–12 September 1978* (Geneva: World Health Organization, 1978); http://www.who.int/publications/almaata_declaration_en.pdf.

3. Tedros Adhanom Ghebreyesus, "All roads lead to universal health coverage," *Lancet Global Health* 5 (September 2017): e839–e840; at e839; http://dx.doi.org/10.1016/S2214-109X(17)30295-4. In a special report on UHC, *The Economist* agreed, noting that "the goal of universal basic health care is sensible, affordable and practical, even in poor countries." "Within reach," *The Economist*, 427 (April 28, 2018): 9; and John McDermott, "Special report—universal health care: an affordable necessity," special issue, *The Economist*, 427 (April 28, 2018); https://www.economist.com/special-report/2018/04/28/both-in-rich-and-poor-countries-universal-health-care-brings-huge-benefits. See also Ariel Pablos-Mendez, Karen Cavanaugh, and Caroline Ly, "The new era of health goals: universal health coverage as a pathway to the Sustainable Development Goals," *Health Systems & Reform* 2 (2016): 15–17.

4. *Tracking universal health coverage: 2017 global monitoring report* (Geneva and Washington, DC: World Health Organization and International Bank for Reconstruction and Development / World Bank, 2017): 14.

5. There is a positive income elasticity of health spending: as gross domestic product increases 1%, health spending goes up by 1.2%.

6. *World health report: Health systems financing: the path to universal health coverage* (Geneva: World Health Organization, 2010); *World health report 2013: research for universal health coverage* (Geneva: World Health Organization, 2013); *Arguing for universal health coverage* (Geneva: World Health Organization, 2013); *Together on the road to universal health coverage: a call to action*, WHO/HIS/HGF/17.1 (Geneva: World Health Organization; 2017); K. Xu, A. Soucat, J. Kutzin, et al., "New perspectives on global health spending for universal health coverage," WHO/HIS/HFG/HF Working Paper 18.2 (Geneva: World Health Organization, 2018); and World Bank, UNICEF, and the Japan International Cooperation Agency, *Business Unusual: Accelerating Progress towards Universal Health Coverage* (Washington, DC: World Bank, 2018).

7. The WHO maintains a data portal on universal health coverage with a wealth of data on country efforts to improve service coverage, financial protection, health system strengthening, health expenditures, and health equity. For an overview of the data, see http://apps.who.int/gho/portal/uhc-overview.jsp. Two other indispensable online resources on country efforts to achieve UHC are the Joint Learning Network, "[a] community of practitioners and policymakers from around the globe as well as a diverse group of international, regional, and local partners who share knowledge and co-develop new tools, guides and resources that address the practical challenges of health systems reform to achieve universal health coverage"; www.jointlearningnetwork.org/about-our-team; and UHC2030, "a multi-stakeholder platform that promotes collaborative working at global and country levels on health systems strengthening, . . .

advocate[s] increased political commitment to UHC and facilitate[s] accountability and knowledge sharing; www.uhc2030.org/about-us.

8. UHC has generated a robust and growing literature by academics, practitioners, and policy professionals. For a guide to this literature through 2016, see *Universal health coverage: an annotated bibliography,* May 2014; *Universal health coverage: annotated bibliography 2.0,* March 2015; and *Universal health coverage: an annotated bibliography 3.0—the new health economy,* May 2016 (all published in Geneva: Graduate Institute Global Health Centre / Rabin Martin / Johns Hopkins Institute for Applied Economics, Global Health, and the Study of Business Enterprise); http://graduateinstitute.ch/home/research/centresandprogrammes/globalhealth/publications/bibliographies.html. We have found the following publications particularly helpful in thinking through the relationships of technical, political, social, and economic factors that shape the path to UHC in each country: Oren Ahoobim, Dan Altman, Laurie Garrett, et al., *The New Global Health Agenda: Universal Health Coverage* (New York: Council on Foreign Relations, 2012); Gina Lagomarsino, Alice Garabrant, Atikah Adyas, et al., "Moving towards universal health coverage: health insurance reforms in nine developing countries in Africa and Asia," *The Lancet* 380, no. 9845 (2012): 933–943; Felicia Marie Knaul, Eduardo González-Pier, Octavio Gómez-Dantés, et al., "The quest for universal health coverage: achieving social protection for all in Mexico," *The Lancet* 380, no. 9849 (2012): 1259–1279; Lara Brearley, Robert Marten, and Thomas O'Connell, *Universal Health Coverage: A Commitment to Close the Gap,* a collaborative report from the Rockefeller Foundation, Save the Children, UNICEF, and the World Health Organization (London: Save the Children, 2013); Nellie Bristol, *Global Action toward Universal Health Coverage* (Washington, DC: Center for Strategic and International Studies, 2014); Naoki Ikegami, ed., *Universal Health Coverage for Inclusive and Sustainable Development: Lessons from Japan* (Washington, DC: World Bank, 2014); Akiko Maeda, Edson Araujo, Cheryl Cashin, et al., *Universal Health Coverage for Inclusive and Sustainable Development: A Synthesis of 11 Country Case Studies* (Washington, DC: World Bank, 2014); Robert Marten, Diane McIntyre, Claudia Travassos, et al., "An assessment of progress towards universal health coverage in Brazil, Russia, India, China, and South Africa (BRICS)," *The Lancet* 384, no. 9960 (2014): 2164–2171; Gilbert Abotisem and Manuela De Allegri, "Universal health coverage from multiple perspectives: a synthesis of conceptual literature and global debates," *BMC International Health and Human Rights* 15 (2015): 17; Rifat Atun, Luiz Odorico Monteiro de Andrade, Gisele Almeida, et al., "Health-system reform and universal health coverage in Latin America," *The Lancet* 385, no. 9974 (2015): 1230–1247; Daniel Cotlear, Somil Nagpal, Owen Smith, et al., *Going Universal: How 24 Countries Are Implementing Universal Health Coverage Reforms from the Bottom Up* (Washington, DC: World Bank, 2015); Julio Frenk, "Leading the way towards universal health coverage: a call to action," *The Lancet* 385, no. 9975 (2015): 1352–1358; David Nicholson, Robert Yates, Will Warburton, and Gianluca Fontana, *Delivering Universal Health Coverage: A Guide for Policymakers,* report of the WISH Universal Health Coverage Forum 2015 (Doha, Qatar: World Innovation Summit for Health, 2015); Michael R. Reich, Joseph Harris, Naoki Ikegami, et al., "Moving towards universal health coverage: lessons from 11 country studies," *The Lancet* 387, no. 10020 (2016): 811–816; Amanda

Glassman, Ursula Giedion, and Peter C. Smith, *What's In, What's Out: Designing Benefits for Universal Health Coverage* (Washington, DC: Center for Global Development, 2017); and Dean Jamison, Ala Alwan, Charles N. Mock, et al., "Universal health coverage and intersectoral action for health: key messages from Disease Control Priorities, 3rd edition," *The Lancet* 391 (March 17, 2018): 1108–1120.

9. Richard Horton and Stephanie Clark, "The perils and possibilities of the private health sector," *The Lancet* 388 (August 6, 2016): 540–541; at 540. For an influential skeptical view of the private sector role in UHC, see Anna Marriott, "Blind optimism: challenging the myths about private health care in poor countries," Oxfam International, February 2009.

10. Jim Yong Kim, "Speech at the 2017 annual meetings plenary," World Bank, October 13, 2017; https://www.worldbank.org/en/news/speech/2017/10/13/wbg-president-jim-yong-kim-speech-2017-annual-meetings-iplenary-session. See also World Bank, *The Changing Wealth of Nations: Measuring Sustainable Development in the New Millennium* (Washington, DC: World Bank, 2018).

11. *Fostering healthy businesses: delivering innovations in maternal and child health*, a report by the Task Force on Sustainable Business Models (New York/Geneva: for the Innovation Working Group in support of Every Woman, Every Child, September 2012); International Finance Corporation, *Healthy Partnerships: How Governments Can Engage the Private Sector to Improve Health in Africa* (Washington, DC: World Bank, 2011); and A. Lin and J. Wilson, *Healthy Markets for Global Health: A Market Shaping Primer* (Washington, DC: Center for Accelerating Innovation and Impact, US Agency for International Development, 2014); https://www.usaid.gov/cii/market-shapingprimer.

12. Simon Szreter, *Health and Wealth: Studies in History and Policy* (Rochester: University of Rochester Press, 2005).

13. Jesse B. Bump, "The long road to universal health coverage: historical analysis of early decisions in Germany, the United Kingdom and the United States," *Health Systems & Reform* 1 (2015): 28–38; Till Bärnighausen and Rainer Sauerborn, "One hundred and eighteen years of the German health insurance system: are there any lessons for middle- and low-income countries?" *Social Science & Medicine* 54 (2002): 1559–1587.

14. Angus Deaton, *The Great Escape: Health, Wealth, and the Origins of Inequality* (Princeton: Princeton University Press, 2013). See also Thomas McKeown, *The Modern Rise of Population* (New York: Academic Press, 1976), for the origins of the modern controversy.

15. See *Declaration of Alma-Ata* (note 2).

16. Felix Dodds, David Donoghue, and Jimena Leiva Roesch, *Negotiating the Sustainable Development Goals: A Transformational Agenda in an Insecure World* (London: Routledge, 2017); and Raj M. Desai, Hiroshi Kato, Homi Kharas, and John W. McArthur, eds., *From Summits to Solutions: Innovations in Implementing the Sustainable Development Goals* (Washington, DC: Brookings Institution, 2018).

17. See the preamble to "Transforming our world," (note 1).

18. Primary healthcare has been defined as "the first level of contact of individuals, the family and community with the national health system bringing health care as close as

possible to where people live and work, and constitutes the first element of a continuing health care process." See *The International Conference on Primary Health Care, Alma-Ata, USSR, 6–12 September 1978, Declaration of Alma-Ata,* for the definition and an explication of primary healthcare; www.who.int/publications/almaata_declaration-en.pdf.

19. On this point, see, for example, D. Sun, H. Ahn, T. Lievens, and W. Zeng, "Evaluation of the performance of national health systems in 2004–2011: an analysis of 173 countries," *PLoS ONE,* 12, no. 3 (2017): e0173346: https://doe.org/10.1371/journal.pone.0173346. The authors comment on the low efficiency of the central planning model and the efficiency effects of "a model that relies more on market competition . . . than central planning and bureaucratic rules."

20. For an informative *Lancet* series, "UHC: markets, profit and the public good," see Maureen Mackintosh, Amos Channon, Anup Karan, et al., "What is the private sector? Understanding private provision in the health systems of low-income and middle-income countries," *The Lancet* 388, no. 10044 (2016): 596–605; Rosemary Morgan, Tim Ensor, and Hugh Waters, "Performance of private sector health care: implications for universal health coverage," *The Lancet* 388, no. 10044 (2016): 606–612; Dominic Montagu and Catherine Goodman, "Prohibit, constrain, encourage, or purchase: how should we engage with the private health-care sector?," *The Lancet,* 388, no.10044 (2016): 613–621; and Barbara McPake and Kara Hanson, "Managing the public–private mix to achieve universal health coverage," *The Lancet* 388, no. 10044 (2016): 622–630.

21. Lord Ara Darzi and his colleagues at Imperial College London have developed a practical tool for measuring the impact of private providers on access and standards of care in health systems: Heather Wadge, Rhia Roy, Arthika Sripathy, et al., *Evaluating the Impact of Private Providers on Health and Health Systems* (London, UK: Imperial College, 2017); http://www.imperial.ac.uk/media/imperial-college/institute-of-global-health-innovation/centre-for-health-policy/public/IMPJ5551-Health-Report-Update-Final-Web.pdf. See also Wadge, Roy, Sripathy, et al., "How to harness the private sector for universal health coverage," *The Lancet* 390 (July 8, 2017): e19–e20.

22. Sources for these examples, and many others, are given in "How the private sector is contributing to universal health coverage: case studies," briefing note by Graduate Institute Global Health Centre (Geneva), Johns Hopkins Institute for Applied Economics, Global Health, and the Study of Business Enterprise (Baltimore) and Rabin Martin (New York), September 2015; http://rabinmartin.com/report/how-the-private-sector-is-contributing-to-universal-health-coverage-case-studies/.

23. Louis Galambos and Jeffrey L. Sturchio, eds., *Noncommunicable Diseases in the Developing World: Addressing Gaps in Global Policy and Research* (Baltimore, MD: Johns Hopkins University Press, 2014).

24. *Reaching a billion—ending neglected tropical diseases: a gateway to universal health coverage,* Fifth Progress Report on the London Declaration on NTDs (2018); http://unitingtocombatntds.org/wp-content/themes/tetloose/app/staticPages/fifthReport/files/fifth_progress_report_english.pdf.

25. Simon Rushton and Jeremy Youde, eds., *Routledge Handbook of Global Health Security* (London: Routledge, 2015).

26. *Working for health and growth: investing in the health workforce*, Report of the High-Level Commission on Health Employment and Economic Growth (Geneva: World Health Organization, 2016).

27. K. Srinath Reddy, "How to define public purpose for a PPP to move beyond marriage of convenience; here is what is critically crucial," *Financial Express,* July 13, 2017; https://www.financialexpress.com/opinion/how-to-define-public-purpose-for-a-ppp-to-move-beyond-marriage-of-convenience-here-is-what-is-critically-crucial/761151/. See also Kent Buse and S. Tanaka, "Global public-private health partnerships: lessons learned from ten years of experience and evaluation," *International Dental Journal* 61, suppl. 2 (2011): 2–10; Kent Buse and A. M. Harmer, "Seven habits of highly effective global public-private health partnerships: practice and potential," *Social Science & Medicine* 64 (2007): 259–71; Michael R. Reich, ed., *Public-Private Partnerships for Public Health* (Cambridge, MA: Harvard Center for Population and Development Studies, 2002); Mark L. Rosenberg, E. S. Hayes, M. H. McIntyre, and N. Neill, *Real Collaboration: What It Takes for Global Health to Succeed* (Berkeley: University of California Press, 2010); Jeffrey L. Sturchio, "Business and global health in an era of globalization: reflections on public/private partnerships as a cultural innovation," in C. Held and H. Moore, eds., *Cultural Politics in a Global Age: Uncertainty, Solidarity, and Innovation* (Oxford: Oneworld Publications, 2008): 270–277; and Jeffrey L. Sturchio and Gary M. Cohen, "How PEPFAR's public-private partnerships achieved ambitious goals, from improving labs to strengthening supply chains," *Health Affairs,* 31, no.7 (2012):1450–1458.

1

Conceptualizing the Health Economy

Ilona Kickbusch and Christian Franz

Universal health coverage has become a central element of achieving the health goals related to the Sustainable Development Goals (SDGs) set forth at the 70th United Nations General Assembly in 2015. In this chapter, we argue that the political momentum of universal health coverage (UHC) among health policy makers needs to reach economic and fiscal policy makers. For that purpose, we propose a simple concept of the health economy consisting of (a) resources needed to establish a health economy, (b) health services and products provided by this health economy, and (c) potential effects from an established health economy. Drawing on evidence from high- and upper-middle-income countries, the chapter illustrates the economic significance of the health sector for the overall economy of a country. A functioning health economy can be a significant share of the total economic activity, has the potential to stabilize economic growth even in phases of an economic downturn, and may drive employment growth.

Why Consider the Economy and UHC Together?

The Political Case Has Been Made, Support Has Increased

Universal health coverage has gained tremendous momentum over the past five years and is now considered the key priority in global health.[1] As target 3.8 of the UN SDGs, it stands at the center of the other 12 health targets and is strongly interlinked with the other 16 SDGs.[2] A wide range of actors is committed to strengthening health systems to reach UHC.[3] The commitment has been made and reiterated by major donor countries (e.g., Germany and Japan); by the leadership of the World Health Organization (WHO), the World Bank, and the Organisation for Economic

Co-operation and Development (OECD); and by many leaders from low-and middle-income countries.[4,5]

This global political push for UHC by governments, international organizations, and civil society has also helped to spell out the vision behind UHC and link it with other key health concepts. In the 2017 joint "Global Monitoring Report" on UHC, the WHO and the World Bank have formulated that "UHC means that everyone—irrespective of their living standards—receives the health services they need, and that using health services does not cause financial hardship."[6] Key policy instruments needed to achieve the objectives within this definition of UHC are summarized under the term *health systems strengthening*: enhancing financing, improving the organization of the healthcare workforce, delivering services and medicines efficiently and effectively, refining health information systems, and improving health security and governance.[7] With the WHO's 13th General Programme of Work (GPW13), the dimension of access to health services is particularly important, because it formulates the goal to have one billion more people enjoying benefits from UHC by 2023.[8] The vision of UHC is not limited to a mere expansion of clinical health services; it also includes the creation of public goods such as clean water, sanitation, and so on. Therefore, the UHC service coverage index of the World Bank and WHO takes into account the extent to which people have access to basic sanitation.[9]

The Case for UHC: Not Just Economics, but Political Commitment

As governments move from political commitments to policy development and implementation, it is evident that additional stakeholders will have to be included in the debate. To keep health and the efforts toward UHC as key policy priorities in any given country, health systems strengthening policies need to correspond to fiscal and economic policy priorities, among others. The decision of how to finance efforts toward UHC—in other words, an expansion of health services coverage—is likely to have far-reaching implications in those policy areas. Making fiscal room for health affects the consumption choices of people, aggregate demand, and eventually the economic activity of the entire country.[10] The unlocked demand for health services triggered by broader coverage needs to be met with an expanded supply of health services and medicines on the one hand, and of public goods such as clean water and sanitation on the other hand. This in turn requires a larger health workforce, mechanisms for strategic purchasing of medicines, and infrastructure investments.

These considerations affect various stakeholders outside of governments too. In many low- and middle-income countries, private sector enterprises (for profit or not-for-profit) provide a major share of the health services. The percentage ranges from below one-third of all outpatient / primary care visits (e.g., in Malawi, China, South Africa) to around one-half (e.g., in Argentina, Sri Lanka), to more than seven out of ten (in India and Nigeria, for instance).[11] Notably, governments in some of those countries are much more involved in health product supply chains than they are in high-income countries, because they often procure drugs and distribute them to health clinics.[12] While there are pros and cons to either variant, both supply-chain mechanisms will have different effects on incentives of actors and on the economics of the health sector.

These examples show that policies that foster UHC in a country (such as health systems strengthening) need to be context-specific and complementary to other policy priorities. Despite broad political commitment and international activities, there has been a lack of acknowledgment of the importance of economic dynamics behind the push for UHC by means of strengthening of health systems. For too long, health has been considered to be a cost factor more than anything else. Today, the importance of health as a macroeconomic factor is beginning to gain relevance.

The Health Economy: How UHC and Economics Interact

The 2013 *Lancet* Commission on Investing in Health made an important case for the effect of health on economic development, estimating that, between 2000 and 2011, 24% of total income growth in low- to middle-income countries (LMICs) was attributable to additional years of healthy life.[13] This argument reflects a shift in how health can be perceived by economic policy planners. The earlier, 2001 report of the Commission on Macroeconomics and Health, chaired by Jeffrey Sachs, was still focused more on questions like "How can we create a healthy population?," and it assumed a reliance on philanthropic donors and "development aid."[14] The message of the 2013 *Lancet* Commission instead viewed health interventions more as investments that would improve the economic well-being of the population in the future.

The global health community has also made significant progress in bringing the economic relevance of healthcare to light. Healthcare is a major economic force: in 2015, the world spent US$ 7.3 trillion on healthcare, which represents almost 10% of the global gross domestic product (GDP). When related services in fields such as nutrition, sports and fitness industries, receipts from over-the-counter medicines, and expenditures on home care services are included, the annual volume reaches US$ 10.7 trillion. By this definition, the contribution of health and healthcare to the global economy accounted for 14.3% of global GDP in 2015.[15] This estimate may still be somewhat limited, because it does not include major economic activities around public health interventions such as investments in water and sanitation infrastructure.

More recently, the work of the UN High-Level Commission on Health Employment and Economic Growth analyzed the pathways from the health system to economic growth and estimated that by 2030 the number of health workers will reach some 67 million—a 55% increase from about 44 million in 2013.[16] Beyond the growth dynamic, health and social work have an important gender component, with women making up more than two-thirds of workers (vs. 41% in total employment).

Building on the three indicative facts above, namely, health as a growth opportunity, health as major contributor to GDP, and health as job creator, this chapter aims to widen the perspective to account for the fact that the health–economy nexus reaches far beyond mere health policies and health outcomes. By conceptualizing a health economy and its importance for UHC-related policies, we aim to position health sector reforms as an integral part of economic and fiscal policies that call for a productive collaboration of actors in the economy—be they from the private or the public sector. By identifying the mechanisms underlying the health economy, the framework of the health economy can guide policy makers not to disregard the significant economic opportunity that lies in investments in health and UHC.

Conceptualizing the Health Economy

The Health Economy as a Market for Products and Services

The notion of the health economy used in this chapter focuses on economic processes that are directly and indirectly concerned with the production, provision, and financing of health-related goods and services in a country. These processes are influenced by national trends (demographic and epidemiological transitions) and global spillovers (health-related trade and international flow of capital and people). As such, studying the health economy enables us to identify and characterize economic effects of those processes that have an impact on the overall economy when greater or fewer resources are allocated to health—for example, through the expansion of health coverage in the population.

As a starting point for conceptualizing the health economy, it is useful to understand efforts of the German government to track the footprint of the health sector by using official statistics (creating a so-called health satellite account). In this perspective, the health economy consists of a core sector and an extended sector (figure 1.1). The former includes health products and services in a narrow sense (such as reimbursable in- and outpatient services, drugs sold over-the-counter, and individual healthcare services). The extended health sector comprises a wider set of health services and products, such as support activities for elderly or disabled people living at home, health research, and vocational training for health personnel. Moreover, the extended health sector includes products and services related to healthy relaxation and healthy food.[17]

By this definition, the German health economy contributed 336.4 billion euros to the country's gross value added, which represented about 12% of the total value added.[18] Put into perspective, the health economy of Germany is as big as the GDP of Austria. Around 20% of final consumption between 2005 and 2012 happened in the health economy.[19]

While those volumes are specific to Germany (the country has the fifth-highest health spending per capita), understanding the health sector as being more than just medicines and care services in hospitals is vital for a concept of the health economy that is applicable to different environments. Independent of a country's financing mechanisms for health, viewing products and services in both a core and an extended market allows policy makers to see consumption patterns and the economic actors behind both the supply and demand side of these markets.

Understanding the Resources and Inputs of the Health Economy

The resources needed to provide health services and products are the main focus of most initiatives of the global health community. In

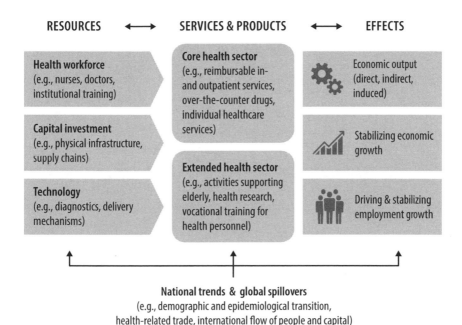

RESOURCES ⟷ SERVICES & PRODUCTS ⟷ EFFECTS

Health workforce
(e.g., nurses, doctors, institutional training)

Capital investment
(e.g., physical infrastructure, supply chains)

Technology
(e.g., diagnostics, delivery mechanisms)

Core health sector
(e.g., reimbursable in- and outpatient services, over-the-counter drugs, individual healthcare services)

Extended health sector
(e.g., activities supporting elderly, health research, vocational training for health personnel)

Economic output (direct, indirect, induced)

Stabilizing economic growth

Driving & stabilizing employment growth

National trends & global spillovers
(e.g., demographic and epidemiological transition, health-related trade, international flow of people and capital)

Figure 1.1. Stylized health economy. Source: Categorization of services and products based on Henke, 2013 (see note 17). Adapted by the authors

general terms, the resources can be separated into the health workforce, capital investments (e.g., the physical infrastructure for healthcare), and technology.

Among those resources, the health workforce is arguably the most crucial one. Research suggests that around 50% of total health expenditure worldwide (both public and private) goes to wages, salaries, and allowances for health workers.[20] However, the policy relevance goes beyond this figure. Creating sufficient training capacities, anticipating the future need for a trained workforce large enough to deliver good service, and shaping the governance framework to increase the efficiency of health workers are all vital elements of the health economy. Despite this importance, the UN Commission on Health Employment and Economic Growth projected a global shortfall of 18 million health workers by 2030.[21] The largest gaps at present and in 2030 will be in Africa and Southeast Asia, accounting for more than half of the global shortfall. But challenges also arise in many western high-income countries. Whereas, in LMICs, shortages of health workers affect population health outcomes (like child mortality)[22] and health systems outcomes (such as child vaccination coverage),[23,24] high-income countries struggle with ensuring access to health services in rural and smaller communities. Political action at the international level is fairly recent: it wasn't until 2017 that the 70th World Health Assembly adopted a five-year action plan for health employment and inclusive economic growth. That same year, the Fourth Global Forum on Human Resources for Health in Dublin initiated a Multi-Partner Trust Fund that will pool funding to finance investments in the health workforce.[25]

Because health systems tend to be highly labor-intensive, it is not surprising that capital investment in health infrastructure, diagnostic, and therapeutic equipment, as well as information and communication technology (ICT), has remained relatively low as compared to other sectors.[26] For example, in 2016, OECD countries invested on average 0.5% of their GDP in the health sector as capital investment. Other sectors such as manufacturing have had much higher capital investment shares. Nevertheless, the past decades have seen a faster growth in health investments than in other sectors in many high-income countries.[27] In low-income countries, development finance institutes have been key to enhancing investments in essential health services.[28]

Technology is crucial for the health economy, but it is one of the most difficult factors to assess. On the one hand, there is tremendous hope that LMICs can attain some leapfrog technologies in healthcare (e.g., using drones for drug delivery,[29] or blockchain technology for more efficient financing mechanisms[30]). On the other hand, the health sector has usually lagged in following megatrends such as the digital transformation.[31] For example, the question of whether the trend to track individual health statistics through health-related wearables (i.e., devices such as watches that track the health status of individuals) remains as unresolved in most countries as does the ultimate question of how to translate digitized knowledge of patients into better health outcomes.[32] Nevertheless, while there is doubt about the cost-effectiveness of some health technologies at the start, it is clear that they represent a major building block for effective healthcare.[33] This building block involves innovation in physical technologies like new drugs, vaccines, medical devices, and diagnostics. It encompasses digital technologies that extend beyond the more speculative technologies mentioned above, such as ICT infrastructure in hospitals and the health system in general that boosts efficiency in patient care. Finally, it looks toward new technologies that might help individual countries, especially LMICs, to leapfrog past some development stages that other countries' health systems may have had to go through in the past.[34] All three aspects of the technology building block can have a profound effect on productivity in the health sector.

Understanding the Effects of the Health Economy

A functioning health economy can have far-reaching effects on the overall economy of a country and its economic prosperity. From a narrow national accounts perspective, three effects can describe the "economic footprint" of the health economy—its effect on economic production, value added, and employment in a country.[35] First, there are the direct effects from the production of health products and provision of health services in the core and extended health sector. Second, there are indirect effects that result from contracting with suppliers for those health goods and services. And third, induced effects, which include "second round"–spending effects from directly and indirectly earned income (including consumption spending resulting from additional employment in the sector), influence the economy. Analysis for the year 2015 for Germany gives an idea of the economic significance of those effects: in total, the economic effect came to around 591 billion euros, of which 324.3 billion euros stemmed from direct effects, 133.4 billion euros from indirect effects, and a nearly equal amount from induced effects.[36]

Beyond those effects on value added, data for a broader set of high-income countries indicate that a functioning health economy can have two more effects on a country's overall economy that actually help in sustaining economic growth. First, empirical evidence from euro-area countries points to a growth-stabilizing effect of the health sector. Figure 1.2 illustrates this by showing the year-on-year change of gross value added in the human and social services sector versus the overall economy from 2001 to 2014. The gross value added of health services increased at a higher average annual growth rate (1.9% vs. 1.0% per annum), but more striking is that the growth rate has never turned negative. That value added from the health sector continues to grow even as the rest of the economy is in decline represents a powerful argument for building a domestic health economy.

The second important effect is that the health economy has proven to be a quite resilient driver of employment growth. Figure 1.3 shows this

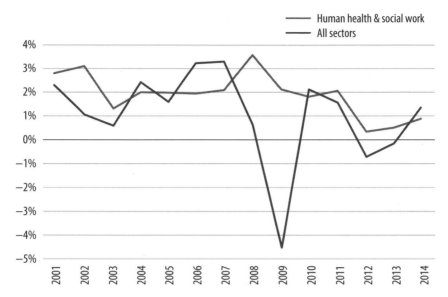

Figure 1.2. Growth of gross value added in 16 euro-area countries, 2000–2014, year-on-year change in percentages. The sample includes 16 euro-area countries for which complete data by sector were available for 2000–2014: Austria, Belgium, Estonia, Finland, France, Germany, Greece, Ireland, Italy, Latvia, Luxembourg, Netherlands, Portugal, Slovak Republic, Slovenia, and Spain.

effect by giving the year-on-year change of employment in the health and social sector and comparing it to the changes in employment across all sectors. Not only does health employment often move against the trend of the overall economy—which makes the sector a stabilizing element during economic crises—the growth of health employment has been consistently higher than the average across sectors. While the job creation dynamics are favorable, pay in the care sector tends to be lower than in the rest of the economy. Women are disproportionately affected by this lower pay, as they represent the large majority among care workers.[37]

Although there are no data available to test those effects for economies in LMICs, there is a growing body of research analyzing health's effect on economic growth more generally. Microeconomic studies have been able to establish a link between the health status of individuals/households and their income levels. For example, a study of malaria prevention interventions among agricultural workers in Nigeria suggests that treatment against ma-

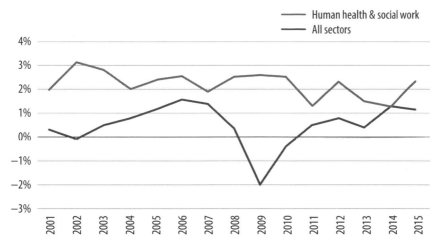

Figure 1.3. Employment growth in selected OECD countries, 2001–2015, year-on-year change in percentages. The sample includes 25 OECD countries for which complete data by sector were available for 2000–2015: Australia, Austria, Belgium, Czech Republic, Denmark, Estonia, Finland, France, Germany, Greece, Hungary, Ireland, Israel, Italy, Japan, Latvia, Luxembourg, Netherlands, Norway, Poland, Slovak Republic, Slovenia, Sweden, United Kingdom, and United States.

larial infection increases both labor supply and productivity and accounts for a 10% increase in earnings among the sugarcane cutters.[38] As labor productivity is a major driver behind economic growth, it seems probable that a scaled-up intervention would contribute to higher economic growth.

Several macroeconomic studies since 2001 show that by improving the health of the population, a country's economic growth should, all other things being equal, increase.[39] These studies identified two major long-term channels. First, health contributes to the human capital of a country, which represents a major determinant of economic growth in the long term. Using a panel data set of 104 countries for growth periods between 1970–80 and 1980–90, Bloom et al. identified a statistically significant effect of life expectancy on growth; namely, a 1% increase in life expectancy increases economic output by 4%.[40] Second, improvements in health usually lead to a sharp decline in death rates (usually among children and mothers first). As families internalize those declines in mortality rates, they decide to have fewer children, which in turn leads to a decline in birth rates. Because there is a time gap between the decline in death rates and birth rates, the population will grow.[41] This population growth produces a "demographic dividend" that can ultimately lead to higher economic growth.

Whether or not this demographic dividend translates into economic growth depends heavily on policies within countries. Empirical evidence from China and India suggests that the major growth drivers behind the increase in economic output were a rise in life expectancy of the population, a rise in trade openness, and increasing share of working-age members among the total population.[42] While India did not increase the life expectancy of its population because of a consequent push for UHC, as K. Srinath Reddy finds (chap. 7, in this volume), the evidence still points to the economic potential of health interventions. More recent research links the two channels above and suggests a two-way relationship between economic growth and human development when measured as health, nutritional, and educational status. Higher economic growth allows more investment into human development to increase human capital, while increased human development in a country also increases the country's growth potential (e.g., through a better-trained labor force).[43]

Given the mounting evidence, state finance and economic ministers, as well as private sector investors, need to take into account the ameliorative effects of the health economy. They should consider four important links: (1) empirical evidence of health's effect on long-term economic growth is increasingly robust; (2) microeconomic research has provided substantial evidence for health interventions having a positive effect on labor productivity; (3) the health economy has the potential to stabilize economic growth in the medium term; and (4) employment growth in the health economy is not just more robust against shocks but is also on average higher than in the rest of the economy.

The effects of the health economy described above deliberately focus on potential macroeconomic effects of a functioning health economy as observed in many high- and middle-income countries. This does not mean that other effects can be neglected. Whether an expansive health economy (and with it probably higher health expenditure per capita) leads to better population health or whether the health system works efficiently remain pressing and necessary questions. After all, the United States represents a clear example of a country with massive economic activity around health and dramatic challenges in improving population health at the same time.[44] Yet, the macroeconomic effects we have discussed are vital when policy makers from policy areas other than health (e.g., finance ministers) have to assess the consequences of a push for UHC in their country.

National Trends and Global Spillovers in the Health Economy

Our conceptualization of the health economy has been limited so far to a purely national perspective. There are, however, important population, health, and economic trends regionally and globally that will have a significant impact on how the health economy functions. While a comprehensive overview of such trends extends beyond the scope of this chapter, some of the key developments should be noted.

International migration of healthcare workers has a profound impact on regional health economies. The reasons behind migration can be diverse, ranging from economic incentives for labor mobility (e.g., earnings opportunities) to forced migration due to conflicts. The health economies in most high-income countries benefit significantly from foreign-trained nurses and doctors. On average, almost 17 out of 100 doctors and 6 out of 100 nurses in OECD countries were not trained in the country where they work now. European economies that already feel the drain in their labor force due to an ever-older population are more and more relying on care workers trained in other countries. The movement is visible in so-called global care chains and might lead to a dramatic shortage of care workers and doctors in the countries of origin. According to the WHO in 2010, there were 4,113 unfilled physician positions and 3,229 unfilled nursing jobs in Poland, a major provider of doctors and nurses to countries such as the United Kingdom and Germany.[45] By 2020, estimates by the Polish ministry of health indicate that the Polish health system will be in need of 60,860 nurses and 4,817 midwives.[46] Similarly, a WHO survey among European ministries of health found that the Romanian health system faces an unfulfilled future need for 20,000 nurses and 4,000 midwives.[47] The financial burden on the governments is also increasing, especially when considering expenditure on medical education. Training medical professionals is both expensive and (from the perspective of the country of origin) inefficient in the context of the existing "brain drain." For example, it is estimated that the Romanian government spends approximately $14,899 to $26,369 per student for the six years of medical training. Estimates from 2013 indicate that the Romanian government spends around EUR 3.5 billion on educating doctors.[48]

From an economic policy perspective, the evaluation of workforce migration can be ambiguous. This can be seen in Sri Lanka: UN estimates in 2015 indicate that between 2009 and 2013, an average of 113,000 women left Sri Lanka to go to the Gulf countries alone, working predominantly as housemaids who also performed care work. While representing a significant disturbance of the local family life, the macroeconomic significance of female migrants is evident in that migrant laborers' remittances contribute significantly to Sri Lanka's foreign exchange earnings, adding up to an equivalent of around 9% of the Sri Lankan GDP.[49]

International trade is likely to significantly affect the supply of health products in a country as well as the resources available (technology, in particular). International trade for health-related goods has dramatically increased over the past 15 years. In total, the global size of the market is around 900 billion USD (up from about 300 billion in 2002).[50] Most countries in the world import more health-related goods than they export. In 2014, only 16 countries in the world had a trade surplus with health-related goods that was above 500 million USD. Among those countries with a trade surplus, India was the only LMIC that exported more than it imported. The country is also an example of how much national policy makers need to shape the institutional framework to ensure that the domestic population benefits from the domestic health economy. India's big trade surplus in health-related goods indicates a globally competitive health industry, having the fourth-highest export surplus in health-related goods globally. At the same time, a large share of India's population suffers from preventable diseases: in absolute terms, communicable, maternal, neonatal, and nutritional diseases caused 120 million years of life lost in 2016. For China, the corresponding figure was just one-tenth of India's disease burden (12 million years of life lost).[51] Beyond national policies, trade agreements can be vital in shaping a country's health economy. There is a continuous need to ensure that those agreements are not implemented in a way that is detrimental to the health system. Development partners, donors, and private sector companies have to ensure fairness in order to encourage further development.[52,53,54]

A third important global force that will likely have a profound impact on the health economy is the commercial determinants of health. These are the dynamic relationships among corporate practices, individual consumption decisions, and market forces in a globalized world.[55] As global corporations increase their outreach into more and more countries with emerging economies, their strategies in marketing, supply-chain management, lobbying, and corporate citizenship influence people's consumption choices and ultimately their health. However, the potential influence of corporate strategies can be detrimental as well as beneficial.[56] For the health economy, this will have an impact on the products and services that the health sector has to provide. Policy makers who wish to shape the health economy need to engage in discussions around consumption taxes and incentives for prevention. Given that the disease burden shifts to noncommunicable diseases as people's incomes rise, the commercial determinants of health will grow in importance.

UHC and the Health Economy

The framework of the health economy we have presented allows policy makers to look at their efforts toward UHC and the policy instruments of health systems strengthening from the perspective of how these policies shape markets, influence characteristics of the health sector, and affect the resources available to the health system. The following section will look more closely at the interaction of UHC-related policies and the health economy.

Financing UHC and the Health Economy

The Sustainable Development Goals and the preceding conferences not only outlined a new set of global goals and indicators until 2030 but also put emphasis on a broader set of sources that would finance the investments needed to achieve those goals.[57,58] Two sources would be most crucial to unlock sufficient investment: (1) domestic finances raised by governments through more rigid tax collection and through the reduction of tax evasion; and (2) investments from the private sector.

Beyond the perspective of raising money, the analysis of healthcare financing policies from a health economy perspective helps us to understand whether a given configuration of institutions supports the growth-stabilizing and employment-driver effect of the health economy. In general, the mix between private and public health expenditure is likely to have a strong effect on this relationship. These effects can best be described by looking at an economy in distress. In a period of economic contraction, tax revenues are likely to decline, thereby putting pressure on governments to cut expenditures across sectors.[59] Governments could also decide to adopt a classical Keynesian approach and implement stimulation packages that try to cushion the effect of falling private investments with public investment in infrastructure. In the former case, health systems would have a procyclical effect on economic growth—in other words, the downturn would be enhanced by the health economy. In the latter case, public health investments would support a stumbling economy and likely stabilize it. With regard to private health expenditure, the case is more straightforward. In times of an economic downturn, households are likely to economize on their health spending and thus emphasize the decline in private consumption. (The opposite is possible with regard to spending on mental health, where one could expect higher expenditures because people seek such help in times of distress, for instance, after losing a job.)

Efforts toward UHC are likely to have a substantial impact on how such economic effects will play out. A key objective of UHC is to reduce the risk of financial hardship when people seek treatment. If that treatment is covered by a health insurance plan independent of someone's current employment or cash situation, they have no reason not to consume health services and products. Out-of-pocket payments would still be reduced, but the overall effect on aggregate consumption would be less severe. Of course, how the health plan or insurance is specified will determine the size of the cushioning effect of the health system. Empirical evidence on the effects of different institutional specifications of national healthcare systems is scarce and hard to provide given the highly country-specific setup of health systems. Nevertheless, a quantitative analysis of 32 OECD countries between 1990 and 2011 shows that there is not just great variation among countries in how economic distress affects health expenditures but also that a simple "Bismarck" versus "Beveridge" dichotomy is insufficient to explain those differences.[60] The results of the analysis indicate that in nine countries, both private and public health expenditures displayed countercyclical patterns; that is, health expenditures went up in times of economic downturns.[61] Among those countries were Canada, France, Germany, Spain, and Switzerland. In another study that analyzed 145 countries from 1987 to 2007, public spending on health and education was found to be procyclical in developing countries and countercyclical in developed countries. Importantly, the degree of cyclicality is higher the lower the level of economic development (measured by income per capita).[62]

Expansion of Health Services and the Health Economy:
The Case of Turkey

Another aspect where it is also useful to look at the health economy in relation to UHC is the provision of services and products. Implementation of UHC-related reforms of national health systems (e.g., expanding coverage) often changes supply and demand structures in the health sector in a fundamental way. The private sector plays a vital role in the provision of services and products and in creating essential parts of the health infrastructure (supply chains, facilities, etc.). Whether the private sector is aligned or incompatible with the objectives of UHC depends heavily on the specific configuration of the health systems policies.

A case in point is Turkey, where the implementation of the far-reaching Health Transformation Program (HTP) started in 2003. The centerpieces of the reform were the Universal Health Insurance Scheme (relying on social insurance contributions and tax-financed government payments for those who are unemployed), a unification of the different health insurance schemes under a single system, and a single-payer insurance agency founded in 2006 which is responsible for purchasing healthcare services from healthcare providers on behalf of the insured population.[63] The reforms delivered results after a remarkably short time period: Between 2003 and 2011, insurance coverage among poor people increased (2.4 million to 10.2 million),[64] primary care visits tripled, and the utilization of hospitals increased.[65] At the same time, the rise in access to healthcare services increased the consumption of pharmaceuticals, which led to an increase in sales from 2.5 billion USD in 2002 to 8 billion USD in 2012.[66] Policies implemented to control pharmaceutical prices seem to have worked; the average cost per prescription decreased from 25 USD in 2009 to 20 USD in 2012.[67]

Given this set of wide-ranging policies, to what extent was the "health economy effect" described above also visible in Turkey? When looking at the country's macroeconomic data between 2000 and 2016, a similar pattern emerges: the gross value added of the health sector grew at an annual rate of 5.5%, whereas the overall economy grew by 4.8% per year. In the same period, the value added never turned negative and thus contributed to economic stability, even when the rest of the economy experienced negative growth rates (in 2009). Employment in the health sector rose from 2.8% of total civilian employment in 2009 to almost 4% in 2015—which represents an increase of employment in the sector of almost 500,000 people in just six years. While the Turkish health system is far from perfect,[68] these figures provide some evidence that the Turkish health economy is supporting and stabilizing economic growth and driving employment.

As do all economic policies—but in particular, ones that reallocate resources to the extent Turkey's health reforms did—the reform packages that pushed toward UHC have effects beyond those described above. One such development is the rapid privatization of hospitals. Between 2002 and 2013 the number of privately owned hospitals doubled and the number of beds in privately owned hospitals tripled.[69] Some analysts point out that private equity firms are increasingly investing in large hospital groups. While not necessarily a negative, this can trigger higher concentration in the market and inequities in de facto access to healthcare.[70]

The private sector has been significant in transforming the Turkish health sector. Particularly notable is the increasing differentiation among service providers. Between 2009 and 2015, health expenditure on private providers rose on average by 13% per year, a growth that was most likely triggered by healthcare reforms. At the same time, the share of those expenditures coming from private payers (either private insurance or out-of-pocket) and not from the Turkish Social Security Institution increased disproportionately, from 43% in 2009 to 58% in 2015. This development needs to be considered together with the fact that private providers tend to perform the majority of "complex surgeries" (such as organ transplants) but not even one out of five doctors' consultations. On the one hand, these two facts imply that private sector providers support the differentiation of provided health services. On the other hand, the data allow the interpretation that it is still the public sector that needs to provide the essential health services.

Conclusion

The concept of the health economy is a useful framework for policy makers to employ when considering policy instruments directed toward achieving UHC from an economic perspective. For that purpose, we outlined a simple concept of (a) resources needed to establish a health economy; (b) health services and products provided by this health economy; and (c) potential effects from an established health economy. It is evident that the health economy in high- and middle-income countries represents a significant share of the total economic activity, has the potential to stabilize economic growth even in phases of an economic downturn, and may drive employment growth.

While the case for UHC is compelling and supports—even goes beyond—the current political commitment, policy makers also need to consider the challenges. First, our study drew on a very simplified concept of welfare, namely GDP and GDP growth. Although highly correlated with many important welfare indicators, GDP remains an ambiguous indicator when used in combination with health. That is, since GDP takes into account only the monetary value and the quantity of services and products, it does not allow for qualitative differences not captured by money. More services and products sold in a country create a higher GDP—whether they are beneficial or detrimental to health. Thus, any health economy also needs to be assessed against the produced health, social, and environmental outcomes.

Second, the concept of the health economy used in this chapter is primarily derived from the experience of high- and upper-middle-income countries. Many institutions that enable a vast market-driven economy and effective redistribution are assumed as given. Although the concept is already idealistic for what is the reality in many high-income countries, many LMICs might have to devise their own way forward to see the benefits of their health economy unfold fully. Nevertheless, the arguments presented here correspond with a point made recently by Russo et al. (2017). They argued that the dependency of several low-income African countries on global commodity prices and external funding through international assistance requires UHC-related policies to be especially suited to crisis situations, since both characteristics make those countries' economies more volatile.[71] Importantly, though, for a functioning health economy to work as a counterforce along the economic cycle rests on mechanisms that require at least moderate fiscal discipline (or creditworthiness). Thus, a high degree of informality in employment and a small tax base are crucial factors that make health system reform more challenging.[72]

Third, building a domestic health industry is extremely challenging, as are all regional development policies. As a recent paper by the German government on health systems strengthening pointed out, local pharmaceutical industries would not only create jobs, attract investment, and trigger research and development, they might also help to make countries more resilient and put pressure on countries to develop their own governance structures for quality control.[73] Building a health research workforce, training pharmaceutical technicians, and establishing policies for both investment in and quality of pharmaceutical companies represents a major task requiring strong political commitment in ministries of health, economic ministries, and ministries of finance.

Definitions of UHC, SDG target 3.8, and SDG indicators 3.8.1 and 3.8.2

Universal health coverage means that all people receive the health services they need, including public health services designed to *promote better health* (such as anti-tobacco information campaigns and taxes), *prevent illness* (such as vaccinations), and to *provide treatment*, *rehabilitation* and *palliative care* (such as end-of-life care) of *sufficient quality* to be effective, while at the same time ensuring that the use of these services does *not expose the user to financial hardship** (emphasis added).

SDG target 3.8: Achieve universal health coverage, including financial risk protection, access to quality essential healthcare services, and access to safe, effective, quality, and affordable essential medicines and vaccines for all.

SDG indicator 3.8.1: Coverage of essential health services, defined as the average coverage of essential services based on tracer interventions—including reproductive, maternal, newborn, and child health; infectious diseases; noncommunicable diseases; and service capacity and access—among the general and the most disadvantaged population.

SDG indicator 3.8.2: Proportion of population with large household expenditures on health as a share of total household expenditure or income.

* WHO and World Bank, *Tracking universal health coverage: 2017 global monitoring report* (Washington, DC, and Geneva: World Bank and World Health Organization, 2017), http://www .who.int/healthinfo/universal_health_coverage/report/2017/en/.

NOTES

1. WHO, *Draft thirteenth general programme of work 2019–2023* (Geneva: World Health Organization, 2017), http://www.who.int/about/what-we-do/gpw-thirteen-consultation/en/.

2. WHO and World Bank, *Tracking universal health coverage: 2017 global monitoring report* (Geneva and Washington, DC: World Health Organization and World Bank, 2017), http://www.who.int/healthinfo/universal_health_coverage/report/2017/en/.

3. WHO and World Bank, *UHC2030: Healthy systems for universal health coverage—a joint vision for healthy lives* (Geneva and Washington, DC: World Health Organization and International Bank for Reconstruction and Development/The World Bank, 2017), https://www.uhc2030.org/fileadmin/uploads/uhc2030/Documents/About_UHC2030/mgt_arrangemts___docs/UHC2030_Official_documents/UHC2030_vision_paper_WEB2.pdf.

4. See, for example, F. Tediosi, A. Finch, C. Procacci, R. Marten, and E. Missoni, "BRICS countries and the global movement for universal health coverage," *Health Policy and Planning*, 31(6), (2016): 717–728, http://dx.doi.org/10.1093/heapol/czv122; and D. McIntyre, M. K. Ranson, B. K. Aulakh, and A. Honda, "Promoting universal financial protection: evidence from seven low- and middle-income countries on factors facilitating or hindering progress," *Health Research Policy and Systems*, 11(1), (2013): 1, https://doi.org/10.1186/1478-4505-11-36.

5. D. Cotlear, S. Nagpal, O. Smith, A. Tandon, and R. Cortez, *Going Universal: How 24 Developing Countries Are Implementing Universal Health Coverage Reforms from the Bottom Up* (Washington, DC: International Bank for Reconstruction and Development/The World Bank, 2015), http://documents.worldbank.org/curated/en/936881467992465464/.

6. WHO and World Bank, *Tracking universal health coverage: 2017 global monitoring report*.

7. WHO and World Bank, *Tracking universal health coverage: 2017 global monitoring report*; and J. Kutzin and S. P. Sparkes, "Health systems strengthening, universal health coverage, health security and resilience," *Bulletin of the World Health Organization*, 94(1), (2016): 2, https://doi.org/10.2471/BLT.15.165050.

8. WHO, *Draft thirteenth general programme of work 2019–2023* [version: 26 January 2018].

9. WHO and World Bank, *Tracking universal health coverage: 2017 global monitoring report*.

10. See, for example, X. Huang and N. Yoshino, "Impacts of universal health coverage: financing, income inequality, and social welfare," *ADBI Working Paper Series* no. 617 (2017), https://www.adb.org/sites/default/files/publication/214481/adbi-wp617.pdf, and K. Cleeren, L. Lamey, J. H. Meyer, and K. De Ruyter, "How business cycles affect the healthcare sector: a cross-country investigation," *Health Economics*, 25(7), (2016): 787–800, https://doi.org/10.1002/hec.3187.

11. M. Mackintosh, A. Channon, A. Karan, S. Selvaraj, E. Cavagnero, and H. Zhao, "What is the private sector? Understanding private provision in the health systems of low-income and middle-income countries," *Lancet*, (388), (2016): 596–605, https://doi.org/10.1016/S0140-6736(16)00342-1.

12. P. Yadav, "Health product supply chains in developing countries: diagnosis of the root causes of underperformance and an agenda for reform," *Health Systems & Reform*, 1(2), (2015): 142–154, https://doi.org/10.4161/23288604.2014.968005.

13. D. T. Jamison, L. H. Summers, G. Alleyne, et al., "Global health 2035: a world converging within a generation," *The Lancet*, (2013), http://dx.doi.org/10.1016/S0140-6736(13) 62105-4.

14. J. D. Sachs, *Macroeconomics and Health: Investing in Health for Economic Development: Report of the Commission on Macroeconomics and Health* (Geneva: World Health Organization, 2001), http://apps.who.int/iris/bitstream/10665/42435/1/924154550X.pdf.

15. WHO, *Together on the road to universal health coverage—a call to action* (Geneva: World Health Organization, 2017), http://apps.who.int/iris/bitstream/10665/258962/1/WHO -HIS-HGF-17.1-eng.pdf?ua=1.

16. R. Horton, E. C. Araujo, H. Bhorat, et al., *High-level commission on health employment and economic growth—final report* (Geneva: World Health Organization, 2016), http:// apps.who.int/iris/bitstream/10665/250040/1/9789241511285-eng.pdf?ua=1.

17. K.-D. Henke, "The economic and the health dividend of the health care system" (presentation at the Health Forum, Vilnius, Lithuania, WifOR Darmstadt, 2013), https:// vitaltransformation.com/sustainablehealth/pdfs/presentations/Klaus-Dirk Henke.pdf.

18. BMWi, *Gesundheitswirtschaft—Fakten & Zahlen* (Berlin: Bundesministerium für Wirtschaft und Energie [BMWi], 2016), https://www.bmwi.de/Redaktion/DE/Publi kationen/Wirtschaft/gesundheitswirtschaft-fakten-zahlen-2016.pdf?__blob =publicationFile&v=16.

19. Henke, "The economic and the health dividend of the health care system."

20. P. Hernandez, S. Dräger, D. B. Evans, T.-T. Edejer, and M. R. Dal Poz, *Measuring expenditure for the health workforce: evidence and challenges* (Geneva: World Health Organization, 2006), http://www.who.int/hrh/documents/measuring_expenditure.pdf?ua=1.

21. Horton et al., *High-level commission on health employment and economic growth—final report*.

22. S. Anand and T. Bärnighausen, "Human resources and health outcomes: cross-country econometric study," *The Lancet*, 364, (2004): 1603–1609, https://doi.org/10.1016/S0140 -6736(04)17313-3.

23. S. Anand and T. Bärnighausen, "Health workers and vaccination coverage in developing countries: an econometric analysis," *The Lancet*, 369(9569), (2007): 1277–1285, https://doi.org/10.1016/S0140-6736(07)60599-6.

24. Y. Hu, L. Shen, J. Guo, and S. Xie, "Public health workers and vaccination coverage in eastern China: a health economic analysis," *International Journal of Environmental Research and Public Health*, 11(5), (2014): 5555–5566, https://doi.org/10.3390/ijerph 110505555.

25. Fourth Global Forum on Human Resources for Health, *Dublin declaration on human resources for health: building the workforce of the future* (Dublin: Fourth Global Forum on Human Resources for Health, 2017), http://www.who.int/hrh/events/Dublin _Declaration-on-HumanResources-for-Health.pdf?ua=1.

26. This section refers to gross fixed capital investment, which covers *only* fixed assets. Fixed assets include land improvements (fences, ditches, drains, and so on); plant, machinery, and equipment purchases; and the construction of roads, railways, and the like, including schools, offices, hospitals, private residential dwellings, and commercial and industrial buildings.

27. In Germany, the United Kingdom, the United States, and Norway, the average annual growth rate of gross fixed capital formation was not just higher than that for the manufacturing sector but also higher than that for the entire economy.

28. I. Massa, M. Mendez-Parra, and D. Willem te Velde, "The macroeconomic effects of development finance institutions in sub-Saharan Africa," ODI 2016, https://www.odi.org/sites/odi.org.uk/files/resource-documents/11182.pdf.

29. K. Makoye, "Buzz as world's biggest drone drug deliveries take off in Tanzania," accessed February 3, 2018, https://af.reuters.com/article/topNews/idAFKCN1B91HV-OZATP.

30. B. M. Till, A. W. Peters, S. Afshar, and J. Meara, "From blockchain technology to global health equity: can cryptocurrencies finance universal health coverage?," *BMJ Global Health*, 2(4), (2017): e000570, https://doi.org/10.1136/bmjgh-2017-000570.

31. McKinsey Global Institute, *Driving German Competitiveness in the Digital Future*, https://www.mckinsey.com/mgi/overview/2017-in-review/whats-next-in-digital-and-ai/driving-german-competitiveness-in-the-digital-future.

32. World Economic Forum, *Value in healthcare: mobilizing cooperation for health system transformation* (World Economic Forum, 2018), https://www.weforum.org/reports/.

33. OECD, *New Health Technologies: Managing Access, Value and Sustainability* (Paris: OECD Publishing, 2017). https://doi.org/10.1787/9789264266438-en.

34. World Economic Forum, *Health systems leapfrogging in emerging economies* (Geneva: World Economic Forum, 2014), http://www3.weforum.org/docs/WEF_HealthSystem_LeapfroggingEmergingEconomies_ProjectPaper_2014.pdf.

35. M. C. Schwärzler and B. Legler, *The economic footprint of the German health economy according to ESA 2010 [Der ökonomische Fußabdruck der Gesundheitswirtschaft in Deutschland nach ESVG 2010]* (WifOR Darmstadt, 2017), https://mpra.ub.uni-muenchen.de/79066/1/MPRA_paper_79066.pdf.

36. Schwärzler and Legler, *Economic footprint of the German health economy*.

37. WHO, *Women on the move: migration, care work and health* (Geneva: World Health Organization, 2017), http://apps.who.int/iris/bitstream/10665/259463/1/9789241513142-eng.pdf?ua=1.

38. A. Dillon, J. Friedman, and P. Serneels, "Health Information, Treatment, and Worker Productivity: Experimental Evidence from Malaria Testing and Treatment among Nigerian Sugarcane Cutters" 8074 (March 2014), http://hdl.handle.net/10986/20645.

39. E. V. Velenyi, "Health care spending and economic growth," in *World Scientific Handbook of Global Health Economics and Public Policy*, ed. R. M. Scheffler (Singapore: World Scientific Publishing, 2016), 1–155.

40. D. E. Bloom, D. Canning, and J. Sevilla, "The Effect of Health on Economic Growth: A Production Function Approach," *World Development*, 32(1), (2004): 1–13, https://doi.org/https://doi.org/10.1016/j.worlddev.2003.07.002.

41. Velenyi, "Health care spending and economic growth."

42. D. E. Bloom, D. Canning, L. Hu, Y. Liu, A. Mahal, and W. Yip, "The contribution of population health and demographic change to economic growth in China and India," *Journal of Comparative Economics*, 38(1), (2010): 17–33, https://doi.org/10.1016/j.jce.2009.11.002.

43. T. Suri, M. A. Boozer, G. Ranis, and F. Stewart, "Paths to Success: The Relationship between Human Development and Economic Growth," *World Development*, 39(4), (2011): 506–522, https://doi.org/https://doi.org/10.1016/j.worlddev.2010.08.020.

44. OECD, "Health at a glance 2017: OECD Indicators: USA" (Paris: OECD Publishing, 2017), https://doi.org/10.1787/health_glance-2017-en.

45. A. Sagan, D. Panteli, W. Borkowski, et al., "Poland: health system review," *Health Systems in Transition*, 2011, 13(8):1–193.

46. Citing the Polish Ministry of Health, Portal of Professional Nurses in Poland, 2012, accessed February 4, 2018, http://www.pielegniarki.info.pl/article/view/id/4109.

47. A. Buscher, *Nurses and Midwives: A Force for Health* (Copenhagen: WHO, 2009), http://www.euro.who.int/__data/assets/pdf_file/0019/114157/E93980.pdf.

48. K. Gillet and M. Taylor, "Romanian health service in crisis as doctors leave for the UK and other states," *The Guardian* (2014), https://www.theguardian.com/world/2014/feb/07/romanian-health-service-crisis-doctors-uk.

49. D. Ratha, C. Eigen-Zucchi, and S. Plaza, *Migration and Remittances Factbook 2016*, 3rd ed. (Washington, DC: World Bank Publications, 2016).

50. M. Helble and B. Shepherd, "Trade in health products: reducing trade barriers for better health," *ADBI Working Paper* no. 643 (ADB Institute, 2017), https://www.adb.org/sites/default/files/publication/224171/adbi-wp643.pdf.

51. C. Franz and S. Deo, "Health from India vs health for India: the financial express," April 7, 2018, https://www.financialexpress.com/opinion/.

52. E. t' Hoen, *Private Patents and Public Health—Changing Intellectual Property Rules for Access to Medicines* (Amsterdam: Health Action International, 2016).

53. V. J. Wirtz, H. V. Hogerzeil, A. L. Gray, et al., "Essential medicines for universal health coverage," *The Lancet*, 389(10067), (2017): 403–476, https://doi.org/10.1016/S0140-6736(16)31599-9.

54. BMZ, *Local production of pharmaceuticals and health system strengthening in Africa* (Berlin: Federal Ministry for Economic Cooperation and Development [BMZ], 2017), https://health.bmz.de/ghpc/evidence_briefs/local_production_pharmaceuticals_health_system_strengthening_africa/EB_Pharma.pdf.

55. I. Kickbusch, L. Allen, and C. Franz, "The commercial determinants of health," *The Lancet Global Health*, 4(12), (2016): 895–896, https://doi.org/10.1016/S2214-109X(16)30217-0.

56. "The commercial determinants of health are those conditions, actions and omissions that affect health. Commercial determinants arise in the context of the provision of goods or services for payment and include commercial activities, as well as the environment in which commerce takes place. Commercial determinants can have beneficial and/or detrimental impacts on health." WHO, Preparation for the third high-level meeting of the General Assembly on the prevention and control of non-communicable diseases, to be held in 2018, report by the Director-General (Geneva: World Health Organization, 2017), http://apps.who.int/gb/ebwha/pdf_files/EB142/B142_15-en.pdf.

57. United Nations, *Transforming our world: the 2030 agenda for sustainable development* (A/RES/70/1), (New York: United Nations, 2015), http://www.un.org/ga/search/view_doc.asp?symbol=A/RES/70/1&Lang=E.

58. United Nations, *Addis Ababa Action Agenda of the Third International Conference on Financing for Development* (New York: United Nations, 2015), https://doi.org/10.1017/CBO9781107415324.004.

59. D. Stuckler, S. Basu, M. Suhrcke, A. Coutts, and M. McKee, "The public health effect of economic crises and alternative policy responses in Europe: an empirical analysis," *The Lancet*, 374(9686), (2009): 315–323, https://doi.org/10.1016/S0140-6736(09)61124-7.

60. The contrast between "Bismarck" and "Beveridge" approaches to health financing derives from the difference between the approach taken in Otto von Bismarck's 1883 social health insurance law in Germany and the United Kingdom's National Health Service (1948), established on principles introduced by William Henry Beveridge in his report on social insurance and allied services in 1942. In a nutshell, Bismarck's approach understood health insurance as a right of labor, funded by private employers and employees, while Beveridge saw health coverage as a fundamental constitutional right of citizenship, funded by general government revenues. Bismarck envisioned social insurance for the workforce, while Beveridge argued for universal health coverage.

61. K. Cleeren, L. Lamey, J. H. Meyer, and K. De Ruyter, "How business cycles affect the healthcare sector: a cross-country investigation," *Health Economics*, 25(7), (2016): 787–800, https://doi.org/10.1002/hec.3187.

62. J. Arze del Granado, S. Gupta, and A. Hajdenberg, "Is social spending procyclical? Evidence for developing countries," *World Development*, 42(1), (2013): 16–27, https://doi.org/10.1016/j.worlddev.2012.07.003.

63. K. Gürsoy, "An overview of Turkish healthcare system after health transformation program: main successes, performance assessment, further challenges, and policy options," *Sosyal Guvence* (2015): 83–112, 10.21441/sguz.2015717913.

64. R. Atun, S. Aydın, S. Chakraborty, et al., "Universal health coverage in Turkey: enhancement of equity," *The Lancet*, 382(9886), (2013): 65–99, https://doi.org/10.1016/S0140-6736(13)61051-X.

65. R. Atun, "Transforming Turkey's health system—lessons for universal coverage," *New England Journal of Medicine Perspective*, 373 (2015): 1285–1289, https://doi.org/10.1056/NEJMp1410433.

66. E. S. Yılmaz, G. Koçkaya, F. B. Yenilmez, et al., "Impact of health policy changes on trends in the pharmaceutical market in Turkey," *Value in Health Regional Issues*, 10(3), (2016): 48–52, https://doi.org/10.1016/j.vhri.2016.07.002.

67. Yilmaz et al., "Impact of Health Policy Changes."

68. A. O. Aktan, K. Pala, and B. Ilhan, "Health-care reform in Turkey: far from perfect," *The Lancet*, 383(9911), (2017), 25–26. https://doi.org/10.1016/S0140-6736(13)62725-7.

69. E. Olcay, "Turkey—medical technology and health IT," 2017, https://www.export.gov/article?id.

70. I. Eren Vural, "Financialisation in health care: An analysis of private equity fund investments in Turkey," *Social Science & Medicine*, 187, (2017): 276–286, https://doi.org/10.1016/j.socscimed.2017.06.008.

71. G. Russo, G. Bloom, and D. McCoy, "Universal health coverage, economic slowdown and system resilience: Africa's policy dilemma," *BMJ Global Health*, 2(3), (2017): e000400, https://doi.org/10.1136/bmjgh-2017-000400.

72. World Bank, *Background paper to the first Universal Health Coverage Financing Forum* (Washington, DC: The World Bank Group, 2016), http://pubdocs.worldbank.org/en/103621460561160053/DRM-policy-note-041216-clean.pdf.

73. BMZ, *Local production of pharmaceuticals.*

2

The Relationship between Health Employment and Economic Growth

Pascal Zurn, Jim Campbell, Jeremy Lauer, Ibadat Dhillon, Tana Wuliji, and Jean-Louis Arcand

The health workforce is at the center of every health system but often turns out to be its weakest link: typically perceived as a cost driver instead of an area for public and private investment. However, with the rise of the new health economy, there is growing recognition that creating jobs for health workers holds the potential to bolster not only population health but also economic growth. The new health economy constitutes a rising economic force, and the health workforce is one of its most important resources. Moreover, the health workforce represents a large and growing share of the total labor force in many countries. Investing in the health workforce leads to significant returns on investment through different economic pathways that improve health outcomes, including the creation of employment opportunities for individuals (particularly for women). These returns on investment contribute to inclusive economic growth, improved social cohesion, and global health security.

Given the needs and challenges of the health workforce in many countries around the world, investment in health employment ought to be significant. Within this context, private sector investments can play a role as well, since, in most countries, private sector workers (in both the formal and informal sectors) are an integral part of the new health economy. Demonstrating the importance of return on investment and attracting enough resources, from both the public and the private sectors, will be critical. To that end, lessons learned from other sectors, notably from the Green

The views expressed in this chapter by its named authors are solely the responsibility of those authors.

Economy, could be very useful. Shifting the paradigm about health employment from one of *cost* to one of *investment* will be key to achieving an effective health workforce in the twenty-first century.

Introduction

The health workforce is at the center of every health system. The knowledge, skills, and motivation of health workers play a crucial role in delivering health services to those in need, which contributes to improving health outcomes and the well-being of the population. Yet, the health workforce often turns out to be the weakest link of the health system and is typically perceived as a cost driver instead of an area for public and private investment. In many countries, policy discussions on health workforce reforms focus on issues of cost containment.

However, with the emergence of the concept of the new health economy, there is a growing recognition that creating jobs for health workers holds the potential to bolster not only population health but also economic growth. Recognizing the new health economy has the potential to transform the health sector and can also have important and positive impacts on other economic sectors. Therefore, this concept plays an increasingly important role in our understanding of the overall economy and in ensuring that economic growth is more inclusive. This emerging shift has been highlighted by the recent work of the UN High-Level Commission on Health Employment and Economic Growth.[1] Health has an economy, an economic footprint, and labor market dynamics all its own.

Building on the recent work of this commission[2] and on *Global Strategy on Human Resources for Health: Workforce 2030,*[3] from the World Health Organization (WHO), this chapter analyzes the key contributions that health employment makes to the overall economy. We discuss the role and importance of the health workforce in the new health economy and the critical link between health employment and economic growth. Then, we shift our attention to lessons learned from the Green Economy that contribute useful insights for the new health economy. Finally, we scrutinize the link between health employment and healthy economic growth.

The Rise of a New Health Economy

The rise of new public health challenges, demographic changes, rapid advances in medical science and technology, the fusion of a wide range of sectors powered by technological advances, and new models of care are all contributing to shape the new health economy, which reaches beyond the health sector to the totality of societal health. Innovative approaches are shaping the new health economy. It is expected to be one of the major growth markets of the future that can drive growth across all sectors of the economy and not merely in healthcare.[4]

The new health economy constitutes an increasingly important economic force simply by reason of its size. When total global health expenditure is used as a proxy for assessing its importance, the health economy amounted to US$ 7.2 trillion in 2012.[5] The health economy also affects the competitiveness of the overall economy in many countries through its effect on labor costs, labor market flexibility, and the allocation of resources, notably the level and allocation of public spending.[6]

The new health economy will also be shaped by global health challenges such as noncommunicable diseases, population aging, global health security, and more generally by policies aimed at achieving universal health coverage and the Sustainable Development Goals (SDGs) adopted by the 70th United Nations General Assembly in 2015. An understanding of the impact and ramifications of the new health economy provides a rationale for investing in health, which can lead to both equitable improvements in health and to economic growth. Within this context, the role of the health workforce is a critical component of the new health economy.

Health Employment Is a Pillar of the New Health Economy

While advances in science and technology are definitely driving the new health economy, it remains very labor-intensive. Employment in health and social services represents a large and growing share of the labor force in many countries. In countries that belong to the Organisation for Economic Co-operation and Development (OECD), health and social work activities constituted around 11% of total employment, on average, in 2014.[7] In countries like Norway, Denmark, and Finland, employment in the health and social care sector as a share of total employment is particularly pronounced (figure 2.1). Employment in the health and social care sector represents more than 16% of these countries' workforces[8] and is projected to rise to 38% in Norway by 2060.[9]

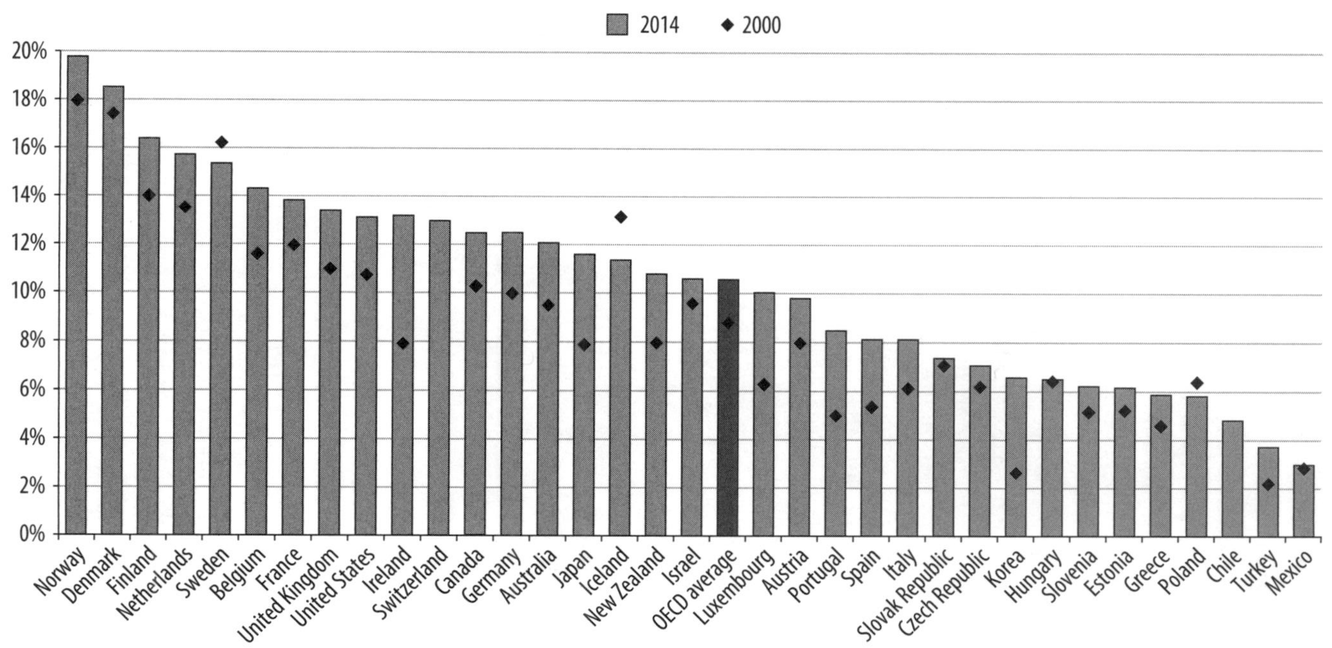

Figure 2.1. Employment in health and social work as a share of total employment in OECD countries, 2004 and 2014 (or latest year available). Sources: OECD.Stat, Annual Labour Force Statistics, Employment by activities and status, 2016, and National Accounts, Detailed Tables and Simplified Accounts, Table 7A. Labour input by activity, International Standard Industrial Classification, revision 4.

In recent years, employment growth in the health sector has also usually exceeded that of other sectors. In the EU-15 (15 countries of the European Union), employment in this sector rose by 5.9 million between 2000 and 2014, corresponding to an increase of 39%, or almost double the rate of growth observed in the service sector (22%).[10] In contrast, over the same period, employment in industry went down as a whole almost everywhere, generating job losses on the order of 6.9 million. Consequently, the share of employed persons in the health and social care sector in total employment rose across the EU-15 from 9.5% to 12.1% between 2000 and 2014.[11]

Employment in the health sector is also resilient, as previous experiences with recession have shown that employment in the health sector tends to be less sensitive to cyclical fluctuations than employment in other sectors.[12] Recent investigations published by the International Labour Organization find a similar employment effect in the wider economy of healthcare at the global level.[13]

According to future projections, the health sector will add many jobs in the next decades. Worldwide, the WHO expects a near doubling in the demand for employment in the health workforce by 2030, with the creation of around 40 million new health worker jobs, primarily in upper-middle- and high-income countries.[14] Each health and social worker job is supported by one to two additional jobs, which in sum may create more than 120 million new jobs worldwide in the health and social sectors by 2030.[15] No doubt, other forms of entrepreneurial growth will be associated with the increase in health employment: training activities, employment centers, and much more will arise as a result. In all, few economic sectors present such opportunities for steady growth (see table 2.1).

In a country like the United States, employment in healthcare occupations is projected to grow 19% from 2014 to 2024, much faster than the average growth for all occupations, and will add about 2.3 million new jobs.[16] Growth is expected to be particularly significant for allied health workers; according to Rush University, more than half of the US healthcare workforce will be employed in an allied health field by 2020.[17] To some extent, a similar trend is anticipated for low- and middle-income countries, as well. For example, India is expected to gain an estimated 7.5 million jobs in the health sector by 2022.[18]

Despite these developments, many countries are still grappling with major health workforce challenges. Critical shortages in the supply of workers,

Table 2.1. Employment by major industry sector in the United States, 2004, 2014, and projected 2024

Industry sector	Number of jobs (in thousands) 2004	Number of jobs (in thousands) 2024	Percentage distribution 2004	Percentage distribution 2024	Annual rate of change 2014–24
Total for all sectors	144,047.00	160,328.80	100	100	0.6
Goods-producing sectors, excluding agriculture	21,815.30	19,227.00	15.1	12	0
Mining	523.2	924	0.4	0.6	0.9
Construction	6,976.20	6,928.80	4.8	4.3	1.2
Manufacturing	14,315.90	11,374.20	9.9	7.1	−0.7
Service-providing sectors	110,646.90	129,904.60	76.8	81	0.7
Utilities	563.8	505.1	0.4	0.3	−0.9
Wholesale trade	5,663.00	6,151.40	3.9	3.8	0.5
Retail trade	15,058.20	16,129.10	10.5	10.1	0.5
Transportation and warehousing	4,248.60	4,776.90	2.9	3	0.3
Information	3,118.30	2,712.60	2.2	1.7	−0.1
Financial activities	8,105.10	8,486.70	5.6	5.3	0.6
Professional and business services	16,394.90	20,985.50	11.4	13.1	0.9
Private educational services	2,762.50	3,756.10	1.9	2.3	0.9
Healthcare and social assistance	**14,429.80**	**21,852.20**	**10**	**13.6**	**1.9**
Leisure and hospitality	12,493.10	15,651.20	8.7	9.8	0.6
Other services	6,188.30	6,662.00	4.3	4.2	0.4
Federal government	2,730.00	2,345.60	1.9	1.5	−1.5
State and local government	18,891.30	19,890.10	13.1	12.4	0.4
Agriculture, forestry, fishing, and hunting	2,111.30	2,027.70	1.5	1.3	−0.5
Agricultural wage and salary	1,149.00	1,307.30	0.8	0.8	−0.6
Agricultural self-employed workers	962.3	720.4	0.7	0.4	−0.5
Nonagricultural self-employed	9,473.60	9,169.50	6.6	5.7	0.7

Source: US Bureau of Labor Statistics, Employment Projections Program, 2015

an inadequate mix of skills in the workforce, and an inequitable distribution of health workers—as well as gaps in the capacity, motivation, and performance of health workers—will seriously affect the future performance of health systems if they are not addressed by bold new measures. Moreover, the dramatic projection of increased demand for new health worker jobs needs to be understood in the context of projected supply shortages of as many as 18 million health workers, primarily in low- and lower-middle-income countries.[19] Reaching an adequate number of jobs—and creating the right type of jobs—requires not only political and social will but also requires significant financial investment. This raises the issue of the return on such investment.

From Health Employment to Economic Growth

The relationship among health, health employment, and the economy is central to the new health economy. While it has long been recognized that increased national wealth is associated with improved health, the contribution of better health to economic growth has only recently become a focal point.[20] The economic effects of population health can be seen both at the individual and at the macroeconomic, or aggregate, level. Improved health boosts personal and national income through its positive effects on education, productivity, investment, availability of resources, and demographics.[21]

Research, including historical case studies, microeconomic studies at the individual or household level, and macroeconomic studies taking different perspectives and approaches, demonstrates that health improvements stimulate economic growth.[22] In particular, both the World Bank's *World Development Report 1993: Investing in Health* and the report of the Commission on Macroeconomics and Health made a strong economic case for investing in health.[23] Although limited primarily to evidence from low- and middle-income countries, these reports helped to prepare the ground for a shift in the paradigm. With this shift, health would no longer be seen as a mere by-product of economic development but as one of several key determinants of both economic development and poverty reduction. In their review of studies, Jamison and colleagues concluded that health improvements have accounted for about 11% of the growth in full income in low- and middle-income countries.[24] More recently, the *Lancet* published *Global Health 2035*, a report by the Commission on Investing in Health, which revisited the case for investing in health and reaffirmed the key role of health in economic growth.[25]

While the health workforce is not the only factor in the overall health of a population, it is a critical factor given its role in service delivery. Its importance is also evident in the large share of total health expenditure made in employing the health workforce. The remuneration of all salaried health workers in the public and private sectors combined was estimated to represent between 35% and 55% of total health expenditure.[26,27] The SDG health price-tag study found that the health workforce is the largest subcomponent of the resources needed to achieve health-related SDGs, constituting nearly 50% of health sector investments.[28]

Therefore, it is important to understand better the economic impact of investing in the health workforce. McPake et al. have thoroughly examined the return on investment of medical education.[29] From this economic perspective, individuals make investment decisions when they choose to undertake a medical education; these are investments in human capital.[30] Unfortunately, human capital has generally been understood as limited to education, whereas, in reality, health status is likewise a form of human capital in the economic sense. Nevertheless, since investment decisions usually incur costs and deliver payoffs over time, we must consider the entire stream of costs and benefits. That is, medical education involves an expenditure of time and money in the near-term future that yields a stream of benefits in the more-distant future. The expected returns on human capital investments (in terms of education) are a higher level of earnings, greater lifetime job satisfaction, and greater appreciation of nonmarket activities and interests. From the human capital approach, the rate of return on education can be estimated: a high and rising average rate of return for a medical profession is expected to attract more individuals to that profession.

A number of estimates have been made on the rate of return for medical education and its net present value (i.e., the value, discounted to the present, of the future stream of benefits). The rate of return provides an easily understood measure of the financial attractiveness of a medical career, since it can be compared with rates of return available from alternative investments and with market interest rates. According to either criterion, in a country like the United States, research has almost always found medical education to be a good investment.[31] However, one limitation of this approach is that it does not account for nonmarket economic benefits, nor does it account for benefits realized beyond the individual (i.e., the impact on productivity for a healthier population that results from having a higher density of health workers). To include a broader range of benefits, both market-valued and non-market-valued benefits, requires a different approach.

Looking at health workforce expenditure from a broader perspective, including all expenses related to the health workforce, the recent work of the UN High-Level Commission on Health Employment and Economic Growth suggests that adequate investment in the health system and its workforce can offer high economic returns.[32] Rather than seeing expenditures on the education and employment of additional health workers as a cost to achieving universal health coverage and SDGs, available evidence suggests that it is a wise investment in the future economic growth of a nation.

The Pathway to Economic Growth

The health workforce contributes to human welfare not only by providing care; it also has additional positive spillover effects. This is illustrated by the framework developed by the UN High-Level Commission on Health Employment and Economic Growth (figure 2.2). This framework presents the multiple pathways from the health system to economic growth, in particular those that involve health employment. The commission identified six main pathways: (i) health, (ii) economic output, (iii) social protection, (iv) social cohesion, (v) innovation and diversification, and (vi) health security.[33]

First, the health pathway—better health leading to longer life expectancy and improved quality of life—not only has a value of its own, but it also allows people to engage in a higher level of (market-valued) activities, which can increase the labor supply and lead to higher levels of productivity.[34] In other words, healthy workers lose less time from work because of ill health and are more productive when they are working; moreover, they have lower rates of early retirement. In this health pathway to economic growth, health is considered to have intrinsic benefit; that is, health has value on its own terms as a fundamental part of well-being. To compare intrinsic benefits with other benefits, health gains are valued with the full-income approach, which incorporates the value of life expectancy gains in monetary terms.

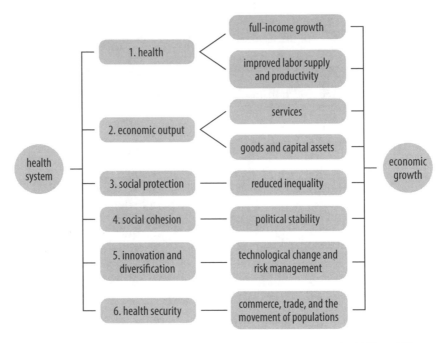

Figure 2.2. Pathways to economic growth. Source: Lauer et al., 2016, p. 176 (see note 33)

Second, as discussed above, the economic outputs of the health sector are large and have been increasing worldwide over the past decades. This trend is expected to continue. In particular, rural areas have benefited directly and indirectly from the economic outputs related to health employment. Evidence shows that health employment is particularly important for rural economic development; in rural communities, a primary care hospital is often one of the largest employers. Health services also have indirect impacts on the rural economy by creating additional jobs and income in other sectors. Studies demonstrate that the primary and secondary impacts on rural community employment and income often account for 15% to 20% of the community's total employment and income.[35] In addition, the literature strongly supports the conclusion that a viable health sector is needed if a rural community wants to attract businesses in other industries.[36] This would, in turn, lead to dynamic economic changes and encourage innovation from the resident population.

Eilrich et al. demonstrate that, in rural areas of the United States, the economic contributions of healthcare services are just as important as the medical contributions.[37] They estimate that a rural physician generates approximately $1.5 million in revenue, $0.9 million in payroll (wages, salaries, and benefits) and creates 22 jobs. Avery et al. show that a family physician practicing obstetrics in rural Alabama adds an additional $488,560 in economic benefit to the community.[38] Added to the $1 million from the physician's practice of family medicine, the total annual benefit is almost $1.5 million. They estimate that of the $616,385 invested by the Alabama Family Practice Rural Health Board, each dollar resulted in a $399 benefit to the community.

The significant economic impact of health employment in rural areas is not limited to physicians. The same study found that physician assistants and nurse practitioners also have an economic effect on the local community.[39] Most of the evidence is from high-income countries, and it is possible that the situation in rural areas differs significantly for low-income countries, notably with respect to their infrastructure, health, and education. Nevertheless, research recognizes similar factors as key elements for rural economic development in low- and middle-income countries.[40] In short, the significant economic contribution of health employment to rural economic development should be central to discussions about improving access to health workers in rural and remote areas.

Third, health employment offers a range of social protection benefits. These benefits reduce the population's economic and social vulnerabilities to poverty and deprivation. In addition, health systems offering protection against the financial consequences of illness represent important positive spillover benefits that contribute to economic growth.[41] Social protection programs also contribute positively to the productivity of the next generation through their impact on upbringing and education.

Fourth, societies are cohesive when they have the capacity to manage collective decision making peacefully. Jobs contribute to social cohesion by nurturing trust in others and reinforcing social capital.[42] Good jobs are needed for economic growth, but they also contribute the most to societal goals—as do jobs in health.[43] Investing in health employment also provides opportunities to increase women's participation in the labor market and to reduce youth unemployment or underemployment (see box below). Currently, the rate of female participation in the labor force is consistently much lower than male participation, and integrating women and youth into the labor force is an opportunity to promote gender equity and bring about social and economic progress.[44,45] The positive economic effects of bringing more women into the workforce is clearly a strong argument in favor of changing investment patterns.

Investing in the health sector generates substantial employment and improves women's participation in the labor market

A recent report by the Women's Budget Group for the International Trade Union Confederation and UN Women shows that investing in the health and social care sector generates substantial increases in employment. The authors estimate that if 2% of GDP were invested in the health and care sector, it would, depending on the country (Brazil, Costa Rica, China, India, Indonesia, South Africa, and Germany) generate increases in overall employment ranging from 1.2% to 3.2%. This would translate into the creation of nearly 24 million new jobs in China, 11 million in India, 2.8 million in Indonesia, 4.2 million in Brazil, just over 400,000 in South Africa, and 63,000 in Costa Rica. In most countries the total quantity of employment generated by investment in health and care is greater than that of an equivalent investment in construction. In addition, across all the countries in this study, the direct effect of public investment in the health and care sector would lead to a greater number of the newly created jobs going to women than if the same level of investment were made in construction. Thus, while public investment in either of these sectors would have a large positive employment effect, if policies aim to create employment for women and reduce the gender employment gap overall, investment in health and care would be the more effective investment.

Source: Jerome De Henau, Susan Himmelweit, and Diane Perrons, *Investing in the Care Economy*, ed. Eva Neitzert and Mary-Ann Stephenson (Brussels: International Trade Union Confederation, 2017).

Fifth, the diversification and innovation pathway illustrates how some countries have invested in their health sectors specifically to promote economic growth. For example, medical tourism is a growing trend, with a growth rate of approximately 15% to 20% annually, amounting to revenues estimated at US$ 50 to 72 billion in 2017.[46] Some of the most important health tourism destinations are Costa Rica, India, Malaysia, Mexico, Singapore, South Korea, Thailand, Turkey, and the United States. Also, the role of technological innovation (3-D imaging in medicine, for example) is important in the new health economy and is a driver of productivity and economic growth.

Sixth, a resilient health workforce contributes to reducing a population's vulnerability to acute public health events that endanger the collective health, both nationally and internationally, according to the WHO. Protection from acute threats to public health is recognized as one of the most important nontraditional security issues.[47] Countries better insulated from disease threats provide safer environments for economic activities. Pandemics without effective responses can devastate public health and the economy. For instance, economic output forgone to Ebola outbreaks in Guinea, Liberia, and Sierra Leone in 2015 was estimated to exceed $1.6 billion, or more than 12% of those countries' gross domestic product (GDP) for the year.[48]

Empirically assessing the overall impact of the health workforce on economic growth is a complex task, however. So determining the specific contribution of the health workforce for each of the above pathways will be challenging. An exhaustive assessment of the impact of health employment on economic growth would require the inclusion of a range of nonmarket benefits beyond those mentioned here. Indeed, many studies estimate growth by using national accounts data, reflecting a market value of goods and services produced in a given period. Excluding nonmarket benefits implicitly undervalues the return on investment; therefore, policy decisions regarding the health workforce may not accurately reflect its true value to society. Within this context, there is a growing global consensus that GDP does not provide a full measure of overall economic performance.[49] The so-called Green Economy provides an interesting additional perspective.

Lessons from the Green Economy

There are parallels between the new health economy and the Green Economy. Both can be seen as contributing to an alternative vision for growth and development, one that generates growth and improvements in people's lives in ways consistent with sustainable development. Although sometimes sustainability and health are postulated as hindrances to economic growth, they are in fact engines of growth because they are net generators of decent jobs.[50]

The Green Economy also highlights the limitations of an economic growth model focused on increasing GDP above all other goals. While this approach has improved incomes and reduced poverty for hundreds of millions, and has contributed to a longer life expectancy, it comes with significant social and environmental costs, which in turn have longer-term

Social return on investment

Social return on investment (SROI) is a tool for measuring social impact that has received a lot of attention in recent years. SROI corresponds to "a process for understanding, measuring and reporting the social, economic and environmental value created by an intervention, policy or organization" (Banke-Thomas et al.). "One of the most critical parts in SROI, methodologically speaking, is the quantitative and especially the monetary capturing of impact" (Centre for Social Investment). In principle, the SROI method can portray the relation between a "social investment" and its social benefits by translating certain aspects of social value into financial values, which result in an SROI coefficient. This monetary component is complemented by an alternative quantitative and qualitative capturing of softer "social" returns.

Sources: Aduragbemi Oluwabusayo Banke-Thomas, Barbara Madaj, Ameh Charles, and Nynke van den Broek, "Social Return on Investment (SROI) Methodology to Account for Value for Money of Public Health Interventions: A Systematic Review" BMC Public Health 15 (2015): 582. Centre for Social Investment, 2013; Centre for Social Investment, Social Returns on Investment (SROI): State-of-the-Art and Perspectives. A Meta-Analysis of Practice in Social Return on Investment (SROI) Studies Published 2002–2012 (Heidelberg: Centre for Social Investment, Heidelberg University, 2013).

economic and social costs that hamper progress toward greater life expectancy and quality of life. In BRICS countries (Brazil, Russia, India, China, and South Africa), economic growth has also brought with it new public health issues and is putting additional pressure on health systems. For instance, pollution, road-traffic injuries, and diseases like diabetes are all increasing. In China, the damage caused by air and water pollution was found to cost the country around 4.3% of its total GDP.[51]

Innovative financing mechanisms: green bonds and Green Climate Fund

Green bonds are innovative financial instruments where the proceeds are invested exclusively in green projects that generate climate or other environmental benefits: projects in, for example, renewable energy, energy efficiency, sustainable waste management, sustainable land use (forestry and agriculture), biodiversity, clean transportation, or clean water. Their structure, risk, and returns are otherwise identical to those of traditional bonds. The International Capital Market Association's Green Bond Principles and the Climate Bonds Initiative's Climate Bond Standards help to determine whether a bond qualifies as green or not. Usually, green bonds must undergo third-party verification or certification to establish that the proceeds are funding projects that generate environmental benefits. The volume of labeled green bonds has grown steadily since 2013, reaching US$ 118 billion in outstanding issuances in 2016.

Source: United Nations Development Programme

The *Green Climate Fund* was created by the UN Framework Convention on Climate Change in 2010. The fund was established by 194 governments to limit or reduce greenhouse gas emissions in developing countries and to help adapt vulnerable societies to the unavoidable impacts of climate change. Initial resource mobilization has raised more than US$ 10 billion and is ongoing. The private sector can engage through the fund's private sector facility.

Source: Green Climate Fund

The inclusion of indicators from the Green Economy is gaining acceptance. Countries such as Finland and the Netherlands are developing nationally adapted indicators to monitor and follow the Green Economy transition. Denmark has developed green production statistics to monitor the future development of green business and its significance for the Danish economy.[52] Governments are no longer relying solely on GDP to measure economic health and growth.

The Green Economy also provides useful insights for measuring non-market-valued benefits. Most environmental goods and services—things like clean air or healthy fish and wildlife populations—are not traded in markets. Their economic value is not revealed in market prices. The only option for assigning monetary values to them is to rely on nonmarket valuation methods. One such method is described in the box on page 54.

Demonstrating that investing in health employment achieves significant returns on investment provides a relevant and powerful argument for investing more in health employment. However, some countries may face fiscal space constraints that would prevent them from adequately raising this investment. In this regard, innovative financing mechanisms such as green bonds, or the new Green Climate Fund, may offer interesting insights for achieving better funding for health employment (see box on page 55).

Funding and Financing Health Workforce Investments and the Role of the Private Sector

While the above elements underline the positive impact of investing in the health workforce, one should also consider how to fund and finance those investments. Such investments, mostly from domestic sources, are achievable in many different country contexts.[53] The exact combination of domestic revenue sources will differ from country to country. However, based on current trends, there will likely be insufficient market demand and fiscal space to create jobs in the health sector to achieve the SDGs in low-income and fragile countries.[54] Since governments have finite resources at their disposal, budgeting is concerned with identifying priorities, assessing the value for money spent, and making decisions.[55] Within that context, it is crucial to achieve value for money spent in the healthcare sector. Investments in the health workforce indeed need to be effective; otherwise, they will undermine public finances. This is particularly important when prioritizing the allocation of public expenditures across sectors, for example, education, infrastructure, and defense. Budget allocation to the health workforce is also likely to be more important if the health workforce is a strategic priority for a country. Beyond public investments, other sources of financing, including private and philanthropic financing, can be instrumental to supporting public policy.

Private healthcare, especially in low-income and middle-income countries, is very extensive and very heterogeneous, ranging from training institutions, to itinerant medicine sellers, and to millions of independent practitioners—both unlicensed and licensed.[56] This heterogeneity is notably illustrated by the importance of informal employment at the community level (roles like traditional healers, home-care aides, or market vendors of various remedies), as well as by the role of nonprofit organizations in some countries. All of these contribute to the new health economy; the difficulty lies in finding the best way to harness informal sector investments to improve health outcomes and economic impact.

Within this context, the private sector can contribute to universal health coverage and to the SDGs. Investment opportunities have been identified for the private sector in the context of the implementation of SDG 3.[57] Defining which approach works best for the private sector will vary substantially, depending on the nature of the health education system, the healthcare product or service, the type of provider, and the level of a country's development in terms of GDP and its health system organization.[58]

Notable private sector investments include medical and paramedical education for the health workforce. The past several decades have seen a rapid expansion in the number of private medical and nursing schools, especially in middle- and low-income countries. In some countries, private medical schools already outnumber public ones. Such a trend has widespread implications for health education, not only for individual nations, but globally as well. The pros and cons of private education for the health workforce are strongly debated, notably in terms of substitution versus additionality. That is, in some cases, private funding substitutes for public funding, such as when it increases the total number of medical schools in places where public finances are limited; in other cases, private funding may produce markedly different, additional outcomes, such as when private institutions ply alternative curricula or feed medical specialties at variance with what public education produces. Private education has often been touted as a means to increase the supply of health workers and thus address shortages in the health workforce, especially in countries where public health education investments are low (like, for example, in India; see chapter 7 by K. Srinath Reddy in this volume). However, the rapid rise of private education raises questions about the quality of training, the relevance of the programs from a public health perspective, the cost of studies, and the lack of social accountability.

Public-private partnership for public goods can play an innovative role: it allows for the possibility of partnerships to exploit the comparative advantages of both parties, as exemplified by the Green Economy. However, one critical issue to consider is how best to align the private sector's financial interests with investing in health while also strengthening progress toward the SDGs, especially to ensure that poorer groups are reached. To that end, governments need to retain sufficient capacity to monitor and enforce the private sector's obligations. The health sector can also learn from other sectors. For example, introducing and adapting criteria like the environmental, social, and governance, or ESG, criteria for health employment could also be an option (see box below).

> ### Environmental, social, and governance criteria
>
> Environmental, social, and governance criteria are a set of standards for a company's operations that socially conscious investors use to screen their investment options. Environmental criteria concern how a company performs as a steward of the natural environment. Social criteria examine how a company manages relationships with its employees, suppliers, customers, and the communities in which it operates. Governance relates to a company's leadership, executive pay, audits and internal controls, and shareholder rights.
>
> Source: Investopedia

Finally, from a governance perspective, the Paris Agreement (COP21 mechanism) could also suggest some interesting directions for how to facilitate international policy dialogue on investing in health employment and to encourage voluntary commitments and innovation.

Toward "Healthy" Economic Growth

For growth to be healthy it needs to be directed to minimizing inequality while maximizing the efficiency of inputs, but it should also leave no one behind.[59] Economic growth is not, however, "distributionally neutral"; it can both increase and decrease inequality in a society. This reflects the prominent efficiency-versus-equity debate. As Arthur Okun has stated, "the conflict between equality and economic efficiency is inescapable."[60] This view has been very influential. Indeed, for a long time scholars thought that more equality could be achieved, but only at the expense of overall economic performance. However, it is now clear that, given the extremes of inequality seen in many countries and the manner in which they have been generated, greater equality and improved economic performance are complements.[61] Far from being either necessary or good for economic growth, excessive inequality tends to lead to weaker economic performance. Recent empirical research by the International Monetary Fund has shown that growth spells tend to be shorter when income inequality is high.[62] This has been supported by other studies.[63,64] Therefore, investing in health employment is instrumental for robust economic growth, since it contributes to decreasing inequalities and is inclusive. Reducing health inequalities not only improves population health, but it also leads to additional social benefits.

Within this context, it is interesting to note that when donors focus on investment in job creation to drive economic growth, they tend not to consider the important link between health employment and healthy economic growth.[65] Accounting for the additional economic and social benefits resulting from investing in health employment should make health employment a more attractive investment for donors.

Equal societies have more social cohesion, more solidarity, and suffer fewer stresses; they offer their citizens a greater range of better quality public goods, more social support, and they accumulate more valuable social capital.[66] Reducing health inequalities also helps economic gains trickle down more efficiently from one social stratum to the next.

Conclusion

The new health economy represents an increasing economic force, and the health workforce is one of its most important resources. The health workforce represents a large and growing share of the total labor force in many countries. As for the future, it is projected that the health sector will add many jobs in the coming decades. With the emergence of the concept of the new health economy, there is a growing recognition that creating jobs for health workers has the potential to bolster not only population health but also inclusive economic growth. Evidence suggests that, rather than seeing the need for additional health workers as a cost, these jobs can be a wise investment for healthy economic growth. Not only are they inclusive; they also contribute to decreasing inequalities. Moreover, international evidence shows that almost no country has sustained rapid growth without also maintaining impressive rates of public investment, notably in infrastructure, education, and health.

Given the needs and challenges for the health workforce in many countries around the world, investment in health employment ought to be significant. Within this context, private sector investments can play a role as well, since, in most countries, private sector workers (in both the formal and informal sectors) are an integral part of the new health economy. The critical questions are how to demonstrate the importance of return on investment and how to attract enough resources from both the public and the private sectors. To that end, lessons learned from other sectors, notably from the Green Economy, could be very useful. Shifting the paradigm about health employment from one of *cost* to one of *investment* will be key to achieving an effective health workforce for the twenty-first century—and to realizing the potential returns to economic growth and health improvement that these investments will drive.

NOTES

1. High-Level Commission on Health Employment and Economic Growth, *Working for Health and Growth: Investing in the Health Workforce* (Geneva: World Health Organization, 2016), http://apps.who.int/iris/bitstream/10665/250047/1/9789241511308-eng.pdf?ua=1.
2. High-Level Commission, *Working for Health and Growth*.
3. World Health Organization, *Global Strategy on Human Resources for Health: Workforce 2030* (Geneva: World Health Organization, 2016).

4. Krisa Tailor, *The Patient Revolution: How Big Data and Analytics Are Transforming the Health Care Experience* (Hoboken, NJ: Wiley, 2016).

5. WHO Health Accounts, "Do Health Expenditures Meet Health Needs?" WHO/HA Policy Highlight no. 1 (Geneva: World Health Organization, 2015), http://www.who.int/health-accounts/Highlight1.pdf?ua=1.

6. Marc Suhrcke, Martin McKee, Regina Sauto Arce, Svetla Tsolova, and Jorgen Mortensen, *The Contribution of Health to the Economy in the European Union* (Luxembourg: European Commission, 2005), http://ec.europa.eu/health/ph_overview/Documents/health_economy_en.pdf.

7. Chris James, *Health and Inclusive Growth: Changing the Dialogue* (Geneva: World Health Organization, 2016), http://www.who.int/hrh/com-heeg/Health_inclusive_growth_online.pdf?ua.

8. James, *Health and Inclusive Growth*.

9. Tyra Merker, Ivar Kristiansen, and Erik Saether, "Human Resources for Health Care in the Nordic Welfare Economies: Successful Today, but Sustainable Tomorrow?," in *Health Employment and Economic Growth: An Evidence Base*, ed. James Buchan, Ibadat S. Dhillon, and James Campbell (Geneva: World Health Organization, 2017), 119–38.

10. Maria Hofmarcher, Eva Festl, and Leslie Bishop-Tarver, "Health Sector Employment Growth Calls for Improvements in Labor Productivity." *Health Policy* 120, no. 8 (2016): 894–902.

11. Hofmarcher, Festl, and Bishop-Tarver, "Human Sector Employment Growth."

12. James, *Health and Inclusive Growth*.

13. High-Level Commission, *Working for Health and Growth*.

14. World Health Organization, *Global Strategy*.

15. World Health Organization, *Global Strategy*.

16. Bureau of Labor Statistics, "Occupational Outlook Handbook: Healthcare Occupations," last modified April 13, 2018, https://www.bls.gov/ooh/healthcare/home.htm.

17. Anna Johansson, "A Look at the Swift Growth in Allied Health Fields," *Huffington Post*, October 17, 2016, http://www.huffingtonpost.com/anna-johansson/a-look-at-the-swift-growt_b_12490054.html.

18. National Skill Development Corporation, *Human Resource and Skill Requirements in the Healthcare Sector*, https://www.nsdcindia.org.

19. Giorgio Cometto et al., "Health Workforce Needs, Demand and Shortages to 2030: An Overview of Forecasted Trends in the Global Health Labor Market," in *Health Employment and Economic Growth: An Evidence Base*, ed. James Buchan, Ibadat S. Dhillon, and James Campbell (Geneva: World Health Organization, 2017), 3–26.

20. World Health Organization, *Macroeconomics and Health: Investing in Health for Economic Development* (Geneva: World Health Organization, 2001).

21. Dean Jamison, Gavin Yamey, Naomi Beyeler, and Hester Wadge, *Investing in Health: The Economic Case*. Report of the WISH Investing in Health Forum 2016. World Innovation Summit for Health, http://globalhealth2035.org/sites/default/files/investing-in-health-economic-case.pdf.

22. Dean Jamison et al., "Global Health 2035: A World Converging within a Generation." *Lancet* 382, 9908 (2013): 439–58.

23. World Bank, *World Development Report.* 1993. (New York: Oxford University Press, 1993), http://elibrary.worldbank.org/doi/pdf/10.1596/0-1952-0890-0; World Health Organization, *Macroeconomics and Health: Investing in Health for Economic Development* (Geneva: World Health Organization, 2001).

24. Dean Jamison, Lawrence J. Lau, and Jia Wang, "Health's Contribution to Economic Growth in an Environment of Partially Endogenous Technical Progress," in *Health and Economic Growth: Findings and Policy Implications*, ed. Guillem Lopez-Casasnovas, Berta Rivera, and Luis Currais (Cambridge, MA: MIT Press, 2005), 67–91.

25. Jamison et al., "Global Health 2035."

26. Patricia Hernandez-Peña et al., "Health Worker Remuneration in WHO Member States," *Bulletin of the World Health Organization* 91 (2013): 808–15.

27. Jeremy Lauer et al., "Paying for Needed Health Workers for the SDGs: An Analysis of Fiscal and Financial Space," in *Health Employment and Economic Growth: An Evidence Base*, ed. James Buchan, Ibadat S. Dhillon, and James Campbell (Geneva: World Health Organization, 2017), 213–40.

28. Karin Stenberg et al., "Financing Transformative Health Systems towards Achievement of the Health Sustainable Development Goals: A Model for Projected Resource Needs in 67 Low-Income and Middle-Income countries," *Lancet Global Health* 5, no. e875–e887.

29. Barbara McPake, Allison Squires, Agya Mahat, and Edson Correia Araujo, *The Economics of Health Professional Education and Careers: Insights from a Literature Review*. A World Bank Study (Washington, DC: World Bank Group, 2015), http://documents .worldbank.org.

30. Ronald Ehrenberg and Robert S Smith, *Modern Labor Economics: Theory and Public Policy*, 11th ed. (Boston: Pearson, 2012).

31. Mircea I. Marcu et al., "Borrow or Serve? An Economic Analysis of Options for Financing a Medical School Education." *Academic Medicine* 92, no. 7 (2017): 966–75.

32. High-Level Commission, *Working for Health and Growth.*

33. Jeremy Lauer, Agnès Soucat, Edson Araujo, and David Weakliam, "Pathways: The Health System, Health Employment, and Economic Growth," in *Health Employment and Economic Growth: An Evidence Base*, ed. James Buchan, Ibadat S. Dhillon, and James Campbell (Geneva: World Health Organization, 2017), 173–94.

34. Lauer, Soucat, Araujo, and Weakliam, "Pathways."

35. Gerald A. Doeksen, Tom Johnson, and Chuck Willoughby, *Measuring the Economic Importance of the Health Sector on a Local Economy: A Brief Literature Review and Procedures to Measure Local Impact*. Southern Rural Development Center, 1997, http://srdc .msstate.edu/publications/archive/202.pdf.

36. Doeksen, Johnson, and Willoughby, *Measuring the Economic Importance.*

37. Fred Eilrich, Gerald A. Doeksen, and Cheryl F. St. Clair, *The Economic Impact of a Rural Primary Care Physician and the Potential Health Dollars Lost to Out-migrating Health Services*. National Center for Rural Health Works, Oklahoma State University, 2007. https://ruralwellness.files.wordpress.com/2007/03/impact_rural_physician1.pdf.

38. Daniel Avery et al., "The Economic Impact of Rural Family Physicians Practicing Obstetrics." *Journal of the American Board of Family Medicine* 27 (2014): 602–10.

39. Fred Eilrich, "The Economic Effect of a Physician Assistant or Nurse Practitioner in Rural America," *Journal of the American Academy of Physician Assistants* 29 (2016): 44–48.

40. Felicity Proctor, *Rural Economic Diversification in Sub-Saharan Africa* (London: International Institute for Environment and Development, 2014), http://pubs.iied.org /pdfs/14632IIED.pdf.

41. Lauer, Soucat, Araujo, and Weakliam, "Pathways."

42. World Bank, *World Development Report 2013: Jobs* (Washington, DC: World Bank, 2012), doi:10.1596/978-0-8213-9575-2.

43. World Bank, *World Development Report 2013.*

44. World Bank, *World Development Report 2013.*

45. Katrin Elborgh-Woytek et al., *Women, Work, and the Economy: Macroeconomic Gains from Gender Equity* (Washington, DC: International Monetary Fund, 2013), http:// www.imf.org/external/pubs/ft/sdn/2013/sdn1310.pdf.

46. Joseph Woodman, *Patient beyond Borders*, 3rd ed. (Chapel Hill, NC: Healthy Travel Media, 2014).

47. David L. Heymann et al., "Global Health Security: the Wider Lessons from the West African Ebola Virus Disease Epidemic," *Lancet* 385, no. 9980 (2015): 1884–901.

48. World Bank, *Ebola: Most African Countries Avoid Major Economic Loss but Impact on Guinea, Liberia, Sierra Leone Remains Crippling* (Washington: World Bank, 2015).

49. Joseph Stiglitz, Amartya Sen, and Jean-Paul Fitoussi, *Report by the Commission on the Measurement of Economic Performance and Social Progress*, n.d., http://library.bsl .org.au/jspui/bitstream/1/1267/1/Measurement_of_economic_performance_and _social_progress.pdf.

50. United Nations Environment Programme, *Towards a Green Economy: Pathways to Sustainable Development and Poverty Eradication*, 2011, https://www.unenvironment.org /explore-topics/green-economy.

51. World Bank, *Cost of Pollution in China: Economic Estimates of Physical Damages*, 2007, http://siteresources.worldbank.org.

52. Danish Energy Agency et al., *Green Production in Denmark—and Its Significance for the Danish Economy*, 2012, https://ens.dk/sites/ens.dk/files/EnergiKlimapolitik/green _production_in_denmark_-_web_111212.pdf.

53. High-Level Commission, *Working for Health and Growth.*

54. High-Level Commission, *Working for Health and Growth.*

55. OECD, *Recommendation of the Council on Budgetary Governance* (OECD, February 2015), http://www.oecd.org/gov/budgeting/Recommendation-of-the-Council-on-Bud getary-Governance.pdf.

56. Maureen Mackintosh, Amos Channon, Anup Karan, Shaktivel Selvaraj, Eleonora Cavagnero, Hongwen Zhao, "What Is the Private Sector? Understanding Private Provision in the Health Systems of Low-Income and Middle-Income Countries," *Lancet* 388, no. 10044 (2016): 596–605.

57. United Nations Conference on Trade and Development, *World Investment Report 2014: Investing in the SDGs; An Action Plan* (New York: United Nations, 2014), http:// unctad.org/en/PublicationsLibrary/wir2014_en.pdf.

58. Dominic Montagu and Catherine Goodman, "Prohibit, Constrain, Encourage, or Purchase: How Should We Engage with the Private Health-Care Sector?," *Lancet* 388, 10044 (2016): 613–21.

59. Peter Baker, "On the Relationship between Economic Growth and Health Improvement: Some Lessons for Health-Conscious Developing Countries." *Radical Statistics*, no. 98 (2009), http://www.radstats.org.uk/no098/Baker98.pdf.

60. Arthur Okun, *Equality and Efficiency: The Big Tradeoff* (Washington, DC: Brookings Institution Press, 1975).

61. Joseph Stiglitz, "Joseph Stiglitz Says Standard Economics Is Wrong. Inequality and Unearned Income Kills the Economy." *Evonomics*, September 9, 2016, http://evonomics .com/joseph-stiglitz-inequality-unearned-income.

62. Jonathan Ostry, Andrew Berg, and Charalambos G. Tsangarides, *Redistribution, Inequality and Growth*. IMF Staff Discussion Note SDN/14/02 (Washington, DC: International Monetary Fund, 2014).

63. Frederic Cingano, *Trends in Income Inequality and Its Impact on Economic Growth*. OECD Social, Employment and Migration Working Papers, no. 163 (OECD Publishing, 2014), http://www.oecd.org/els/soc/trends-in-income-inequality-and-its-impact -on-economic-growth-SEM-WP163.pdf.

64. Markus Brueckner and Daniel Lederman, *Effects of Income Inequality on Aggregate Output*. Policy Research Working Paper, no. 7317. World Bank Group Latin America and the Caribbean Region, Office of the Chief Economist, 2015, http://documents .worldbank.org/curated/en/291151468188658453/pdf/WPS7317.pdf.

65. Department for International Development, *Economic Development Strategy: Prosperity, Poverty and Meeting Global Challenges* (DFID, 2017).

66. Angus Deaton, "Health, Inequality, and Economic Development," *Journal of Economic Literature* 49 (2003) 113–58.

3

Engagement of the Private Sector in Advancing Universal Health Coverage

Understanding and Navigating Major Factors for Success

Nathan J. Blanchet, Adeel Ishtiaq, and Cicely Thomas

Even in countries with large, robust public health delivery systems, people still use private health services extensively, and there is growing recognition of the potential private sector contribution to universal health coverage (UHC). Achieving UHC and the Sustainable Development Goals as established at the 70th United Nations General Assembly in 2015 will thus require strong public capacity to steward mixed health systems and engage private sector providers to deliver high-quality health services. This chapter briefly explains the rationale for engaging the private sector, offers a framework for mapping the complex array of factors that may facilitate or more often block such engagement, and proposes several key principles for deliberative processes that can help navigate those factors.

Introduction

Given the substantial utilization of private health services in many countries, there is growing global recognition that achieving UHC and the Sustainable Development Goals will require governments to engage and oversee the private sector that uses innovative delivery systems to provide high-quality health services.[1,2,3,4] The theoretical rationale for engaging the private sector in a country's pursuit of UHC can be strong, and effective empirical examples of such engagement are increasing.[5,6,7] Yet the private sector is still often perceived with distrust, and even policy makers who wish to engage the private sector struggle with how to proceed.

There are several theoretical benefits to engaging the private sector to advance UHC. First, all countries, but especially lower-income countries, have limitations in the extent to which their public sector health infrastructure and providers can deliver the care their populations need. Most fall short of universal delivery and have few options in the short or medium term for major public sector expansion. Private providers can augment this capacity, increasing access to care for certain geographic areas, subpopulations, or specialty services. Second, private providers may increase technical efficiency of service delivery through competition, though the record of the private sector's effect on systemwide technical efficiency is mixed.[8] Promoting such efficiency and continually increasing health value for always-insufficient money is a key part of the successful stewardship required for UHC. (Stewardship involves defining strategic directions for the system, setting and enforcing rules, and balancing the interests of key actors such as purchasers, providers, and patients.[9])

Third, the private sector can be a source of quality-enhancing innovation and of responsive, consumer-oriented services, as shown by many of the examples in chapter 4 of this collection, by Dimovska and Campbell, and elsewhere (of course, private providers can also have negative effects on quality). Public providers also innovate, but private providers can leverage diverse features of scale, organization, financing, or legal mandates that simply differ from those available to government, and therefore enlarge a country's enabling environment for innovation.[10,11,12] Finally, engaging private providers can improve equity, but only if such engagement occurs alongside financing mechanisms that allocate care based on patient need rather than ability to pay.[13,14] As countries move to improve access, efficiency, quality, and equity on the road to UHC, an effectively engaged private sector could make major contributions.[15,16]

The empirical case for private sector engagement in UHC has been developing for some time. There is undeniably extensive use of private health services in many countries, including in countries with large, robust public health delivery systems such as Malaysia, India, and Ghana.[17] Several high-income countries regarded as having achieved UHC rely on some form of private service delivery in their publicly financed and stewarded health systems (including Canada, general practitioners in the United Kingdom, and Taiwan), and more recent national health insurance systems in several low- or middle-income countries (LMICs) do the same (as in Ghana, Rwanda, and India).[18,19,20,21,22]

Recent global experience in the pursuit of UHC and the adoption of UHC as SDG 3.8 likely bolster the case for private sector engagement.

Governments have recognized that reforms focusing primarily on financial protection (or coverage) against the risk of needed healthcare are necessary but insufficient for UHC.[23] Typically, simultaneous or precursory expansion and improvement in the supply of services is also required, and this, given limitations to public sector expansion in the short term, implies engaging the private sector in new ways. Malaysia is a case in point, where the government's recent health system transformation initiative quickly recognized that, with the private sector dominating use of outpatient services, transformation toward UHC would require much more robust engagement with and stewardship of that sector than exists today.[24,25]

Despite a strong rationale for private sector contributions to UHC in publicly stewarded health systems and useful examples of such engagement, most private health sectors in LMICs remain largely fragmented, weakly stewarded, and insufficiently engaged toward the pursuit of UHC.[26,27] Why is this, and what can be done?

The authors have recently supported public and private sector actors from six African and four Asian countries in seeking greater public-private engagement in pursuit of UHC. Based partly on this experience, we suggest that the success of public-private engagement efforts is influenced by four major categories of factors: political, organizational, economic, and legal. We propose five key principles for deliberative processes that can help raise awareness of and navigate this complex set of factors—with illustrations of one process driven by policy makers in public sector health financing and the other by networks of private health providers.

Factors Affecting Private Sector Engagement: More Than a Contract Negotiation Problem

Engaging the private sector in new and substantial ways in pursuit of UHC should be informed by a clear understanding of the political, economic, organizational, and legal/regulatory factors that influence outcomes in individual countries (figure 3.1). Simply raising policy makers' and providers' awareness of these factors could improve the planning, design, and results of efforts to increase private sector engagement. It should at least help them avoid contracting solutions that ignore such factors and are therefore unlikely to be adopted or sustained. Beyond awareness, progress will stem from deliberative processes of analysis and dialogue between public and private actors.

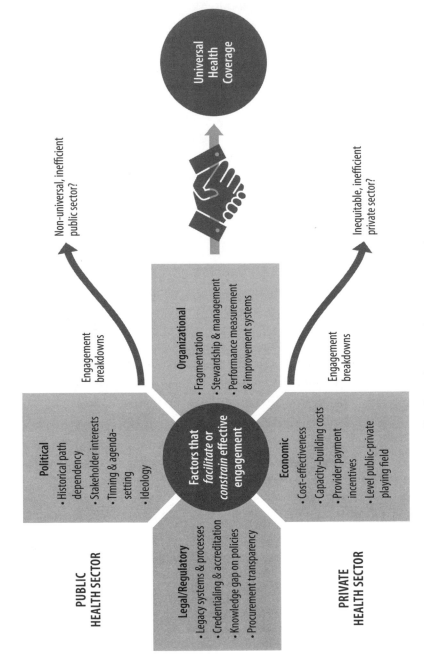

Figure 3.1. Navigating major factors for effective private sector engagement.

Political Factors

HISTORICAL PATH DEPENDENCY

Increasing or changing the role of the private sector in achieving UHC is an inherently political endeavor (as are all major health system reforms). Approaches to private sector engagement will be shaped by the historical roots of a given health system and the path dependency created by past opening or narrowing of public-private cooperation. Path dependency entails that actors are constrained by existing institutions and structures created by previous decisions and thus channeled toward certain policy outcomes, making substantial changes to the status quo difficult.[28]

In Tanzania, for example, there is little precedent and still a good deal of mistrust among public sector policy makers in engaging for-profit private sector providers in health service delivery—a legacy of the country's socialist past. A 2009 government policy promoting new public-private partnerships (PPPs)[29] trains the focus instead on basic dialogue about how public and private actors can benefit from each other, foundational policies and laws for PPPs, and time-intensive processes of negotiating and experimenting with new engagements. As such, Tanzania's national government has undertaken a process of launching public-private health forums (PPHFs) in each of the country's regions, bringing together key public and private stakeholders to advance this agenda and create new openings for public-private cooperation.

STAKEHOLDER INTERESTS

Health system stakeholders are among society's most politically influential people. Every prime minister has a personal physician, a nurses' strike can bring hospitals and clinics to life-threatening halts, and health workers' professional associations have a proven ability to thwart reforms that are contrary to their political, economic, or ideological interests.[30,31] Unionized public sector workers, for example, may strike to protest public funding for private sector providers lest it affect resources for public sector salaries, pensions, and equipment. Private sector providers may also be uninterested in public engagement, fearing loss of autonomy and unfair pricing, especially where competition between public and private providers does not account for the subsidization of infrastructure that public providers typically receive. There are also common suspicions of motivations and capacities on both sides of the public-private divide: public actors suspect

private providers of seeking profits above public welfare and delivering in-
ferior quality, and private providers fear public actors' ability or willingness to deliver promised goods and pay fair prices in a timely manner. Private providers in Ghana have had such fears confirmed, as the country's
National Health Insurance Authority has historically failed to pay claims
within the contractually obligated period of time from submission of
claims.[32] These are just a few of the most common stakeholder barriers;
many more have been documented. Stakeholder analysis and strategic communications are vital first steps in health reform that change the roles, responsibilities, and resource flows among influential stakeholders.[33]

TIMING AND AGENDA SETTING

Beyond preexisting starting positions and stakeholder interests,
efforts to engage the private sector in pursuit of UHC must also contend
with the universal challenge of agenda setting and the timing of policy reform. As Kingdon's widely applied theory of agenda setting holds, reform is
likeliest to occur when three policy-making "streams" converge with a "window of opportunity" for change—including a "problem" identification
stream, a "policy" solution stream, and a "politics" calculus stream.[34] For private sector engagement, the first "problem" stream could be, for example,
when broad societal complaints about healthcare conditions sharpen, perhaps spurred by prominent events or media coverage, into a widely recognized and specific problem relevant to private sector service delivery (such
as an acute gap in coverage for a high-priority need like maternity care). In
that same case, the second "policy" stream requirement could be a known
mechanism to leverage the private sector to deliver needed maternity care—
such as a successful voucher program in a neighboring region or country.
The third "politics" stream would then need to hold some rational motivation for action by political leaders, such as a campaigning parliamentarian
wanting to secure votes in the affected region and subpopulation affected.
When a clearly defined and felt problem converges with a feasible policy solution and a political motivation to connect the two, actors can seize "win-
dows of opportunity"—a new government or a financial crisis, for example—
to make change. Analyses of historical starting points, stakeholder interests,
and other timing considerations, some of which can be influenced or even
engineered, can help create effective strategies for greater engagement of
the private sector.

IDEOLOGY

Deeply held ideological beliefs are another potentially powerful political factor affecting governments' engagement of private providers in service of UHC. In many LMICs, governments may be wary of the private healthcare sector, which they perceive as profit-oriented, costly, or even corrupt. They may therefore shun the private sector or engage with it selectively. For instance, governments may choose to engage only private not-for-profit (PNFP) providers, which are typically faith-based, profess a social mission, and enjoy considerable trust among the population.

The Christian Social Services Commission (CSSC) in Tanzania is an apt example. It organizes the largest network of private facilities in the country—comprising about 900 providers—and claims to deliver 40% of healthcare services.[35] The government of Tanzania routinely contracts with CSSC facilities, ranging from individual church-run dispensaries to secondary and tertiary care hospitals (often selected officially as Designated District Hospitals or Regional Referral Hospitals) and even specialist teaching hospitals at the national level. This contrasts sharply with the case for private for-profit (PFP) facilities, which may at best receive some in-kind support for priority government programs. Similarly, in Uganda the faith-based "medical bureaus" providers receive block grants for their facilities from the government under loosely regulated memoranda of understanding to deliver primary healthcare (PHC) services. These grants often sustain these facilities as private not-for-profit concerns, but are not available to private for-profit providers.[36,37] The authors found further examples of ideological barriers to public-private interaction in Cambodia. Officials there express deep distrust of the private for-profit sector, evidenced by comments such as "the private sector is profit-oriented, offers limited services, and refers to the public sector" and is "motivated by profit and only really offers coverage to richer Cambodians."[38]

These examples show that engaging the private sector can be hard when governments view the private (especially for-profit) sector with suspicion. Developing trust, aligning with public goals, and using evidence to show the efficiency and equity-enhancing aspects of engaging private providers is essential to overcome such views.[39]

Organizational Factors

HEALTH SYSTEM FRAGMENTATION

Health system fragmentation is an organizational barrier that results in the lack of purchasing regimes that include both public and private providers, deficiencies in capacity and experience at all levels of the system, and a dearth of unified information technology (IT) systems that can track patient data and monitor quality. While public providers are organized within government health systems, few private sector aggregating bodies exist in LMICs to help create similar sector representation and engagement platforms, especially among small-scale private providers. This limits public sector ability to identify private sector providers and understand the types and quality of services they offer. Public officials must identify and engage individual providers using separate contracts, making engagement time-consuming and costly.

Decentralization of the planning, financing, delivery, and governance of primary healthcare can pose further challenges for public-private engagement at subnational levels of government. Tanzania's case is particularly instructive, where planning, financing, delivery, and monitoring of services at the primary and secondary levels (and some tertiary care) is delegated to local government authorities (LGAs) and regional administrations.[40] Recent efforts to promote a newly developed PPP policy in these subnational jurisdictions by the national health ministry through a PPHF have found widely varying capacities, experiences, and appetites for engaging the private sector among local and regional authorities.[41] For instance, private for-profit providers at the local levels are typically excluded from both LGA "Comprehensive Council Health Planning" processes and legacy systems of contracting with private providers. Overall, a tapering away of public sector capacity and experience at local levels in decentralized settings creates hurdles in the way of effective PPP engagements for more robust PHC service delivery.

Further, fragmented health systems also lack integrated health IT mechanisms, which facilitate communication across the health system and monitoring of patient data, access to care, and quality of care. While public sectors in most countries operate health management information systems (HMISs) and require public providers to provide data through these channels, private providers are not necessarily captured in these mechanisms because their inclusion is not prioritized by the government, they lack the capacity to contribute to the HMIS, or they do not wish to contribute to the system. For instance, in Cambodia the national government has successfully implemented an electronic, integrated, and standardized HMIS in the public sector with near 100% compliant monthly reporting at primary, secondary, and tertiary care hospitals (though some basic care "Health Centers" are still being connected); the government uses the resulting data for quarterly and annual reviews, performance monitoring of contracting arrangements internally with public providers, budgeting, and other purposes. But private providers are not included in the HMIS, though private pharmacies and outpatient clinics are often the first point of care for many Cambodians. Only a few private facilities are provided training, but these may not have computers and internet to link to and routinely use the HMIS.[42] This means that the public sector is unable to factor in private sector capabilities and activities in planning and coordinating service delivery for citizens. Similarly, it cannot hold private facilities accountable to standards of care applicable to (or at least more readily monitored for) public sector providers.

STEWARDSHIP AND MANAGEMENT

Public and private sectors do not typically collaborate in facilitating optimal functioning of the health market by identifying market failures (such as underprovided or underperforming services) and carrying out joint planning and resource allocation to address them.[43] This is in part because mechanisms to facilitate such "health market development" at the national and subnational levels do not exist, which causes private providers to be excluded from key health system governance and organization initiatives and reduces their stake and ownership. Just one manifestation of this is hostility to (often widespread) *dual practice*,[44] such that government healthcare workers are compelled (or at least incentivized) to keep their private healthcare practice outside of routine monitoring, regulatory, and purchasing regimes.[45] Finally, there is often limited community engagement in health system decision making, preventing adequate reflection of the community's health-seeking behavior in decision making and leading to the exclusion of or inadequate focus on privately provided services.

Economic Factors

In addition to political and organizational factors impeding closer cooperation between the public and private sectors in delivering on UHC goals, the following economic challenges may constrain collaboration if not adequately analyzed and addressed.

COST-EFFECTIVENESS

Leveraging the private sector should offer clear advantages in the cost-effectiveness of delivering a minimum package of healthcare benefits to the population, but comparing cost-effectiveness between the public and private sectors is not straightforward. Policy makers may lack data indicating the unit costs of delivering priority services in the private sector (and/or the public sector), utilization rates for these services among the population, and the efficacy of many services offered in the public sector that patients will expect to access at private providers. For example, recent analysis in South Africa of current costs and potential future resource needs for priority primary healthcare services delivered by public providers highlighted the challenges posed by poor availability and quality of data, absence of consistent costing methodologies, and the need to invest in better data systems that may facilitate the future National Health Insurance regime for UHC.[46] Such constraints hinder policy makers' motivation to procure services from private facilities to complement those available in the public ones.

PUBLIC SECTOR CAPACITY-BUILDING COSTS

Integrating private sector providers within public sector UHC mechanisms will require investment in systems for financing, service delivery, and governance. The government's health planning and pooling-purchasing entities will need to develop strategies for outreach and engagement; invest in capacity building to identify providers, negotiate contracts, and monitor service delivery and compliance with contract terms; implement IT systems for integrating routine information and reporting from the private sector into the public sector health information systems; and routinely process and release payments. These large upfront investment costs for systems and capacities may make engaging the private sector relatively inefficient compared to scaling up the delivery of priority services in the public sector.

For instance, under Chile's Regime of Explicit Health Guarantees (Plan AUGE) healthcare reform, the government prioritized the delivery of an increasing set of prescribed minimum benefits (raised from 25 in 2005 to

80 in 2013) via public sector facilities under guarantees of service quality, affordability, timeliness, and access.[47] While the share of citizens covered under the public sector insurer Fonasa with access to this minimum package has increased, the share of payments by Fonasa to the private sector has remained low (under 15% in 2012). Hence, even as services, coverage under prepaid-pooled UHC schemes, and overall health spending increase, public purchasers may choose to direct resources toward the existing public sector infrastructure rather than incurring additional costs to incorporate an increasing number of private sector providers.

PROVIDER PAYMENT INCENTIVES

Additionally, incorporating private providers into UHC systems requires instituting purchasing mechanisms that may create adverse incentives for service providers and/or require broader facilitating conditions for successful implementation. For priority PHC services in particular, the chief provider payment mechanisms tend to be budget or block (or in-kind) transfers, capitation payments, and fee-for-service. The various benefits and challenges for each of these methods, summarized in table 3.1, can complicate closer cooperation between the public sector and private providers—as illustrated in several examples given below.[48]

Fee-for-service payments: In Tanzania, private providers often have to wait up to six months to be paid by the country's National Health Insurance Fund (NHIF) for PHC services delivered to enrollees, while claims can be rejected for clerical errors such as forgetting to add the date or failing to get a patient's signature.[49] This requires considerable administrative effort on the part of under-resourced private PHC facilities—often run by an individual physician, nurse practitioner, or midwife—on claims processing and review and follow-up with the NHIF for payment, imposing significant costs and causing uncertainty in revenue.

Capitation payment: Capitation payment schemes are commonly used to reimburse providers for PHC service provision. In such schemes, providers "are paid, in advance, a predetermined fixed rate to provide a defined set of services for each individual enrolled with the provider for a fixed period."[50] Capitation payments to private facilities to cover PHC services for social health insurance beneficiaries under Tanzania's National Social Security Fund amount to a little over $1 per month per beneficiary, which the facilities consider very low and against which they are unable to

Table 3.1. Potential benefits and challenges of selected provider payment methods

Provider payment method	Potential benefits	Potential challenges
Fee-for-service payment (Providers can charge the purchaser a previously agreed price for specific services delivered to individuals covered under prepaid-pooled UHC financing mechanism)	■ Can encourage greater volume of service provision ■ Can easily enable care seeking in any location and type of provider; useful for geographically mobile patient populations ■ Can facilitate easy tracking and monitoring of services, especially for target populations/geographies	■ **No incentives for efficiency but incentives to over-provide** services, causing high and unpredictable costs ■ **No incentive for prevention** because providers do not get paid for averting the need for pricey services ■ **Unpredictable costs** for the payer and **unpredictable revenue** for providers ■ **High administrative costs** of claims processing and verification
Capitation payment (Providers "are paid, in advance, a predetermined fixed rate to provide a defined set of services for each individual enrolled with the provider for a fixed period."*)	■ Incentives for a holistic approach to primary healthcare ■ Predictable spending for the purchaser ■ Low administrative costs for both payer and provider ■ Incentives on part of providers for prevention and efficiency	■ **Registration of enrollees** with the particular facilities receiving capitated budgets for outpatient services ■ Sufficient **data on patient characteristics** to develop a risk-adjusted capitation payment ■ **Incentive for under-provision** ■ Managing care and monitoring outcomes for **geographically mobile patients** ■ Requires providers to have **full/defined array of PHC services**

Budget transfers, block payments, or in-kind support (The public sector may transfer block grants, equipment and drugs, and even health workers to private providers to cover the delivery of certain priority services such as vaccinations, family planning, and other maternal and child health services)	■ Leverages existing public financial management systems for allocation, transfer, and financial control of budget payments	■ **Inability to target service provision** to key PHC priorities
		■ **Reduces provider autonomy and doesn't incentivize or facilitate**
		  □ Efficiency gains and management improvement
		  □ Service delivery improvement
		  □ Transparency in resource use

* John C. Langenbrunner, Cheryl Cashin, and Sheila O'Dougherty, "How-to Manuals: Designing and Implementing Health Care Provider Payment Systems" (Washington, DC, 2009), https://openknowledge.worldbank.org/bitstream/handle/10986/13806/48599.pdf.

provide a guaranteed minimum set of services (hence, no such minimum set of services applies). Similarly, under Nigeria's National Health Insurance Service, capitation payments to accredited private facilities are about $2.40 per month per beneficiary, for which a set of primary care services—including facility-based deliveries but not any drugs—must be covered by providers.[51]

Budget, block, or in-kind transfers: LGAs in Tanzania provide sexual and reproductive health commodities at no cost to private providers but require that they provide services free of charge to users.[52,53] However, this leaves uncovered operational costs such as facility rents, expenses on utilities, and salaries of healthcare workers, which a private provider must cover out of its own resources. This deters public-private collaboration in the absence of (1) adequate supply-side financing for private providers, (2) capacity to forecast and plan for utilization of resources, and (3) contractual safeguards and guarantees to support sustainable provision of contracted services.

LEVEL PUBLIC-PRIVATE PLAYING FIELD

A final challenge related to payment mechanisms is that public sector purchasers must negotiate reimbursement rates or the terms for supply-side financing for private providers such that there is a "level playing field" between public and private providers, with arrangements that are financially viable for private providers. Output-based purchasing from public sector providers under prepaid-pooled financing mechanisms for UHC typically reimburses only the variable costs incurred by facilities, separate from other supply-side funding that facilities receive through recurring government health spending on infrastructure and salaries. Private providers, who do not benefit from such supply-side funding, need reimbursement rates that would cover the full costs of service provision. For instance, private providers in Uganda receive routine immunization supplies from the public sector, but they must cover from their own resources the transportation charges for these supplies as well as utility bills and healthcare workers' time for administering free immunization services, putting them at a disadvantage compared to public facilities. By contrast, reimbursement rates for private providers under the Mandatory Health Insurance Fund in Kyrgyzstan include the cost of health worker salaries, which helps significantly in creating equity between public and private providers. However, private providers are still subject to tax burden on their revenues, which may undermine their viability relative to public providers. Plans are being discussed to exempt private providers from taxation in order to provide them with a level playing field.[54] Failing to take such conditions into account may stop private providers from participating in prepaid-pooled funding mechanisms for UHC.

Legal and Regulatory Factors

Legal and regulatory factors also influence cooperation between the public and private sectors. In many countries, legacy systems for budget-based transfers of grants, commodities, equipment, or health workers may exist, particularly for higher-level private not-for-profit providers. However, new arrangements to purchase PHC services from private providers—particularly using routine supply-side healthcare budgets—are often treated as formal public-private partnerships that can be either stalled for lack of needed regulation or stifled by a tendency toward overregulation and lengthy bureaucratic procedures. For example, the Kampala Capital City Authority (KCCA) in Uganda uses about $224,000 from its annual health budget to make grants for PHC services to about 33 hospital-level, private, not-for-profit facilities within the Greater Kampala region.[55] The KCCA would like to use these funds strategically to "decongest" the provision of maternal health services in public facilities using output-based purchasing from the more than 2,000 private healthcare providers in the city. It is constrained, however, by a lack of autonomy to alter how these PHC grant funds are deployed and by a revamped—but still to be fully implemented—public-private partnership policy requiring approvals from several national ministries and departments. As a result, the KCCA is unable to recruit the many smaller, cheaper, and well-staffed private providers in Kampala to expand maternal health services for a growing population. This illustrates how channeling public funds—particularly budget-based funding—to private providers can be overly burdensome, if not plainly disallowed. And even where allowed, public sector purchasers may have limited ability to solicit, negotiate, and execute contracts in a transparent and competitive manner.

Credentialing and accreditation of private providers for compliance with standards and regulations can also be lengthy, cumbersome, and expensive for private providers. In Kenya, for example, all health facilities must be registered with the Kenya Medical Dentists and Practitioners Board, and private specialty facilities must also register with individual professional boards, which results in multiple licensing fees for providers.

Regulatory mechanisms and regulatory actors often have overlapping roles, creating contradiction and duplication in the system and an increased burden on the private sector, who feel "over"-regulated. In Ghana, several government agencies are responsible for licensing and credentialing facilities. The Health Facilities Regulatory Agency registers and regulates private providers, but the National Health Insurance Authority, as purchaser, also credentials private providers to determine their eligibility for receiving payment through the scheme. Such lack of clarity between roles and the duplication of efforts can cause the purchasing relationship to break down between public systems and private providers.

Private providers and subnational implementers often lack knowledge of regulatory mechanisms and processes, as national regulatory mechanisms are often not effectively implemented at the subnational level. In Nigeria, smaller-scale maternity clinics—often run by nurses or trained midwives—must initiate, pay for, and await accreditation by the National Health Insurance Scheme without guidance on accreditation procedures or support in meeting minimum standards and requirements.[56] Private providers themselves may lack the motivation to pursue accreditation because of the requisite investments in facilities and structural quality, as well as lack of awareness and/or financial resources.

Navigating the Labyrinth: Deliberative Processes Driven by Public and Private Sector Actors

Successful engagement of the private sector requires navigating a labyrinthine array of political, organizational, economic, and legal/regulatory factors. This helps explain why "off-the-shelf" models from elsewhere—a particular form of public-private partnership, a way of organizing providers, a payment mechanism, an IT innovation for monitoring or regulation—do not replicate easily. And it explains ultimately why the private sector in many countries remains largely separated from public efforts to finance and deliver services universally.

The authors propose that multifaceted, deliberative processes that raise awareness and identify solutions through analysis and structured dialogue among key stakeholders are the best way to navigate the "labyrinth" and yield new forms of engagement. Such processes can be initiated by both public officials, especially those responsible for systemwide health financing and service delivery reform, and private health providers, especially those seeking to enhance the sustainability and equity of their financing. Neutral facilitators can support both sides to structure their approaches, conduct analyses, facilitate dialogue, and timeously source relevant models from elsewhere that may be adapted to the local context. Based on our recent (and ongoing) experience playing such a facilitator role, we hypothesize that such processes should hold to several principles to work effectively, as described below and shown in figure 3.2.

Be demanded and led by local stakeholders with the ability and authority to create new tools, rules, and roles. Ensuring that local stakeholders with suffi-

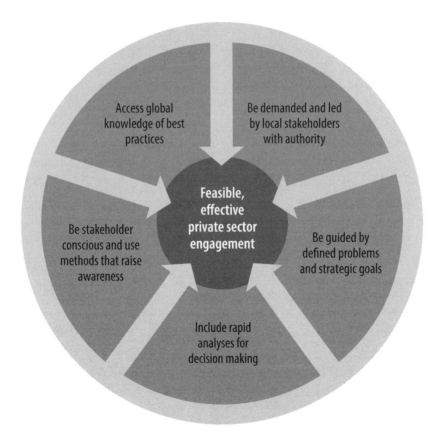

Figure 3.2. Principles of deliberative processes for new private sector engagement. Source: Results for Development (www.R4D.org)

cient authority demand and lead new engagement processes helps in three ways: (1) it taps into a wealth of tacit knowledge of local context, such as the kind required to navigate historically set institutions and current (and often undocumented) political incentives; (2) it organically develops local owner-ship and support for any follow-on actions once a new engagement is de-signed; and (3) it more quickly and accurately identifies the new operational-level tools, rules, and roles needed to make a new engagement work.

Be guided by clear problem definitions, strategic goals, and a practical, step-by-step "roadmap." Planning processes for new public-private engagements are complex and often time-consuming, so clear problem definitions and strategic goals (e.g., lowering maternal mortality by improving access to quality care by a marginalized subpopulation) are key to maintain direc-tion and evaluate potential engagement options. Actors that need to lead such processes do not have time to digest and translate global experience on best practices—including sequencing of actions, one of the biggest chal-lenges. Guides, manuals, or step-by-step "roadmaps" that are written in ac-cessible, operations-oriented formats therefore help actors decide where to focus first, how to maintain progress, and where to look for tools to adapt.

Include rapid analyses that produce just-in-time evidence needed for decision making. A variety of analyses are typically needed throughout planning processes to define problems clearly, understand the baseline context and constraints, and to evaluate multiple options proposed for new engage-ments. We have found that the most helpful analyses are relatively rapid (taking weeks or months, not years), conducted by "insider" stakeholders independently or with assistance from outside facilitators in a participa-tory fashion, and scoped to produce fit-for-purpose evidence just in time for the next step in planning, such as generating options for engagement, evaluating those options, or building persuasive cases for particular decision makers.

Be "stakeholder conscious" and use implementation methods that raise aware-ness while also generating needed evidence. Every step of planning a new en-gagement must be "stakeholder conscious." This does not mean that every possible stakeholder needs to be equally involved in every step, which can lead to paralysis, but rather that the positions, power, and possible actions and reactions of relevant stakeholders should be considered and managed from beginning to end of any new arrangement (i.e., from initial dialogue, through analyses and options creation, and onward in implementation).

Careful method choice can help with this by raising awareness with key stakeholders at appropriate times while simultaneously gathering needed evidence. An example is using key informant interviews with insiders rather than only conducting document review to gather baseline information (even if this is duplicative from a data collection perspective) and beginning to discuss potential new arrangements in those discussions. The goal of being stakeholder conscious is to design new engagements that are technically sound and also deemed acceptable and feasible by stakeholders who can make or break their adoption.

Access global knowledge of best practices and enable optional adaptation of known models—often but not necessarily through peer learning. We propose deliberative planning processes dominated by local stakeholders from the initial demand to address a problem to the final design and implementation. However, global best practices and models from elsewhere are still relevant and can improve outcomes. To do so, the planning process needs to have ways to access such knowledge at just the right times—often within days or weeks of a specific decisional need being identified. And to be able to access knowledge in the right formats—more often in the form of short memos or presentations, less often in more formal and lengthy literature reviews. When promising models from elsewhere are identified as potential solutions (e.g., a mobile platform to pay and monitor the quality of delivery by private providers), it is best to have operational details such as costs, human resource needs, and hardware/software requirements available, either through written descriptions or—even better—a (preferably local) expert, who can quickly explain and advise on which elements of the model can be changed. Such global knowledge and models can be integrated through external facilitators with technical expertise, by means of various global health knowledge aggregations platforms, and/or by external facilitators with technical expertise.

Table 3.2 illustrates how these principles were embodied in two different efforts to promote private sector engagement, where the authors served as technical facilitators. The first is the Joint Learning Network for Universal Health Coverage's[57] (JLN) Private Sector Engagement Collaborative, through which public officials joined together to harness experiences and develop practical advice for public sector implementers to support private sector engagement. Recognizing the complex factors that influence private sector engagement, the collaborative avoided recommending particular

Table 3.2. Two public- and private-led initiatives that fulfill principles of deliberative processes for private sector engagement

Principle	Public-sector-led example (JLN)	Private-sector-led example (SIFPO2)
Be demanded and led by local stakeholders with the ability and authority to create new tools, rules, and roles.	■ A recommended approach to engage the private sector was jointly developed by country director-level public officials with current responsibility and authority to better leverage and regulate the private sector. These included heads of primary healthcare units and private sector engagement units within a ministry of health and heads of contracting directorates in a national health insurance authority.	■ Private social franchise managers expressed demand / self-selected to get support in creating new strategies to leverage public financing. ■ Franchise managers and staff contributed to every step of analysis, options creation, and options evaluation; a senior management team of the organization made final decision on whether and how to proceed.
Be guided by clear problem definitions, strategic goals, and a practical, step-by-step "roadmap."	■ Process (documented in a practical guide) calls for first understanding and detailing the rationale and goal for the engagement and actively listening to the private sector. ■ For each step, the guide provides information on why the step is important and how to do it.	■ A guide written for private network managers and staff helps them structure and conduct various analyses and options-generation steps to develop a feasible strategy for leveraging public financing. ■ Guide includes practical tips and tools, such as key informant interview guides, templates for documenting and analyzing data, and rubrics for options creation and evaluation.
Include targeted analyses that produce just-in-time evidence needed for decision making.	■ Major analytic component focuses on provider mapping, generating evidence that is needed to create feasible payment, contracting, and regulatory mechanisms (based on experience from Ghana and Malaysia). ■ Options for regulation of private providers will be based on six country-led implementation assessments of private PHC regulation in Ghana, Indonesia, Kenya, Malaysia, Mongolia, and Morocco.	■ Three core analyses are conducted in first phase—analyses of platform needs, health financing system, and health market of relevant goods and services—in order to create feasible options for the platform. ■ Follow-up work targets further research to design and propose public-private partnership modalities, drawing upon, for instance, the specific requirements of a regional or local government, other relevant mechanisms from within or outside the country setting, and mapping of attendant costs and operational prerequisites.

(continued)

Table 3.2. (continued)

Principle	Public-sector-led example (JLN)	Private-sector-led example (SIFPO2)
Be "stakeholder conscious" and use implementation methods that raise awareness while also generating needed evidence.	▪ Approach calls for dialogue and consensus on shared value propositions between public officials with authority to purchase/finance health services and private providers with interest and potential capacity to deliver services with public funding. Provides examples of some easy, low-cost possible engagements. ▪ Provider mapping steps include guidance on disseminating results to a broad audience of health system stakeholders. ▪ Approach to private sector regulation emphasizes strategic communications efforts between public and private sectors and consumers. ▪ Stakeholder analysis explicitly integrated into all steps.	▪ Process systematically identifies key stakeholders to interview early in analytic phase and explicitly maps political feasibility in final phase of ranking options. ▪ Key stakeholders targeted in the follow-up phase of implementing options for partnership, consultation, or technical or funding involvement via direct outreach and collaboration, engagement through consultative forums, and advocacy.
Access global knowledge of best practices and enable optional adaptation of known models—often but not necessarily through peer learning.	▪ Peer learning across numerous country cases and experiences to elucidate the guidance, as well as operational templates used for documenting rationales for engagement, conducting provider mapping, and actual contracts used in contracting private providers. ▪ Workshops guided by expert technical facilitators.	▪ Rapidly sourced models of "intermediary organizations" from operations research conducted by the Center for Health Market Innovations. ▪ Tapped expert knowledge of health financing and social franchise options from facilitators.

policy solutions and instead co-developed a deliberative, five-module sequence that policy makers in any country could follow to better identify and seize opportunities for greater private sector engagement.

The second example is an effort under a US Agency for International Development project, Support for International Family Planning Organizations 2: Strengthening Networks (SIFPO2). Under SIFPO2, primary healthcare provider networks affiliated with Population Services International in Cambodia, Nigeria, Tanzania, and Uganda implemented a deliberative process—detailed in a written guide—to plan ways of improving sustainability and equity, primarily through greater connection to public financing.[58] Typically reliant on unsustainable donor financing and inequitable out-of-pocket payments, the process helps these networks identify and capitalize on domestic financing opportunities such as new national health insurance programs or other public-private partnerships.

There are many other instructive, proactive efforts by networks of private PHC providers to engage with government and leverage public health financing. Various networks are developing options to (1) tap into sources of prepaid-pooled financing to mitigate financial barriers to service utilization by patients and to fund provider support activities, and (2) play an intermediary[59] role at the interface of public and private sectors, helping governments map, monitor, and manage private providers in service to UHC goals. Under one initiative through the African Health Markets for Equity (AHME) program (supported by the Bill & Melinda Gates Foundation and the UK Department for International Development), private primary healthcare providers in Kenya are being organized under a network management organization (NMO). The NMO can play a variety of intermediary roles on behalf of public and commercial purchasers—helping to monitor quality, manage claims, electronically channel service delivery information, and aggregate providers for easier accreditation, negotiation, and contracting. Further, private intermediaries in India are co-developing with the government in Uttar Pradesh state an online platform for accrediting facilities and managing claims. This will allow them to strategically purchase family planning services from private providers that are closer to women for whom farther flung and more crowded public facilities are out of reach.[60] The Hausala Sajheedari Program has helped to replace traditional—and tedious—paper-based accreditation and payment mechanisms, enabling more robust partnerships, financing, and stewardship.

Most of these initiatives are in early stages, surfacing concrete options to connect public and private sectors, unpacking the challenges to their implementation, and facilitating innovative engagement and partnership modalities. Overall, the approaches advance efforts to connect private provider networks with financing sources—particularly public ones—that may enhance sustainability, equity, and health system coordination. Importantly, they are opportunities to raise awareness of and mitigate barriers such as those highlighted in this chapter—including, for instance, public financial management systems that impede supply-side contracting between the public and private sectors, high costs of accrediting or paying private providers, or fragmented information management systems that preclude effective government stewardship of the private healthcare sector.

Conclusion

Achieving universal health coverage will require effective engagement of private sector health providers in some form and to some extent in nearly all countries. In some countries, the need for such engagement is clearer and more urgent in the short to medium term, such as where a public sector expansion large enough to meet all needs is simply not feasible. This chapter has shown, however, that a theoretical rationale for engaging the private sector is far from sufficient for actually doing so. A dizzying array of political, organizational, economic, and legal/regulatory factors—often but not always constraints—must be recognized and context-specific solutions devised. We have found that deliberative processes with analysis, structured dialogue among local stakeholders, and several other key principles are perhaps the best approach to navigating complex factors toward new engagements. These can be initiated by public or private sector leaders with or without support from external facilitators. We call for increased peer learning about such processes globally, increased sharing of adaptable solutions those processes create, and continued research into optimal balances between government and market forces in support of health system goals.

ACKNOWLEDGMENTS

The authors gratefully acknowledge their colleague Ms. Neetu Hariharan, Senior Program Associate at Results for Development, for her excellent research assistance for this chapter. They also thank all the coauthors and editors of this volume for their review, discussion, and suggested improvements to earlier drafts.

NOTES

1. Gina Lagomarsino, Stefan Nachuk, and Sapna Singh Kundra, "Public Stewardship of Private Providers in Mixed Health Systems" (Washington, DC, 2009).

2. Tanya Caulfield and Krishna Hort, "Governance and Stewardship in Mixed Health Systems in Low- and Middle-Income Countries," Working Paper No. 24 (Melbourne: Nossal Institute for Global Health, 2012).

3. International Finance Corporation, "Healthy Partnerships: How Governments Can Engage the Private Sector to Improve Health in Africa" (Washington, DC, 2011).

4. Cicely Thomas, Marty Makinen, Nathan J. Blanchet, and Kirsten Krusell, eds., *Engaging the Private Sector in Primary Health Care to Achieve Universal Health Coverage: Advice from Implementers, to Implementers* (Washington, DC: Joint Learning Network for Universal Health Coverage Primary Health Care Technical Initiative).

5. Barbara McPake and Kara Hanson, "Managing the Public-Private Mix to Achieve Universal Health Coverage," *The Lancet* 388, no. 10044 (2016): 622–30.

6. Donika Dimovska and John Campbell, "Innovative Initiatives from the Private Sector: What Have Been the Experiences? What Opportunities Lie Ahead and How Can They Be Harnessed More Effectively?," in *Universal Health Coverage and the New Health Economy*, ed. Christian Franz et al. (Washington, DC: Johns Hopkins Bloomberg School of Public Health, n.d.).

7. Thomas, Makinen, Blanchet, and Krusell, eds., *Engaging the Private Sector in Primary Health Care.*

8. Rosemary Morgan, Tim Ensor, and Hugh Waters, "Performance of Private Sector Health Care: Implications for Universal Health Coverage," *The Lancet* 388, no. 10044 (August 2016): 606–12, doi:10.1016/S0140-6736(16)00343-3.

9. Christopher J. L. Murray and Julio Frenk, "A Framework for Assessing the Performance of Health Systems," *Bulletin of the World Health Organization: Evidence for Health Policy* 78 (2000): 717–731.

10. Edith Patouillard et al., "Can Working with the Private For-Profit Sector Improve Utilization of Quality Health Services by the Poor? A Systematic Review of the Literature," *International Journal for Equity in Health* 6, no. 1 (November 2007): 17, doi:10.1186/1475-9276-6-17.

11. Karen Schlein et al., "Private Sector Delivery of Health Services in Developing Countries: A Mixed-Methods Study on Quality Assurance in Social Franchises," *BMC Health Services Research* 13, no. 1 (January 2013): 4, doi:10.1186/1472-6963-13-4.

12. Babar Tasneem Shaikh, "Private Sector in Health Care Delivery: A Reality and a Challenge in Pakistan," *Journal of Ayub Medical College Abbottabad* 27, no. 2 (2015): 496–98.

13. Sanjay Basu et al., "Comparative Performance of Private and Public Healthcare Systems in Low- and Middle-Income Countries: A Systematic Review," ed. Rachel Jenkins, *PLoS Medicine* 9, no. 6 (June 19, 2012): e1001244, doi:10.1371/journal.pmed.1001244.

14. Guy Stallworthy et al., "Roundtable Discussion: What Is the Future Role of the Private Sector in Health?," *Globalization and Health* 10, no. 1 (June 2014): 55, doi:10.1186/1744-8603-10-55.

15. Sarah Thurston et al., "Establishing and Scaling-Up Clinical Social Franchise Networks: Lessons Learned from Marie Stopes International and Population Services International," *Global Health: Science and Practice* 3, no. 2 (June 12, 2015): 180–94, doi: 10.9745/GHSP-D-15-00057.

16. "Healthy Markets for Global Health: A Market Shaping Primer" (Washington, DC, 2014), https://www.usaid.gov/sites/default/files/documents/1864/healthymarkets_primer.pdf.

17. International Finance Corporation, "Creating Markets Annual Report 2017" (Washington, DC, 2017), http://www.ifc.org/wps/wcm/connect/c40f7054-55c5-4606-8612-811edb34f73f/IFC-AR17-Full-Report-Vol-1-v2.pdf?MOD=AJPERES.

18. Maureen Mackintosh et al., "What Is the Private Sector? Understanding Private Provision in the Health Systems of Low-Income and Middle-Income Countries," *The Lancet* 388, no. 10044 (2016): 596–605.

19. K. Srinath Reddy et al., "Towards Achievement of Universal Health Care in India by 2020: A Call to Action," *The Lancet* 377, no. 9767 (2011): 760–68.

20. Shankar Prinja, Manmeet Kaur, and Rajesh Kumar, "Universal Health Insurance in India: Ensuring Equity, Efficiency, and Quality," *Indian Journal of Community Medicine: Official Publication of Indian Association of Preventive & Social Medicine* 37, no. 3 (2012): 142.

21. Nathaniel Otoo et al., "Universal Health Coverage for Inclusive and Sustainable Development: Country Summary Report for Ghana," in *Japan–World Bank Partnership Program for Universal Health Coverage (91299), Health, Nutrition and Population Global Practice, World Bank Group Report*, 2014.

22. Julie Rosenberg and Rebecca Weintraub, "Four Countries' Experiences of Universal Health Coverage Implementation: Lessons for the Future," *The Lancet Global Health* 3 (2015): S8.

23. "SDG 3: Ensure Healthy Lives and Promote Wellbeing for All at All Ages," World Health Organization, 2017, http://www.who.int/sdg/targets/en/.

24. Mishra Ramesh and Xun Wu, "Realigning Public and Private Health Care in Southeast Asia," *The Pacific Review* 21, no. 2 (2008): 171–87.

25. World Health Organization, "Malaysia Health System Review" (Manila, Philippines: WHO Regional Office for the Western Pacific, 2012).

26. Thomas, Makinen, Blanchet, and Krusell, eds., *Engaging the Private Sector in Primary Health Care*.

27. Gina Lagomarsino et al., "Moving towards Universal Health Coverage: Health Insurance Reforms in Nine Developing Countries in Africa and Asia," *The Lancet* 380, no. 9845 (2012): 933–43.

28. David Wilsford, "Path Dependency, or Why History Makes It Difficult but Not Impossible to Reform Health Care Systems in a Big Way," *Journal of Public Policy* 14, no. 3 (1994): 251–83, http://www.jstor.org/stable/4007528.

29. Prime Minister's Office, United Republic of Tanzania, *National Public Private Partnership (PPP) Policy* (Dar Es Salaam, Tanzania: Prime Minister's Office, 2009).

30. Michael R. Reich et al., "Moving towards Universal Health Coverage: Lessons from 11 Country Studies," *The Lancet* 387, no. 10020 (2016): 811–16.

31. Amanda Glassman and Kent Buse, "Politics, and Public Health Policy Reform," *International Encyclopedia of Public Health* 5 (2008): 163–70, https://www.brookings.edu/wp-content/uploads/2016/06/09_public_health_glassman.pdf.

32. Philip Ayizem Dalinjong and Alexander Suuk Laar, "The National Health Insurance Scheme: Perceptions and Experiences of Health Care Providers and Clients in Two Districts of Ghana," *Health Economics Review* 2, no. 1 (July 2012): 13, doi:10.1186/2191-1991-2-13.

33. Nathan J. Blanchet and Ashley M. Fox, "Prospective Political Analysis for Policy Design: Enhancing the Political Viability of Single-Payer Health Reform in Vermont," *Health Policy* 111, no. 1 (2013): 78–85.

34. John W. Kingdon, *Agendas, Alternatives, and Public Policies* (Pearson, 2010).

35. "In-Person Interviews with Christian Social Services Commission Staff" (Dar es Salaam, Tanzania, 2015).

36. "In-Person Interviews with Kampala Capital City Authority Officials" (Kampala, Uganda, 2015).

37. "In-Person Interviews with Uganda Muslim Medical Bureau Staff" (Kampala, Uganda, 2015).

38. "In-Person Interviews with Ministry of Health Officials" (Phnom Penh, Cambodia, 2017).

39. Shankar Prinja, "Role of Ideas and Ideologies in Evidence-Based Health Policy," *Iranian Journal of Public Health* 39, no. 1 (March 31, 2010): 64–69, http://www.ncbi.nlm.nih.gov/pmc/articles/PMC3468969/.

40. James White et al., *Private Health Sector Assessment in Tanzania*, World Bank Studies (The World Bank, 2013), doi:doi:10.1596/978-1-4648-0040-5.

41. Organized in the Shinyanga, Iringa, Mbeya, and Morogoro regions (and several local councils and districts) in 2016, and involving stakeholders from a wide cross section of the public and private healthcare sectors.

42. World Health Organization, "The Kingdom of Cambodia Health System Review" (Manila, Philippines, 2015), http://www.wpro.who.int/asia_pacific_observatory/hits/series/cambodia_health_systems_review.pdf?ua=1.

43. Lagomarsino, Nachuk, and Kundra, "Public Stewardship of Private Providers in Mixed Health Systems."

44. "Dual practice" refers to public healthcare workers who simultaneously work in the private healthcare sector. This can be seen as a threat to quality, dedication, and access to services in the public sector and, in such instances, may be discouraged, penalized, or regulated by ministries of health.

45. Karolina Z. Socha and Mickael Bech, "Physician Dual Practice: A Review of Literature," *Health Policy* 102, no. 1 (2011): 1–7.

46. Neetu Hariharan et al., "Synthesis of PHC Cost Estimates from South Africa's Primary Health Care Costing Task Team" (Washington, DC, 2016).

47. Ursula Giedion et al., "Health Benefit Plans in Latin America: A Regional Comparison" (Inter-American Development Bank, 2014).

48. "Using Data Analytics to Monitor Health Provider Payment Systems: A Toolkit for Countries Working toward Universal Health Coverage" (Washington, DC, 2017).

49. "In-Person Interviews with National Health Insurance Fund Officials and Providers" (Abuja, Nigeria, 2016).

50. World Bank and USAID, *Designing and Implementing Health Care Provider Payment Systems: How-To Manuals* (Washington, DC, 2009), 33–34.

51. "In-Person Interviews with National Health Insurance Fund Officials and Providers."

52. "In-Person Interviews with Local Government Authority Officials" (various, Tanzania, 2015).

53. "In-Person Interviews with Local Government Authority Officials" (various, Tanzania, 2016).

54. Ainura Ibraimova et al., "Kyrgyzstan Health System Review," *Health System in Transition* vol. 13, no. 3 (European Observatory on Health Systems and Policies, 2011).

55. "In-Person Interviews with Kampala Capital City Authority Officials."

56. "In-Person Interviews with National Health Insurance Fund Officials and Providers."

57. The Joint Learning Network for Universal Health Coverage (JLN) is a demand-driven community of policy makers and practitioners that co-create practical "how to" knowledge to accelerate country progress toward UHC. The Primary Health Care Initiative is one of several initiatives under the JLN, focused on co-production of tools and resources that can help accelerate progress toward UHC by orienting health systems toward high-quality PHC services.

58. Neetu Hariharan et al., "Linking Private Primary Health Care Networks to Sustainable Domestic Financing: A Practical Guide for Network Managers." Washington: Results for Development and Population Services International, 2018.

59. Intermediaries are defined as organizations that form networks between small-scale providers to interact with governments, patients, and vendors. These organizations can perform key health systems functions that are typically more challenging for individual private providers to do on their own. Examples include professional organizations, social franchise networks, health maintenance organizations (HMOs), etc.

60. Deepti Mathur et al., "Ushering in a New Era of Public-Private Family Planning Partnerships in Uttar Pradesh, India | The Challenge Initiative," *Johns Hopkins Bloomberg School of Public Health*, 2017, https://tciurbanhealth.org/.

4

Innovative Initiatives from the Private Sector

What Have the Experiences Been? What Opportunities
Lie Ahead, and How Can They Be Harnessed
More Effectively?

Donika Dimovska and John Campbell, Jr.

The landscape of private sector involvement in improving health
systems in low- and middle-income countries (LMICs) is rapidly evolving.
Untapped opportunities exist in certain market segments, areas where,
despite existing or latent demand for services, there are few innovative
models operating at scale to meet the demand. Using the Center for Health
Market Innovations (CHMI) database, we characterize innovative models
of care delivery that respond to four emerging market opportunities in
mixed health systems: (1) de-fragmentation of delivery, (2) improvement
in care coordination and service integration, (3) standardization of operating processes and procedures, and (4) the application of technology to
improve the management and delivery of care. Key obstacles to scaling
such innovative approaches lie in a suboptimal balance between looking
for novel solutions and scaling existing models, in addition to various operational and funding challenges that limit the ability of innovations to
grow and adapt in new settings. In this chapter we point to three ways of
addressing barriers to scaling for the innovations we discuss in an effort to
promote lasting systems-level change.

The global movement toward universal health coverage means there is
a greater need for more healthcare providers to achieve full population
coverage. The new Sustainable Development Goal for health, established
by the 70th UN General Assembly in 2015, has placed a renewed focus on
improving the quality and quantity of healthcare provision globally. However, the successful delivery of effective health interventions and advancement toward universal health coverage in LMICs depends on the existence
of well-functioning health systems that embrace innovation and mitigate

system-level challenges. The health systems in many LMICs can be characterized as "mixed," in which centrally planned public health services operate alongside private markets for similar or complementary products and services.[1] Addressing the persistent challenges of scant availability, uneven quality, and the lack of affordable key health services in many such systems requires effective government stewardship of the entire mixed health system combined with a thriving local ecosystem for innovation that nurtures promising models stemming from the private sector.[2]

Investment in strengthening health systems and expanding health services has long been a focus of concern for governments and multilateral organizations. As countries and multinational agencies work to improve access, quality, efficiency, and equity through their commitment to strengthening health systems, there has been increasing recognition of the potential of private actors to complement the public provision of services in a mixed health system. How to harness these private-sector-led models most effectively has been the subject of continuous debate, especially over the past decade or so, as the size and scope of the private sector has continued to grow and has begun to attract increasing attention from both governments and global development actors.[3] With these questions in mind, health systems, nongovernmental organizations, and social entrepreneurs around the world have started experimenting with new, disruptive forms of healthcare delivery. LMICs have proven to be especially fertile ground for these innovations, as they are less shackled by legacy practices and infrastructure. This chapter looks at some of the most compelling models, with a particular emphasis on how they provide step-function improvements in cost, quality, and access and so are fundamentally changing the traditional model of healthcare delivery. This chapter also examines how the principles and lessons from successful models can be adapted for use in other countries, focusing on the supportive role that critical stakeholders must play to leverage fully the transformational potential of these innovations and accelerate the progress toward achieving universal health coverage in LMICs.

Depending on the country and context, the private sector's involvement in the provision of healthcare encompasses a complex range of activities carried out by various nonstate actors. These can include for-profit organizations, social enterprises, not-for-profit entities such as nongovernmental organizations and faith-based organizations, corporate entities, and informal sector actors such as traditional healers, birth attendants, and individual medicine sellers. Several common factors have contributed to the growing significance of the private sector, including (i) scantly available and overcrowded public services that, when combined with growing populations, have opened up new market opportunities for private providers; (ii) demand by consumers for affordable and accessible services; (iii) new technologies, particularly information communication technologies (ICTs), that have contributed to the proliferation of new private sector business models; and (iv) explicit policies by development partners that have begun to create stronger linkages to and more funding for private sector models.[4]

Owing to the increased number of global and country-level efforts focused on better understanding the size, scope, and potential impact of private-sector-led interventions, the global health community now knows more than ever before about the nature of private sector provision: who accesses care from private providers and what the quality of that care is.[5] This improved access to information and collective knowledge has highlighted the many complexities and challenges that countries face in effectively engaging the private sector, including sector fragmentation and the lack of consolidated capacity across many small-scale private providers, uneven quality across the range and types of providers, and, not least of all, the numerous practical difficulties of implementing public-private partnerships.[6,7]

Therefore, despite the increased availability of data, evidence, and practical experience, the promise of private sector solutions to contribute to countries' efforts toward universal health coverage has yet to reach its full potential. The global momentum to harness promising innovations stemming from the private sector, however, continues to grow, encouraged by the widespread recognition that they can have a positive impact on the broader health system.[8] And while the evidence gap for the scale, scope, and results of such models is still significant, many of the current issues that systems face pertain to the question of *how* to integrate promising private sector solutions most effectively into health systems for increased collective impact.[9]

A Changing Landscape

Over the past decade or so, a vast number of new private sector actors have begun to explore ways of improving how mixed health systems function through the introduction of new approaches to healthcare delivery and financing.[10] A large array of health market innovations—defined as programs, policies, and practices that have the potential to improve the quality and affordability of healthcare—have been conceived and launched.[11] Results for Development's CHMI captures information on over 1,300 health market innovations across 130 countries covering areas such as service delivery, financing, policy and regulation, technology, processes, and products.[12]

Many of the innovations documented by the CHMI have been launched in the last 10 years, spurred by both perceived demand for improved and more accessible services and by a strong interest from social entrepreneurs and funders viewing these innovations as potential stepping-stones to system-level improvements. The diversity of approaches is great, covering a broad spectrum of interventions that address specific challenges present in many LMICs, including reducing the fragmentation of private providers (franchises and provider networks), changing provider incentives and improving monitoring (accreditation and licensing models and insurance or voucher programs), and providing subsidies for targeted populations and high-impact interventions (risk-pooling programs).[13] In addition, several models work on the demand side of health systems by educating patients to seek out the most beneficial health services (social marketing and conditional cash transfer programs). Others apply innovative uses of ICT to expand access to care (telemedicine solutions and electronic medical records and databases).[14] A common characteristic is also the focus on nimble models of care delivery that respond to market gaps, such as restricted outreach to rural areas, the presence of spurious drugs in the market, limited availability for consumers to make informed medical decisions, and few financing options that enable low-income communities to afford healthcare.[15] While some attempt to address the challenges of providing good-quality, affordable healthcare, others try to provide basic services at scale or introduce new healthcare solutions through disruptive innovations (e.g., new ICT models).[16]

The CHMI database reveals how health market innovations in LMICs have evolved over the last decade.[17] Analysis of the information points to several emerging trends that characterize the nature and results of the health market innovations documented by the CHMI. For example, perhaps unsurprisingly given the demand for these services, the top three health areas of focus for health market innovators are maternal, newborn, and child health (MNCH); primary care; and reproductive health and family planning. These priority areas have remained fairly consistent over the years, while others have emerged more recently and have grown rapidly: for example, pharmacy services, emergency care, dentistry, and noncommunicable diseases are all areas that have attracted increased attention from private sector providers because of a growing demand for these services and the perceived market opportunities they present. Furthermore, a large percentage (58%) of programs in the CHMI database focus their efforts on opportunities around process improvement (including the application of ICT, new diagnostics or products, supply chain enhancements, and so forth). Another subset of programs (51%) prioritize efforts around changing behaviors (such as consumer education or provider training). Service delivery innovations (approximately 30% of programs include this function) often combine their approach with the use of innovative technologies (like telemedicine) and other complementary approaches (e.g., changing behavior strategies). It is important to note that the primary source of funding for programs continues to be donor assistance, followed by self-sustaining revenue that is generated by the programs from consumers paying for services.

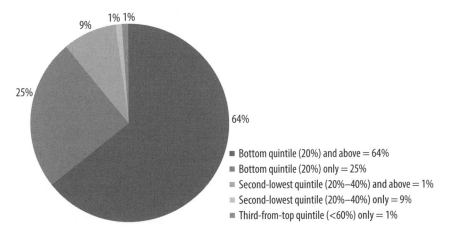

Figure 4.1. Healthcare social enterprises show promise in reaching markets at the bottom of the pyramid. The pie chart shows the percentage of CHMI programs serving each wealth quintile.

A more in-depth analysis of CHMI data on target populations revealed that while many programs begin with the aim of providing services to the poorest, pressure to be profitable prompts them to focus on segments of the population that have the ability to pay, as well as bear the indirect costs associated with healthcare. Hence, the target population for 90% of CHMI-profiled programs are bottom-of-the-pyramid markets; however, of these, 65% serve the bottom quintile and other income segments, and only 25% of programs focus on just the bottom quintile. Recent evolution in the global health field is changing the funding landscape and increasing the complexity of the fund-raising process for nonprofit and for-profit global health social enterprises. These programs continue to cite access to financing as a primary barrier to growth, in spite of both increasing government interest in innovations that can drive health outcomes and reported increases in capital available from a variety of sources seeking financial return as well as social impact. One critical differentiator in raising funds is whether the program is for-profit, not-for-profit, or a hybrid of both. This determines the primary sources of funding that programs access and, within that, the different financial instruments available to them. An analysis of CHMI-profiled programs based on their legal status shows the growth of for-profit enterprises—from 13% of profiled programs in 2010 to 31% in 2018.

Another new dimension is the rise of disruptive-technology-enabled models. Disruptive uses of technology have emerged as a major influence on services provided by programs launched in the last decade, rapidly opening new interventions such as telemedicine, call centers, and healthcare hotlines to connect remote rural populations to medical advice from specialists, who were not always available to them. The proportion of programs utilizing virtual technology has more than doubled for programs launched in the 2010–2018 period when compared to programs launched prior to 2010 (figure 4.2).

To date, close to 460 programs have provided self-reported results across performance dimensions like quality, efficiency, and sustainability.[18] In figure 4.3, 155 organizations reported improvements in health outputs (such as the number of health services provided), 47 reported changes in the health status of a given population as a result of their efforts, and 115 reported improvements in the affordability of the health services or products they provide. However, very few programs (a little over 5%) shared

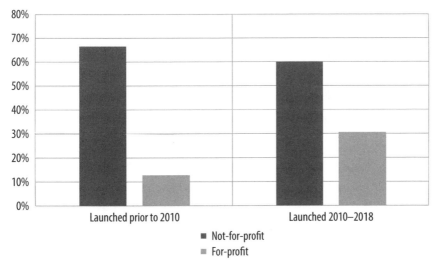

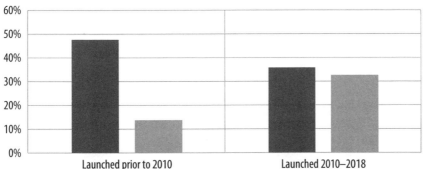

Figure 4.2. A changing landscape in health markets. The top panel shows an increase over time in for-profit programs profiled in the CHMI database. The bottom panel shows an increase over time in virtual healthcare programs profiled in the CHMI database.

externally validated evidence that speaks to their effectiveness, pointing to an important evidence gap for evaluating the impact of health market innovations. Still, although it can be difficult to assess the net impacts these approaches have had in strengthening the overall health system, it is clear that most programmatic innovations align with the core aims of strengthening systems to promote quality, access, and equity through the expansion and improvement of services.

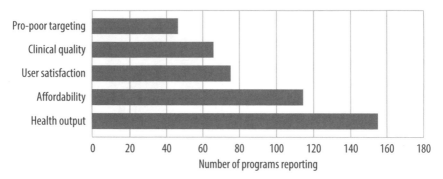

Figure 4.3. The CHMI's Reported Results Initiative tracks programs' impact. The bar graph shows the number of programs that reported results in key performance dimensions.

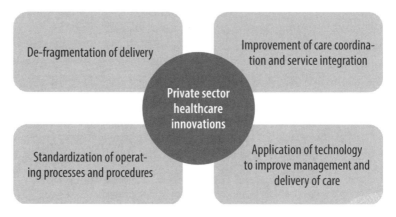

Figure 4.4. Emerging private sector healthcare innovation trends with high growth and impact potential in mixed health systems.

To better understand the current landscape of innovative health programs in LMICs, we utilized the CHMI database, the most comprehensive resource on private sector health market innovations in developing countries. As we examined the characteristics of private sector models in the CHMI database, we observed four clusters of innovation that are attracting interest among private sector providers, entrepreneurs, and other partners in developing countries and emerging markets (figure 4.4). These are discussed in the next section, with illustrations of some of the more instructive practical solutions and salient trends (table 4.1). While this review is the most expansive landscape analysis to date of health innovations, it is

Table 4.1. Four major health market innovation trends with examples of private sector innovator solutions

Innovation trend	Description	Examples of innovator solutions
De-fragmenting delivery	Healthcare innovators are aggregating the supply of health services into networks to create economies of scale that allow for lowered costs and increased access to quality care for underserved populations.	PurpleSource LifeNet International Christian Health Association of Malawi (CHAM)
Integrating services	Delivery innovations appear to have the most impact when they operate within a system of integrated care where information and incentives are aligned so that all providers collaborate in the best interests of patients. The integrated model delivers a dramatic reduction in costs while raising patient satisfaction and clinical quality.	Possible Health Clínicas del Azúcar Salud Cercana
Standardizing operating procedures	The operating procedures of many effective innovations are highly standardized, allowing for the elimination of waste, the improvement of labor and asset utilization, and the raising of clinical quality.	Aravind Eye Care NephroPlus
Deploying proven technologies disruptively	Healthcare technologies are emerging as a key enabler of care delivery. Innovative models often use proven technologies in new ways, repurposing rather than reinventing. They bring together low-cost screening and diagnostic devices connected by information technology and software systems that store, manage, analyze, and monitor data from patients and caregivers, leading to faster, cheaper, and convenient diagnosis of patients and the provision of point-of-care decision support.	ClickMedix doctHERs

neither exhaustive nor representative of the full range of inventive models of care delivery, financing, systems support, or products and technology that seek to bring about improvements in access, affordability, and/or quality in resource-limited settings.

Many of the models highlighted on this list are not necessarily new or groundbreaking; in fact, a number of them utilize well-established strategies and approaches (e.g., task-shifting, para-skilling, one-stop-shop clinics, or social franchising). The main reason for highlighting them is to draw attention to the potential they hold, not necessarily as individual models but as a collective of organizations that are all iterating, experimenting, and improving on their approaches with the goal of addressing pressing challenges in mixed health systems like care fragmentation, lack of affordability, and poor quality.[19] The secondary reason is to demonstrate that the field of health market innovation has matured as a sector over the last decade, with many more players (second movers) entering the market and building on previous ideas and solutions. Along with the market's maturation, the level of experimentation and creativity continues to be high—a sign that we can expect more innovation in the future, especially in areas such as new business models, cost reduction strategies, and technology use.

By demonstrating the range of ways in which health innovations can be harnessed along the path to achieving universal health coverage, as illustrated by select case examples to highlight exemplary models, we hope to (1) stimulate and inform greater uptake of health innovations that show promise and (2) initiate a larger dialogue about opportunities to support the scaling and adaptation of successful innovations in healthcare in an effort to strengthen systems and promote quality, access, and equity through the expansion and improvement of services.

Models That De-fragment Delivery to Enable Enhanced Engagement at Scale

Despite the presence of government-provided healthcare services in most LMICs, many patients turn to private sector providers, who are often perceived as providing higher-quality, more convenient services. These private small-scale providers include a vast range of entities, including nonprofit and for-profit health clinics, faith-based organizations, drug shops, informal (village) providers, and traditional healers. This proliferation of small-scale providers helps in meeting patient needs and demands, but it also contributes to confusion and further fragmentation in mixed health systems, making it difficult for governments to monitor and regulate their entire health system and engage with private sector providers, through methods such as the strategic purchasing of services.

Over the last decade, a number of new models have emerged to address some of the challenges associated with the delivery of care; the CHMI database identifies over 400 programs working on improving how patients access care. Of these, many seek specifically to address challenges stemming from high levels of fragmentation: including a lack of proactive population management and continuity of care; lack of quality care that is safe, effective, and patient-centered; lack of long-term management capacity; and lack of integration of providers into larger systems for payment.

For example, PurpleSource, operating in Nigeria, has developed a model to de-fragment and scale the capacity of the healthcare system. PurpleSource aggregates private healthcare providers and deploys finance, management, quality certification, capacity building, and technology solutions to integrate care across practices, bringing sole proprietorships into consolidated health systems. PurpleSource provides the platform required to scale medical enterprises and optimize their clinical, financial, and operational processes to deliver affordable, quality healthcare to patients and value to payers. The PurpleSource model is focused on primary healthcare, preventive services, and care management. Importantly, PurpleSource fosters knowledge sharing among its member clinics, adapting to new learning by encouraging member clinics to take up innovative approaches.

Another example, LifeNet International, integrates existing healthcare providers into a franchised network to improve quality of care. Working in Burundi and Uganda, LifeNet International partners with church-based health centers that have strong community reputations and provides the selected franchisees with three benefits: (1) standardized training for staff, (2) pharmaceutical supply delivery, and (3) growth financing. The LifeNet International training curriculum is adapted to the unique context and needs of each country and includes units on evidence-based clinical practices as well as financial management skills. Franchisees who successfully participate in training and meet certain quality indicators can order pharmaceutical supplies through the franchise and can also access favorably structured financing to purchase new equipment or expand operations. The LifeNet International model is designed to fill critical gaps in continuing medical education and growth financing for small clinics serving low-income populations.

The Christian Health Association of Malawi (CHAM), a network comprising 180 church-owned health facilities, exemplifies the potential benefits of such models. The presence of CHAM allows the government of

Malawi to purchase health services strategically from one service-level agreement with CHAM, rather than contracting with each of the 180 facilities. CHAM manages the contract and ensures that providers receive their payments, while providing quality monitoring and training on clinical guidelines. The ability to access government funding is a strong incentive for the providers to maintain high levels of quality and meet all necessary standards. From the government's perspective, this partnership allows them to harness existing capacity and improve system efficiency and effectiveness.

The existence of these various models working to de-fragment the provision of care reveals an increasing recognition of the potential of "intermediary" models, defined as "organizations that form networks between small-scale private providers to interact with governments, patients, and vendors while performing key health systems functions that are challenging for individual private providers to do on their own."[20] Recent research conducted by the CHMI points to the potential of these various models for enabling public sector engagement with small and fragmented private providers. While very few existing intermediary models currently perform all necessary functions to engage effectively with government (like proactive population management, quality improvement, management capacity, integration of payment systems, and universal health coverage), these existing structures may hold the potential to de-fragment private sector provision effectively and have a positive impact on mixed health systems if they are strengthened and encouraged to evolve.[21]

Models That Improve Care Coordination and Service Integration

Integrating care delivery has increasingly been advocated as a strategy for advancing healthcare for the poor in LMICs.[22] While the definition of what *integration* means varies across contexts and organizations, integrated care generally refers to organizing care delivery through better service coordination to improve patient care.[23] There is no agreement, however, about what it means to have integrated services, about which services should be integrated, or where integration should happen. While the concept of integrated care has been the focus of several studies internationally, confusion persists as to the overall nature of the concept and to its relationship to improved patient outcomes.[24,25]

A number of organizations documented by the CHMI have begun to experiment with new models of delivery that seek to integrate services more effectively. A common case of service integration is among providers working in areas such as MNCH and primary care. The University of Toronto's Health Organization Performance Evaluation team and the CHMI recently completed research to better understand the motivation for private primary care organizations to include MNCH services as part of their package. The research identified what models have worked best for primary care organizations and determined how to share that knowledge with other organizations that are either interested in integrating from scratch or in integrating MNCH and primary care services more effectively.[26] Findings indicated that organizations integrate MNCH service with primary care for three main reasons: patient and community demand, financial incentives, and the provision of a one-stop shop for their patients.

In rural Nepal, Possible Health's bundled primary and maternal healthcare delivery model provides integrated care through a hub-and-spoke model that connects government facilities and community health workers at and across the points of delivery, from hospital to home. Possible Health's innovative approach integrates three evidence-based approaches for MNCH focused on the "golden 1000 days" from conception through age two: (1) group antenatal and postnatal care to improve the institutional birth rate and reduce mortality among children under age two; (2) a community health worker model of home-based care to monitor and increase the utilization of services, maternal and neonatal health knowledge, self-efficacy, social support, and emergency planning among mothers; and (3) a mentoring approach to quality improvement targeted at government clinic providers in the study population. This model is supported financially through a partnership with the Nepali government's Safe Motherhood Program, where both pregnant mothers and Possible Health receive payments for making prenatal care visits and delivering in a health facility.

In addition to MNCH and primary care, integration can also be found in the area of chronic disease. Due to the growing chronic disease burden in many LMICs, many providers are looking for opportunities to prevent and manage chronic diseases through the integration of services that would typically be provided at different levels of the healthcare systems (e.g., primary care and diabetes management).

Clínicas del Azúcar, based in Mexico, provides patient-focused diabetes management targeting low- and middle-income populations. It serves as a one-stop shop, providing easy access to an array of services for patients with diabetes. Patients receive care at successive diabetes "stations," where the provider deploys evidence-based care algorithms that assess the patient's readiness to change and the patient's experience of disease, modifying the message at subsequent stations based on patient response. Fixed-cost membership fees make care available to more people at a reduced cost by allowing patients to plan for the cost of care and the clinic to spread costs across members, and facilitated diabetes support groups help patients manage their care. Clínicas del Azúcar's one-stop-shop clinics offer a comprehensive set of services on-site, including clinical consultations and assessments, lab testing, and access to medicine, so that patients do not need to travel to multiple places to manage their diabetes. This integrated services model reduces costs to patients by dramatically reducing the number of trips patients need to make.

Other programs take advantage of new technologies to integrate services. Salud Cercana in Mexico is a digital patient-management platform that integrates primary care and chronic disease services and accompanies patients throughout their care. Salud Cercana's digital platform allows patients, primarily those with cardiovascular diseases, to access a primary care network of doctors that are certified and use Salud Cercana's electronic prescriptions software, as well as a referral network of specialists. To help achieve their best health, patients receive care coordination, nutritional and psychological support, and notifications and reminders, all through the platform.

While these examples of integrated models remain relatively few in number, such programs are charting the way for new models that consider various integration approaches and point to potential ways that healthcare delivery platforms may evolve in the future.

Models That Standardize Operating Processes to Improve Care Efficiency and Affordability

A number of innovators seek to adopt precisely defined target populations and clinical processes that allow them to develop highly focused and cost-effective operations (for example, human capital strategies). This is particularly critical for providers focused on a select number of services (e.g., eye care, cardiac care, and deliveries in childbirth), as it allows them to achieve economies of scale, quality improvements, and a successful transfer of knowledge across their organization.

Given the imperative of cost reduction and low customer margins, business models for inclusive healthcare often achieve profitability and sustainability primarily through the scale effect. For instance, India-based Aravind Eye Care exploits the scale benefit quite effectively; this allows it to provide quality eye care to the maximum number of patients at minimum cost. The basis of Aravind clinics is standardization by adopting an assembly-line model to deliver eye care services efficiently (such as engineering cataract surgery for high-volume production). At Aravind Eye Care, employees (primarily women from the rural villages in which Aravind operates) are trained extensively in discrete skills, and they perform all levels of administrative work, diagnostics, nursing, and assisting. Professionally trained ophthalmologists and surgeons make initial diagnoses, verify the results of routine tests done by Aravind-trained employees, and perform repetitive assembly-line-style surgeries.

This process allows Aravind to tap the latent human resources of the communities in which it resides at the same time that it utilizes the most trained and highest paid professionals in its employment at their maximum capacity. However, central to the success of the model are the economics. The key is in the volume: Aravind averages 2,000 cataract surgeries per doctor per year compared to roughly 400 in standard Indian clinics. This high productivity is achieved by significant innovations in processes that are driven by a close analysis of the time spent delivering value-adding services. Of considerable importance is the fact that Aravind's treatment is not provided at low cost by compromising on quality. A key statistic in medical care is infection rate, and the Aravind system consistently performs better than many Western hospitals.

In concert, Aravind also leverages a financing innovation that is based on a customer's willingness and capacity to pay. Aravind has created differentiated products or experiences for varying levels of patients. The same operation can be priced very differently (ranging from free to a little more than US$ 1,000) according to the accommodations for the surgery and the type of lens implanted. These innovations in differentiated offerings—allowing patients to elect a level of services and accommodations based on their preference and ability to pay—effectively discover the willingness-to-pay of a broad spectrum of clients, from the poorest of the poor to the quite wealthy. It also ensures that Aravind is extracting optimal value from each transaction. In practice, one paying patient can subsidize the no-frills surgeries and pre- and postoperative care of two nonpaying patients. Cross subsidy along these lines, on top of Aravind's high productivity, accounts for its massive scale and effective delivery of services to the poorest communities.

In India, NephroPlus manages a chain of kidney care clinics specializing in high-quality, affordable kidney care, including kidney dialysis, at-home dialysis, removal of kidney stones, and other minor urological surgeries, as well as nutrition and kidney care education for patients. A patent-pending 56-step process innovation and standardized clinical protocols and operating procedures help prevent cross-infections. Another priority for NephroPlus is achieving and maintaining profitability, which has long been a challenge for Indian dialysis providers plagued by inefficient operations. From its inception NephroPlus has kept operational costs low through several measures:

- *Lean staffing.* While hospitals in India mostly use nurses to perform all tasks, including lower-skilled, nonmedical tasks, NephroPlus created new staffing categories such as a dialysis therapist for medium-value-adding tasks and a dialysis assistant for low-value-adding tasks. Nurses are then able to provide clinical care of high value and perform tasks related to medical complications, reducing the number of nurses needed to manage a single clinic. At the same time, NephroPlus trimmed overall staffing costs through a differentiated pay scale commensurate with skill and training level.
- *Virtual supervision.* NephroPlus introduced a centralized patient monitoring system that enabled medical staff at its headquarters to monitor patients at service centers through closed-circuit television. The company also created an online portal to collect patient data to support virtual supervision.
- *Bulk and demand-based procurement.* NephroPlus purchased consumables and equipment in bulk, allowing the company to negotiate prices 15% to 20% lower than large corporate hospitals. In addition, a management information system helped staff share and monitor their use of

consumables and equipment across centers. This ensured an optimal distribution of resources and avoided waste.

Together, these measures represent the critical building blocks for Nephro-Plus's low-cost service model, one that it has been replicated in over 75 centers across India.

Models That Harness Proven Technologies in New Ways

Technology solutions in emerging markets are increasingly being used in both product and process innovations to increase healthcare coverage in scalable and cost-efficient ways and to engage patients in a user-friendly manner. Nearly 56% of the programs that the CHMI profiles rely on technology to deliver affordable, quality care. Common ways of utilizing technology include improving health providers' ability to diagnose and treat patients, enhancing communications between providers and patients outside traditional office visits, and streamlining overall data collection and analysis.

For example, through innovative mobile technologies, ClickMedix has enabled low-cost health services as well as high-quality healthcare diagnosis and treatments to reach over 700,000 underserved patients in 15 countries. ClickMedix provides an innovative smartphone-enabled technology platform that connects medical providers and patients without the physical presence of a doctor. The ClickMedix application can either be installed on a smartphone or accessed through a web browser, allowing for end-to-end healthcare delivery and care management from frontline health workers, physicians, and remote specialists. Community-based health workers act as the hands and eyes of remote doctors, transmitting descriptions of symptoms using best-practice disease assessment protocols, diagnostic devices, images, and video recordings of the patient through the Click-Medix platform. Upon receiving a medical consultation request with advance symptoms information about the patient, the doctor provides diagnosis and treatment instructions to the community health professional, who then administers appropriate treatment and continues to provide follow-up care to the patient. The ClickMedix model creates value for all involved and achieves major improvements in health systems. Underserved patients with diabetes, heart conditions, cancer, and HIV/AIDS are able to receive high-quality individual care and treatment earlier than ever before (in less than three days instead of months or sometimes years, as previously). Meanwhile, health workers can increase their incomes and improve their skills, and doctors can treat more patients.

In Pakistan, doctHERs is a digital health platform that connects female doctors to millions of underserved patients in real time through online technology. This enables doctHERs to circumvent sociocultural barriers that restrict women to their homes, while correcting two market failures: access to quality healthcare and inclusive employment for qualified female health professionals. Home-based female doctors remotely access patients via high-definition, nurse-assisted video consultation using a cloud-based telemedicine system that includes electronic medical records, an online referral system, and the application of peripheral diagnostic tools such as blood pressure sensors, pulse oximeters, and electronic thermometers and ophthalmoscopes. Lower-middle-income frontline health workers (community health promoters, nurses, and midwives) are recruited, trained, and equipped with the necessary hardware, software, and Wi-Fi with broadband connectivity. They are then deployed in corporate offices, factories, retail clinics, and ambulances, where they are able to connect health consumers (especially female workers who otherwise have highly restricted access to women's healthcare) to remotely located female doctors who assist in the physical assessment of patients at point-of-care. These trusted intermediaries are trained to conduct sophisticated diagnostic and interventional procedures under the supervision and guidance of a remotely located (home-based) female doctor. By creating a more agile workforce on the supply side, doctHERs is able to match the underutilized capacity of female doctors to the unmet needs of millions of underserved Pakistanis, including those in corporate value chains (smallholder suppliers, distributors, retailers, and micro-retailers, including their spouse, children, and parents).

As these examples illustrate, the main purpose for which programs use ICT can vary. CHMI-led research on how programs are using ICT found six primary purposes: (1) extending geographic access, (2) facilitating patient communications, (3) improving diagnosis and treatment, (4) improving data management, (5) streamlining financial transactions, and (6) mitigating fraud and abuse. These various uses frequently overlap and are used together. They also demonstrate that technology is often used in conjunction with other nontech innovations that position the technology as an enabler and amplifier of the overall program's approach.[27]

Experts recognize the potential of technology-driven innovations and expect the rapid growth of these innovations to continue as more and more organizations become increasingly focused on technology.[28] A number of these new healthcare technologies hold the potential to drive efficiencies and improve care delivery processes by integrating all parts of the healthcare value chain; for example, they may be well placed to help mitigate many of the current challenges faced by health systems, such as the shortage of health workers in rural areas, the variable quality of care, lack of patient compliance, and fraud. It will be crucial to continue to track which of these purposes are being successfully fulfilled by technology and what devices and use cases are most effective in attaining them.

What's Next: Creating Opportunities That Promote Lasting Systems Change

The health market innovations we highlighted in this chapter have the potential for broader impact, but many face various operational and funding challenges, which limit their ability to grow and adapt in new geographies. To date, only 52 CHMI-profiled programs have reported scaling up (out of 103 programs in total that have shared evidence of their impact through comprehensive self-evaluation or progress reports), either by offering clients a wider range of services, adding facilities within their countries, increasing the number of people served, or replicating/adapting in a new country. Many of the barriers are specific to the individual business model—for example, poor population targeting, issues of affordability of services, uneven quality, or inadequate financing—while other barriers are broader and pertain to the particular environment in which programs operate, conditioned by factors such as government policies and regulations.

Despite these challenges, many encouraging developments point to potential ways of addressing system-level barriers to scaling. The global development community is increasingly directing its attention to building effective innovation ecosystems, both globally and locally, that identify, support, and nurture promising solutions and develop pathways for their uptake. Also encouraging is that national governments are starting to direct increased public investment to private sector models with the potential to meet national health priorities (through, for example, new platforms that purchase services from private providers, and new progressive policies and regulations). The stewardship of governments is also key to ensuring that the private sector models that do scale up and get integrated into the broader health system are the ones optimally focused on improving the quality, affordability, and accessibility of services, especially for the poor.

These promising developments can be further amplified with targeted investments in efforts to promote lasting change to health systems:

- *Increase investment in iteration and adaptation of existing models to scale their impact.* Many of the innovative private sector models that have emerged over the last few years build on previous ideas and approaches—few are entirely novel and disruptive. However, many of the funding opportunities available have focused on identifying novel approaches and perhaps have missed opportunities to support existing models that require some extra help in their refinement to land on a solution that works at scale. A related challenge is the lack of comprehensive understanding of the various potential pathways to scale for different models.[29] For example, in many contexts, scaling up has been defined as the process of growing the services or size, or both, of individual organizations; therefore, measuring how well models are scaling has been defined by the rate of success of stand-alone organizations.[30] Given how difficult (or inappropriate, in some cases) it is for individual organizations to scale, and the fact that very few are replicable in their entirety, expanding the definition of scaling may be useful for differentiating *scaling impact* from *scaling out*: the "process of taking ideas far beyond their original progenitors"[31] (scaling out) and of "finding ways to scale an organization's impact without scaling its size"[32] (scaling impact). Systems leaders can consider investing in targeted learning efforts that promote peer-to-peer engagement for program implementers with the lessons and solutions they generate being shared broadly with others who stand to benefit from their knowledge, by adapting and building on existing models. This can be complemented with targeted opportunities for rapid experimentation or "adaptive learning,"[33] which can be invaluable to programs in allowing them to test and compare different iterations of service design and delivery.

- *Support the effective integration of innovations that address priority health challenges.* To function effectively, mixed health systems require the introduction of a range of innovations with the potential to optimize the use of resources and ensure that government funding is spent where it is needed most, in underserved communities. Innovations such as new private-sector-led technologies or specialty health services can be identified and introduced into systems to meet specific system challenges and priorities. Such models can be harnessed more effectively by identifying who their innovators are, supporting them to further prove their model, and linking them to potential funding sources to enable their expansion. Eventually, some of these models may be funded through government financing or may continue to operate as privately funded businesses offering services directly to consumers at an affordable price. What is key is that such models operate within a strong framework of stewardship set out by the government, whereby the government puts forth core system priorities that private sector providers can respond to and align with.

- *Encourage positive market shaping and de-fragmentation of the private delivery system.* A key challenge for many countries is the highly fragmented and disorganized nature of the private sector, characterized by numerous small-scale providers, making it difficult for governments to engage. Governments are unable to monitor the quality of services across private sector providers and cannot ensure that private providers align with national health priorities in terms of their service packages, comprehensive care management, costs to consumers, and other variables. To address some of these challenges around fragmentation, systems leaders can support the development of innovative intermediary models that de-fragment private sector provision by harnessing existing structures (or introducing new ones); these can include clinic chains, social franchise networks, professional associations, and health management organizations. Over time, these stronger delivery systems can be well positioned to respond to government purchasing demand.

Although unable to transform health systems as stand-alone interventions, health market innovations, if harnessed effectively, can complement key elements of countries' healthcare financing and delivery platforms. At the same time, the global health industry is in the midst of a transformation that is unlocking many new opportunities and forcing organizations both new and traditional to rethink their places within it. The result will be a more innovative, equitable, and valued-driven new health economy, one better able to fulfill one of humankind's most fundamental needs—to be and stay well.

NOTES

1. Maureen Mackintosh et al., "What Is the Private Sector? Understanding Private Provision in the Health Systems of Low-Income and Middle-Income Countries," *Lancet* 388, no. 10004 (2016): 595–605.
2. Gina Lagomarsino, Stefan Nachuk, and Sapna Singh Kundra, *Public Stewardship of Private Providers in Mixed Health Systems* (Washington, DC: Results for Development Institute, 2009).
3. David Bishai and Karampreet Sachathep, "The Role of the Private Sector in Health Systems," *Health Policy and Planning* 30, issue supplement 1 (2015): i1.
4. Catherine Olier, *The Role of the Private Sector in Health Care: Challenging the Myths* (Brussels: Oxfam, 2012).
5. Bishai and Sachathep, "Role of the Private Sector in Health Systems."
6. Oliver Wyman Health Innovation Center, *Convergence: Opportunities for Innovation in the New Health Economy* (New York: Oliver Wyman, 2014).
7. May Sudhinaraset et al., "What Is the Role of Informal Healthcare Providers in Developing Countries? A Systematic Review," *PLoS One* 8, no. 9 (2013).
8. Junaid Ahmad et al., *Decentralization and Service Delivery*. World Bank Policy Research Working Paper no. 3603, 2005.
9. Bishai and Sachathep, "Role of the Private Sector in Health Systems."
10. Onil Bhattacharyya et al., "Innovative Health Service Delivery Models in Low and Middle Income Countries—What Can We Learn from the Private Sector?," *Health Research Policy and Systems* 8 (2010): 1–11.
11. Donika Dimovska et al., *Innovative Pro-Poor Healthcare Financing and Delivery Models* (Washington, DC: Results for Development Institute, 2009).
12. "Center for Health Market Innovations," Results for Development Institute, last updated March 7, 2018, http://healthmarketinnovations.org.
13. Duncan Green, *Fit for the Future? Development Trends and the Role of International NGOs*. Oxfam Discussion Paper, 2015.
14. World Bank Group, *Digital Dividends*. World Development Report (Washington, DC: World Bank Group, 2016).
15. Natalia Agapitova, *Leveraging Inclusive Innovations for Sustainable Results at the BoP* (Washington, DC: World Bank Group, 2015).
16. IBM Institute for Business Value, *Healthcare 2015 and Care Delivery: Delivery Models Refined, Competencies Defined* (Somers, NY: IBM Global Business Services, 2015).
17. "Center for Health Market Innovations," Results for Development Institute.

18. "Reported Results," Center for Health Market Innovations, Results for Development Institute, last updated March 7, 2018, http://healthmarketinnovations.org/about/reported-results.

19. Sarah Murray, "Innovative Fever Breaks Out as Development Landscape Shifts," *Financial Times*, June 18, 2014.

20. Center for Health Market Innovations, *Intermediaries: The Missing Link in Improving Mixed Market Health Systems?* (Washington, DC: Results for Development Institute, 2016).

21. Patricia Odera et al., *Healthcare Innovation in East Africa: Navigating the Ecosystem* (Durham, NC: Social Entrepreneurship Accelerator at Duke, 2016).

22. Zulfiqar A. Bhutta et al., "Interventions to Address Maternal, Newborn, and Child Survival: What Difference Can Integrated Primary Healthcare Strategies Make?" *Lancet* 372, no. 8642 (2008): 972–89.

23. Sara Shaw, Rebecca Rosen, and Benedict Rumbold, *What Is Integrated Care? An Overview of Integrated Care in the NHS* (London: Nuffield Trust, 2011).

24. Dennis L. Kodner, "All Together Now: A Conceptual Exploration of Integrated Care," *Healthcare Quarterly*, January 1, 2009.

25. Ashwin Vasan et al., "Integrated Care as a Means to Improve Primary Care Delivery for Adults and Adolescents in the Developing World: A Critical Analysis of Integrated Management of Adolescent and Adult Illness," *BMC Medicine* 12, no. 6 (2014).

26. Onil Bhattacharyya, "Assessing Health Program Performance in Low- and Middle-Income Countries: Building a Feasible, Credible, and Comprehensive Framework," *Globalization and Health* 11 (2015).

27. Trevor Lewis et al., "E-health in Low- and Middle-Income Countries: Findings from the Center for Health Market Innovations," *World Health Organization Bulletin* 90, no. 5 (2012): 332–40.

28. Harvey Koh, Nidhi Hedge, and Ashish Karamchandani, *Beyond the Pioneer: Getting Inclusive Industries to Scale* (Deloitte Touche Tohmatsu India, 2014).

29. Gina Lagomarsino, "Joint Learning—a Model for Future Success in Global Development," *Huffington Post*, November 16, 2016.

30. Harvey Koh, "Scaling Out," *Stanford Social Innovation Review*, February 23, 2017.

31. Jeffrey Bradach, "Scaling Impact," *Stanford Social Innovation Review*, Summer 2010.

32. Koh, "Scaling Out."

33. Aline Kramer, Clara Péron, and Tendai Pasipanodya, *Multiplying Impact: Supporting the Replication of Inclusive Business Models* (Endeva, 2014).

5

Healthy Women, Healthy Economies

Essential Facets of Universal Health Coverage

Felicia Marie Knaul, Belén Garijo, Christine Bugos,
Héctor Arreola-Ornelas, and Yasmine Rouai

Empowering women, improving women's health, and addressing gender inequalities are moral imperatives that figure prominently throughout the Sustainable Development Goals (SDGs) that were established at the 70th United Nations General Assembly in 2015. Improving working conditions, economic opportunities, and gender diversity for both paid and unpaid healthcare work is necessary for producing more health and economic growth for all, particularly in the context of the new industrial revolution and the increasing importance of knowledge-related work. Further, women are both consumers and providers of healthcare and are central to the success of universal health coverage (UHC).

This chapter focuses on the multiple linkages between women, health, and the economy, applying a framework that promotes the health of women and men as part of UHC. To address the needs of women and girls as both users and providers of healthcare, we apply a women-and-health approach and identify opportunities to improve their health and ensure that they are supported and valued in their multiple roles.

The chapter also presents a case study of a public-private partnership, Healthy Women, Healthy Economies, that reflects and implements the women-and-health approach. The case highlights how the private sector can have a catalytic role in implementing and promoting the health and empowerment of women in the context of UHC and describes the participation of Merck KGaA, Darmstadt, Germany, in Healthy Women, Healthy Economies.

Introduction

Empowering women, improving women's health, and addressing gender inequalities in health and other realms of life are moral imperatives.[1] They are also smart economic investments.[2,3] The relationships between health, gender equality, and economic development are intertwined and mutually reinforcing as both gender parity and health are key to sustainability and economic growth.[4] Evidence demonstrates that when allowed to reach their full potential, girls and women make significant contributions to their own, their family's, and their community's health and well-being and become key actors in achieving sustainable development, including UHC and SDG 3.[5,6,7]

Adopting and applying a gender lens to UHC is critical.[8] UHC is about the health of all people, and the production of healthcare is undertaken by both men and women, yet gender disparities in health needs, access to healthcare, and labor market participation make a focus on women particularly important in improving health for all. Actions to improve gender equity and to address women's rights to health count among the most direct and potent ways to reduce health inequities and ensure effective use of health resources.[9] UHC cannot be achieved if women are marginalized and their health is not prioritized, both because of the loss of their own health and because women are integral to the world's capacity to produce health and healthcare, and this drives the women-and-health approach.

At the same time, a focus on "whole of government" and "whole of society" approaches—the spirit of SDG 17—is also critical to achieve gender equality and better health outcomes.[10] The private sector, which depends on an educated, a healthy, and a diverse workforce, has much to gain from gender-inclusive economic and social policies. Moreover, the private sector has a key role to play in delivering gender transformative health and economic programs that benefit women's health and their economic empowerment.

In this chapter, we apply a "women-and-health" lens, drawing on the work of the *Lancet* Commission on Women and Health.[11] This novel approach considers the multifaceted ways in which women and health interact, including how these interactions are mutually reinforcing and undervalued contributions to economic development. It takes account of a fact that has been largely ignored in healthcare provision: that women, as well as men, are essential providers of healthcare who can and must contribute to the success of UHC. To move beyond a narrow focus on women's health to one that addresses the roles of women as both users and providers of healthcare, the women-and-health approach promotes innovative, all-of-society initiatives to improve the health of women and girls and their families, as well as to ensure that women and girls are supported and valued in their multiple roles as providers of care.

We begin by describing the important synergies between women's well-being, health, and economic growth. We then apply a women-and-health lens to the emerging challenge of chronic and noncommunicable diseases (NCDs),[12] focusing on how this will increase the demand for women's time as paid producers of healthcare and as unpaid producers of caregiving, and the impact that the changing burden of disease is having on women's health. After presenting data on the value of women's contributions to healthcare, we discuss some gender-transformative policy platforms that can improve the visibility of these contributions and mitigate the barriers to gender equality in the labor market. We then consider how the private sector can be harnessed to better respond to women's health priorities, while also promoting the empowerment of women as providers of healthcare through public-private partnerships. The accompanying case study focuses on the international Healthy Women, Healthy Economies program, and especially the role of Merck KGaA, Darmstadt, Germany, and their work in low- and middle-income countries (LMICs). This is an example of how the private sector can engage in multi-institutional programs focused on UHC, in this case by promoting the health and empowerment of women in ways that stimulate economic growth.[13] In the conclusions, we highlight some general lessons and call for additional research to evaluate the effectiveness of this and other projects.

Women, Health, and Economic Growth

Health is intrinsically valuable, but it is also an investment in economic growth as well as in reducing poverty and in human development. Improvements in health increase the productivity of education and of the workforce. The opposite is also true: a lack of health reduces the potential for economic growth and drags families and countries into a vicious cycle of poverty.

Decades of studies (historical, microeconomic, and macroeconomic) have traced and quantified these links. For example, improvements in health and nutrition explain about 30% of the growth in the gross domestic product (GDP) of Great Britain between 1780 and 1979.[14] The analysis of more recent data reinforces this historical analysis. A 10% increase in life expectancy generates a 0.4% increase in economic growth,[15] reductions in mortality account for about 11% of recent economic growth in LMICs, and, between 2000 and 2011, approximately 24% of total income growth was the result of increases in years of healthy life.[16] From a microeconomic perspective, differences in health can explain 17% of the variance in productivity of a workforce.[17] Employees with health conditions or who are at risk for health problems can have productivity costs up to $1,601 more per year than employees without these conditions, which can result in substantial losses for employers with many employees.[18] Further, research shows that improvements in health catalyze investments in other sectors, especially in education, which is key to the production of human capital and hence workforce productivity.[19]

Women play a key role in this dynamic of health, economic growth, and well-being (figure 5.1). Yet, there are two possible scenarios linking economic growth and health with a focus on women: a virtuous cycle and a vicious circle. Both can apply to families, communities, and workplaces, in public and private spheres, and to countries, regions, and indeed the entire world.

The starting point is the health of women. More health and less illness produce healthier families and workers, and more economic growth helps lift families, including the women themselves, out of poverty. Finally, if economic growth is invested in cost-effective and context-appropriate health interventions, the virtuous cycle continues. The vicious circle—of low investment in the health of women, lower earnings and labor force participation, less production of health inside the home and in the labor market, and less economic growth and more poverty—is what countries and families must avoid through policies that encourage and facilitate investment in health and especially in the health of women. This poverty trap is also bad for health systems and derails efforts to achieve UHC.

Healthy women are more productive in all their activities. They can learn more and better, and work more and earn more, in the health sector

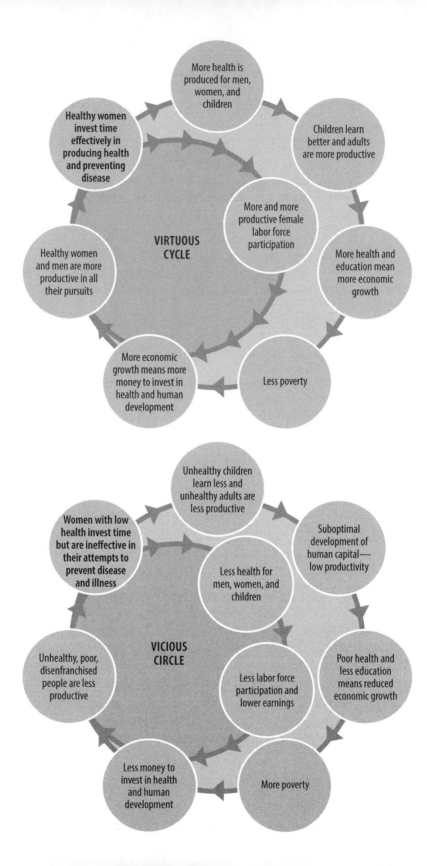

and elsewhere. Their contributions to healthcare have a multiplier effect because health is an investment that drives productivity as well as economic and human development for families and for countries.[20] If women and their children are healthier, their ability to contribute to more productive and better-educated societies is greater.[21] Indeed, recent research shows that investing in the health of women increases economic growth and accelerates demographic transition facilitating economic takeoff.[22] Thus, women are key recipients and drivers, both within and outside the paid health labor force, of the virtuous cycle between health and economic growth and well-being. Investing in the health, education, and empowerment of girls and women is thus an economic, intrinsic, and ethical imperative.[23] A large body of literature also shows that increased female labor force participation spurs economic growth.[24] Women tend to invest a large part of their earnings in their families, on average 90% worldwide (as compared with only 30% to 40% invested by men).[25,26] As participants in the labor force, they also pay taxes and contribute to overall economic growth.

Thus, the huge, virtually worldwide increase in the labor force participation of women (more than half a billion women have joined the paid workforce since 1980, and women now account for more than 40% of the world's workforce[27]) is a driver of economic progress. A 2015 McKinsey Global Institute report, "The Power of Parity," indicates that under a full-potential scenario in which female participation in labor markets is identical to that of men, the additional contribution of women in 2025 would be $28 trillion, or 26% of global annual GDP.[28] This corresponds to the current size of the US and Chinese economies, combined, in terms of GDP. Under this scenario, the global average participation rate by women of prime working age would rise by about 30% to almost 95%. A "best in region" scenario—if each country were to bridge its gender gaps at the same rate as the fastest-improving country in its regional peer group—could still add as much as 11% to GDP in 2025. Countries in Latin America would close the gap at Chile's annual rate of 1.9%, while countries in East and Southeast

Figure 5.1. Women's contributions to health and the economy—the choice: Do we aspire to a virtuous cycle or a vicious circle? Source: Adapted from Julio Frenk et al., "Economía y salud: propuestas para el avance del sistema de salud en México," Informe Final (México, DF: Fundación Mexicana para la Salud, 1994): 144–45.

Asia would do so at Singapore's rate of 1.1% per year. At these rates of progress, global average labor force participation rates would reach 74% by 2025. Each of these positive scenarios depends on gender equality in labor markets and assumes that women can participate in the world of work in ways that are at least similar to men. Increasing the labor force participation of women accounts for the majority of the impact; working more hours and fewer part-time jobs are also important, as is transitioning women from lower productivity sectors, such as agriculture, to higher productivity sectors, such as business services.

Women's labor force participation is estimated globally to be just over 60%, well below that of men.[29] Further, data from the World Economic Forum (WEF) suggest that the gap between women and men in economic participation is large and widening, although other areas such as education have improved. Given current trends, the economic gender gap (measured by labor force participation, wage and income equality, and occupational equality) will not be closed for 217 years.[30] The economic gender gap is particularly concerning in the context of the new industrial revolution in which there is less emphasis on physical strength and knowledge-related work is increasingly important.

Many factors contribute to gender disparities in labor markets. We consider three of them: shortfalls in women's health, gender bias in the provision of unpaid healthcare and caregiving, and discrimination in women's work in the healthcare sector.

Emerging Health Challenges and the Health of Women
Chronic and Noncommunicable Diseases

With population aging, the number of frail elderly people increasing, and chronic diseases and NCDs becoming increasingly common, the need for caregiving will grow. At the same time, the needs for healthcare and demands placed on health systems throughout the world will become increasingly complex and costly. NCDs (such as cancer, dementia, cerebrovascular disease, lung disease, and mental illness), as well as some diseases of infectious origin for which medical care has greatly increased the possibility of cure and of extending life expectancy (most notably HIV/AIDS and several cancers), will be responsible for an ever-increasing proportion of the burden of disease worldwide, including in LMICs.

Population aging will affect almost all aspects of life. Between 2015 and 2050, the over-60 population is projected to more than double, while the over-80 group will more than triple.[31] Further, these changes will be especially rapid, and hence challenging, in LMICs, which have the weakest health and social infrastructure. Between 2015 and 2030, the fastest population growth is expected in Latin America, the Caribbean, Asia, and Africa. By 2050, about 25% of the world's population will be 60 or older, and 77% of older people will live in LMICs.[32]

The world is facing a huge and increasing burden of chronic diseases and NCDs that is part of a prolonged and protracted epidemiological transition, linked to the demographic transition.[33] In 2016, NCDs accounted for more than 70% of deaths and 60% of the global disease burden (in disability-adjusted life years, or DALYs), compared with 58% of deaths and 44% of DALYs in 1990.[34] By 2030, NCD-related deaths are projected to account for almost 70% of DALYs.

Clearly, the impact of chronic diseases and NCDs on caregiving, health, and healthcare, as well as on economies, is significant and will grow.[35] Globally, almost half of these deaths occur in people of productive working ages, implying that governments and employers are adversely affected by lost productivity, lost human capital, and rising healthcare costs.[36] In 2009 and 2010, the WEF listed chronic diseases among the top five global risks in terms of likelihood. In its most recent report, the WEF classified them as a "trend"—a long-term, evolving pattern that could amplify and modify other global risks—because increasing rates of chronic diseases lead to rising costs of long-term treatment and threaten recent societal gains in life expectancy and quality.[37]

Chronic diseases and NCDs affect women in many ways. First, their direct impact on women's health and the increasing need for healthcare pose a significant challenge to health systems. Second, these diseases will greatly increase the demand for caregiving, which is still largely met by women (often younger or older women who may have to withdraw from school or the workforce). Finally, chronic diseases and NCDs dramatically change the demand for healthcare, and women are the majority of professional healthcare providers in the world. Each of these three pathways is analyzed below.

The Health of Women

Despite the important contributions women make to the well-being of their families and communities, hazards to their own health are among the key factors holding women back and limiting the health of societies, efforts to improve the overall condition of women, and economic growth. Women face a 10.4% higher rate than men of years lived with disability across all conditions, standardized for age.[38] Also, the health of women today hinges on the serious and growing threat of NCDs.[39]

The world has witnessed remarkable transformations over the past few decades in the health challenges faced by women. These are largely a product of the overall epidemiological transition, which will bring about rapid change in other areas of women's lives such as education and labor force participation. Still, women face a complexity of health challenges. The women's health agenda must continue to focus on the equity-imperative of reducing the burden of preventable mortality associated with childbirth, under-nutrition, and communicable diseases, which is increasingly concentrated among the poorest women. Simultaneously, the agenda must expand its capacity and dedication to addressing the burden of NCDs in order to achieve the goals of improved health, increased female empowerment, economic growth, and poverty reduction, all leading toward UHC.[40]

An effective response must address the multiple health challenges that currently threaten girls and women throughout their lives—as children, adolescents, mothers, and grandmothers and as producers of health and economic, social, and human development.[41,42,43] A focus on the health needs of women does not exclude the needs of men, but rather encompasses a population-wide approach while seeking to identify and correct disparities. The response must be anchored in an expanded concept of women's health that incorporates health challenges before, during, and beyond their reproductive years. It must also prioritize the health challenges that women share with men, because the manifestations and impact of disease and ill health are often especially severe due to biological, gender, and other social determinants (including discrimination) that disproportionately affect women. Female deaths and disability may also trigger higher child and infant mortality, food insecurity, disruption in children's school attendance, increased school dropout, increased childhood workload, and a loss of assets.[44] Women also face gender-specific issues of illiteracy, poor education, low socioeconomic status, cultural burdens and limitations, familial responsibilities and workload, and the costs of seeking care.[45] WHO Global Health Observatory data suggest a higher risk among women globally for many of the lifestyle-related NCDs risk factors.[46]

Significant progress has been made in combatting infectious disease and in specific areas of women's health such as maternal mortality.[47] The global maternal mortality ratio (MMR), for example, has fallen 30% since 1990; in 2016, so-called maternal disorders accounted for 7.7% of deaths and 3.9% of DALYs among women aged 15 to 49.[48] As a result, maternal disorders as a cause of DALYs moved from fifth place in 1990 to eleventh in 2016.[49] With notable and concerning exceptions in the lowest income countries and for the poorest in many parts of the world, these gains have been global. While successes were the result of many factors, several stand out. First, this problem gained global recognition, and United Nations Millennium Development Goals (MDGs) established clear global targets for tackling this and related issues. Second, governments, civil society, international organizations, and the private sector accelerated a range of efforts to raise funds, set country targets, and implement a variety of partnerships, many embedded in overall efforts to strengthen health systems through UHC.

By contrast, and in line with overall health transitions, the burden of NCDs has risen and now dominates the burden of disease for women. In 2016, 51% of global mortality for women aged 15 to 49 was due to NCDs, compared to 44% in 1990.[50] According to the Institute for Health Metrics and Evaluation, 18 million women worldwide die annually from NCDs, such as cardiovascular disease, diabetes, thyroid disease, autoimmune disorders, and cancers.[51] Also, chronic conditions such as multiple sclerosis affect twice as many women than men.[52]

Cardiovascular disease (CVD) ranks as the primary cause of death for women globally and accounts for one-third of deaths registered among women annually.[53] Further, women face specific challenges. For example, the risk of disability due to stroke is higher in women than in men.[54] Also, certain CVD-specific barriers make women particularly vulnerable, as some symptoms specific to women tend to be neglected in diagnosis and treatment guidelines, leading to under-diagnosis and under-treatment.[55]

Diabetes is the ninth leading cause of death among women globally and affects a large share of women 40 to 60 years old.[56] Diabetes is also an important and critical maternal health issue: gestational diabetes targets women and their offspring. It not only causes perinatal complications but also leads to an increased risk for mother and child to develop type 2 diabetes later in life.[57] Unlike for men, the all-cause mortality and cardiovascular mortality rates for women with diabetes have not declined over the past 30 years.[58]

By 2025, it is estimated that globally more than half of annual deaths from cancer will be among females (4.8 million out of 8.9 million deaths), and the share will be higher in less-developed regions of the world (68%).[59] Cancers that exclusively or almost exclusively affect women and are associated with reproductive health (breast, uterine, ovarian, and cervical) total 1.5 million deaths annually.[60] This significant burden of cancer in women, and especially poor women, is also highly amenable to prevention and early detection.[61]

Breast cancer is the second most common cancer overall, the most frequently diagnosed cancer among women globally, the leading cause of death from cancer among women in LMICs, and the second leading cause of death from cancer among women in high-income countries and many middle-income countries. The incidence of breast cancer, and NCDs, is likely to increase dramatically in LMICs over the coming decades, making early detection and access to treatment a high priority.

Cervical cancer—often classified as an NCD but in fact of infectious origin—ranked as the fourth leading cause of death among women in 2012 globally. An estimated 0.53 million new cases of cervical cancer occurred in 2012 worldwide,[62] and a strikingly high share of deaths (more than 90%) occurred in LMICs.[63] Weak health system infrastructure and challenges related to access to care in LMICs constitute huge current obstacles to screening and treatment.[64] Safe and effective access to the HPV vaccine can prevent many future cases of cervical cancer. However, access to treatment for women who develop the disease is essential from both a health and equity perspective.

Women as Paid and Unpaid Producers of Health and Healthcare

Women produce most of the world's healthcare, both inside the home as caregivers and as members of the professional healthcare workforce. The total value of these direct contributions is estimated to be at least 5% of global GDP.[65] Further, both the paid and unpaid contributions of women exceed those of men when valued at the same wages for similar work. Evidence from Mexico shows that, after adjusting for gender discrimination in wages, the value of women's contributions to health is approximately double that of men. Unpaid contributions are three times more, and paid contributions of women are 1.6 times the value of those of men.[66]

Unpaid Work in Health

According to the Organisation for Economic Co-operation and Development, women in every part of the world spend more time on unpaid work than men do.[67] This inequality hinders not only women and their families and communities but also individual businesses and global economies. The SDGs recognize that reducing the gender gap in unpaid work is critical to achieving gender equality.[68] In addition, the increased burden of chronic diseases and NCDs and aging will increase the need for caregiving, and under current scenarios this translates into a larger burden of unpaid work for women. Shortages in the supply and quality of human resources for health induce demand for unpaid or informal care, which eventually creates a disproportionate workload for the female population. A striking example is from Spain, where 88% of all health work is unpaid.[69] In Canada and the United States, around 70% to 80% of elderly care is carried out by family members.[70]

The unpaid healthcare work carried out by women, at home and in community settings, is a hidden subsidy to health systems and societies. Since women's healthcare work is mostly unrecognized and unaccounted for in GDP, one can conclude that countries in fact invest much more in health systems than has been reported.[71] This hidden subsidy is very conservatively valued at almost 2.4% of global GDP, including only the hours spent entirely and specifically on healthcare. This estimate does not include the promotion of health through domestic work, which would add several percentage points to the current estimate. Estimates suggest that 75% of the world's total unpaid care (such as child care, elder care, cooking, and cleaning) is undertaken by women and is valued conservatively at $10 trillion, equivalent to 13% of global GDP.[72]

Women's unpaid work in health and caregiving is undervalued, unrecognized, and often invisible, and in most countries there is no professional training or legislation around hours or working conditions. Gender-transformative policies can correct this and enable women to function to their full potential and contribute to sustainable development as healthier, valued, and empowered individuals. Examples of such policies include adequate caregiver support policies, including training, offering access to enabling technologies, and providing for fair compensation and paid leave. These benefits and protections are not gender-specific and should apply equally to men and women.[73]

Several countries have adopted gender-transformative policies around unpaid caregiving. For instance, Norway's right to four months of paternity leave encourages women's workforce participation and at the same time promotes shared parenthood. In Costa Rica, family members of patients with a terminal illness have the right to paid caregiving leave and access to psychological and social worker support.[74]

Paid Work in Health

Globally, women are the majority of healthcare professionals and paid providers. Nurses represent about 80% of the healthcare workforce worldwide and the vast majority—over 90% in many countries—are women, as are the overwhelming majority of community health workers and midwives. Further, while the modern medical profession has traditionally been dominated by men, women's participation has rapidly increased and women now predominate in medical school student bodies in many countries and at all income levels. In 2017, more than 50% of incoming medical school students in the United States were women, and the figure was also over 50% in Mexico.[75,76]

However, despite the remarkable share of female employment in the health sector, there are serious problems of gender imbalance. First, occupational segregation affects wages: as an occupation becomes feminized, wages tend to fall. The care economy is an important example of a sector where the lack of gender diversity leads to lower wages.[77] Second, women's representation in senior professional, high-ranking, and decision-making leadership positions is insufficient. The UN 2015 Women in Politics map indicates that among 191 countries, only 51 have female ministers of health.[78] The field of medicine is illustrative of many of these challenges. While women enter medical school in growing numbers, they are less likely to practice medicine, less likely to participate in the professional activities and specialized training that are associated with highest wages, and more likely to be unemployed given the difficulties of work-life balance. Further, female physicians tend to earn less than their male counterparts.[79]

Workplace training and education practices for physicians have been heavily criticized for paying little attention to the family-work balance. Many women who study medicine (in countries of all income levels) are forced to choose not to pursue specialized education and residencies, forgo professional advancement, and take part-time work or career breaks that often mean permanently leaving the profession. A recent study of Mexico showed the earnings difference between men and women is at least 30%, and that 80% of men who train as physicians work full time in their profession compared to less than 60% of women.[80]

Policies to redress the undervaluation of female healthcare providers are crucial to improve health sector effectiveness and retain workers, especially in the face of human resource shortages. These can include flexible schedules and leadership development and mentoring programs, as well as policies and employment guidelines to ensure equal compensation for equal work.[81] These need to be established alongside national policies to provide gender-neutral support for caregiving.

Harnessing the Private Sector to Promote Women and Health

Public-Private Partnerships

Sustainable Development Goal 17 is intended to revitalize the global partnership for sustainable development by promoting partnerships and coordinated action among governments, the private sector, and civil society at the global, regional, national, and local levels. The United Nations, as part of the goal, urges immediate action "to mobilize, redirect, and unlock the transformative power of trillions of dollars of private resources to deliver on sustainable development objectives."[82]

The private sector can provide dynamism and resources to solve some of the most urgent and complex health challenges and has multiple skills that can be leveraged by both the global community and governments. Among them are market discipline, regulatory harmonization, innovation, technological solutions, media and communications, logistics and supply-chain management, education and training for medical workers, human resources management and employment policy, and project management.[83]

Public-private partnerships (PPPs) can be an important modality to achieve these goals; they are proven mechanisms to achieving better health outcomes in many countries around the world.[84] PPPs can contribute to evidence-building and more effective decision and policy making, promote knowledge sharing, and enhance policy dialogues around health system solutions. Health system strengthening through these partnerships potentially addresses the challenges concerning women's health and reveals their untapped potential for the overall economy.

In the face of the health and economic implications of aging and the rise of chronic diseases and NCDs, companies should use the many platforms at their disposal to facilitate an effective global response. To achieve this, the WEF suggests that the private sector first identify and take stock of all relevant assets and capabilities, and then match these assets with trends and developments in the relevant ecosystem to both implement changes within the company and promote transformative change.[85]

The Healthy Women, Healthy Economies initiative is a growing PPP. This international initiative is dedicated to strengthening health systems, increasing access to healthcare for women, facilitating gender-transformative policies, increasing female labor force participation, and supporting better caregiving opportunities for men and for women. The case study that follows describes the initiative and the work accomplished to date.

Case Study: The Healthy Women, Healthy Economies Initiative

In 2014, the governments of the United States and the Philippines, in partnership with Merck KGaA, Darmstadt, Germany,[86] launched Healthy Women, Healthy Economies as a PPP under the auspices of the Asia-Pacific Economic Cooperation (APEC) forum.[87,88] This PPP is an effort to explicitly link the issue of women's health and well-being with economic growth within the APEC region and beyond. Healthy Women, Healthy Economies brings governments, employers, and other stakeholders together to address barriers for women to access the labor force and builds a foundation of data to make a stronger case for the need to address healthcare and work-life integration barriers to unleash women's economic potential. Additionally, Healthy Women, Healthy Economies provides a monitoring and evaluation framework that can help countries achieve UHC and the SDGs.

As the private sector leader of Healthy Women, Healthy Economies, Merck KGaA, Darmstadt, Germany, has worked both as a company and with external partners to advance policies around the world that support women's abilities to join, thrive, and rise in their communities and workplaces. The company's rationale for engaging in Healthy Women, Healthy Economies stems from the company's origins and ethos, as well as from the concerns and commitments of its executive leadership.

In addition, it reflects the company's recognition of the importance of promoting gender diversity as a strategy to strengthen financial performance and corporate growth and success.[89,90,91] Businesses with gender-diverse leadership are 15% more likely to report above-average financial returns,[92] and in one study a 1% increase in gender diversity correlated with a 3% gain in revenue.[93] Companies with the highest proportion of women board members had 42% higher return on sales and 66% higher return on investment.[94]

The Healthy Women, Healthy Economies strategy focuses on how health and prosperity are intertwined for women, with an emphasis on the private sector's leading role in promoting effective policies and fostering workplace cultures that equally support women and men. The strategy is also designed to promote, recognize, and invest in the importance of the public and private sectors working together to achieve public policy goals.

Implementation of Healthy Women, Healthy Economies takes several forms: with awareness- and capacity-building projects, through engagement with countries, and directly within the company, and by supporting applied research to strengthen the evidence base. Examples of specific activities are detailed below.

To build awareness and capacity, the Healthy Women, Healthy Economies toolkit was released in 2015 as a collaborative project between APEC and Merck KGaA, Darmstadt, Germany. The toolkit was produced by a multisectoral expert group composed of representatives from APEC economies and ministries of health, gender, and labor; the private sector; international organizations such as the World Bank and the International Labour Organization; academia; and civil society organizations.

The toolkit takes a whole-of-society approach and emphasizes the need to strengthen health systems to ensure universal access to healthcare, eliminate or reduce the financial barriers to health services, and develop health policies, services, and programs better targeting women's health needs. It includes suggestions and recommendations on how to improve women's health and encourage and expand women's participation in the economy.[95] The toolkit provides a menu of options to public, private, and nonprofit actors so that they can pilot, implement, and scale up policies and programs applicable to local needs and conditions in five areas:[96]

- *Workplace Health and Safety*: Review occupational safety and health (OSH) laws to make sure they address women's needs, expand OSH laws to protect vulnerable workers, develop guidelines for how to accommodate pregnant and lactating women, and train healthcare workers to detect and diagnose workplace injury and illness common in women.
- *Health Access and Awareness*: Conduct gender-based research and analysis, identify sex-specific gaps in data sets, train health practitioners on diseases common in women and the associated risk factors, and develop health policies and services that target women's health.
- *Sexual and Reproductive Health*: Reduce financial barriers to women accessing services, strengthen healthcare worker training, and assess the legal environment.
- *Gender-Based Violence*: Develop, implement, and monitor anti–sexual harassment legislation, create support mechanisms to address workplace sexual harassment, conduct seminars on legal rights for female migrant workers, and disseminate information to prevent intimate-partner violence.
- *Work-Life Balance*: Establish and strengthen sick and paid time off policies, caregiving leave, and parental leave, with attention given to gender-equity, improve family care options through the development of protective parental leave laws and policies, introduce supportive policies for breastfeeding, and raise awareness regarding women's double burden of paid and unpaid work.

As the private sector leader of Healthy Women, Healthy Economies, Merck KGaA, Darmstadt, Germany, works on a continuing basis with the APEC economies and other interested countries to implement the recommendations and activities proposed in the toolkit and facilitates cross-country learning-exchange opportunities.[97,98] To facilitate learning among the 21 member countries, an annual implementation workshop based on the toolkit has been held alongside APEC meetings since 2015.

Several country-specific, multi-institutional collaborative initiatives have emerged from the Healthy Women, Healthy Economies initiative. For example, within six months of launching the toolkit, Merck KGaA, Darmstadt, Germany, formed a partnership with the Philippine Department of Health and Philippine Thyroid Association to advance health awareness and education on thyroid disease. This project has a three-pronged approach: to provide expertise and know-how to develop and strengthen national policy, training, and public awareness campaigns; to provide technical expertise on timely diagnosis; and, with the Philippine Thyroid Association, to support medical associations, pharmacists, and other healthcare professionals to improve the patient journey. Based on the lessons learned from the experience in the Philippines, the company partnered in 2016 with the Royal Health Awareness Society of Jordan to launch a thyroid awareness campaign to educate patients, most of whom are women, and health practitioners on the importance of diagnosis and treatment.[99]

As of 2017, the company has been launching collaborations to increase awareness and understanding of the health barriers that prevent women from joining, thriving, and rising in the workplace and to advocate for change. These collaborations are designed to highlight the importance of public policies such as paid family and caregiving leave, to improve maternal health and birth outcomes, and to increase the recognition of caregivers as a critical element of the healthcare continuum. For example, Embracing Carers™ is a global initiative to recognize and raise awareness of the crucial role of unpaid caregivers. The Embracing Carers™ International Survey was released at the International Carers Conference in Australia in 2017, providing evidence of the strong, global need for increased support to caregivers, whose well-being is often overlooked.[100] The company now is working with several leading caregiving organizations around the world to help implement better support systems for caregivers.[101] In addition, a three-year alliance has been initiated with the US March of Dimes to promote research into the relationship among economic and employer policies, women's health and productivity, and childbirth. The March of Dimes will also expand its Healthy Babies Healthy Business® workplace wellness program, which supports health benefits and policies for strong moms and babies.[102]

The company and its leadership recognized the importance of "walking the talk"—that the company's ability and credibility to encourage others in both the public and private sectors to adopt Healthy Women, Healthy Economies policies depends on its own efforts to foster an equitable workplace, where talented men and women can thrive and excel without sacrificing their health or family well-being. The company developed a plan to integrate the Healthy Women, Healthy Economies mission into its core commitments, based on three pillars: (1) all women should have access to health solutions and awareness of the options available to them to advance their health and well-being; (2) detriments to women's health caused by trying to balance family and workplace responsibilities must be reduced; and (3) public and private organizations have a responsibility to create equitable workplaces. Internally, the company has conducted a rigorous root cause analysis, informed by focus group work, of the key drivers for women to achieve leadership parity. The results of that work led to the establishment of a global Women in Leadership program with key action plans to advance more women into senior roles. Workstreams include having women on interview slates and involved in succession planning; supporting flexible work arrangements; establishing a peer-to-peer employee resource group for caregivers; fostering gender balance in leadership training programs; and working with senior leaders to help eliminate gender bias through unconscious bias training.

To make a strong case for policies that support equal participation of women in the workplace, the Healthy Women, Healthy Economies strategy includes a robust and rigorous evidence base. Merck KGaA, Darmstadt, Germany, is supporting research that quantifies the health and economic impact of women's work as producers of both paid and unpaid healthcare in the labor market, the community, and the home. Building on the methods mentioned above and first presented in the report of the *Lancet* Commission on Women and Health,[103] in-depth country-specific research and policy analysis is underway in several countries, including Mexico, Peru, Canada, Chile, and China. This research strengthens the evidence that women produce the majority of healthcare and has identified key policy responses related to gender parity. Collaborating researchers come from a range of research institutions and policy think tanks, including the University of Miami, Harvard University, and the Mexican Health Foundation, and collaborate with local experts in each of the countries. To share knowledge and promote its translation into action, the research program includes a component for disseminating findings in each country,[104] as well as through key international fora such as the APEC meetings and Women Deliver.[105]

In summary, the private sector has played a crucial role in the progress of the Healthy Women, Healthy Economies initiative. Merck KGaA, Darmstadt, Germany, is the private sector co-chair of the initiative with APEC. The firm has exerted a strong convening role and facilitated policy dialogue, contributed to the development of the policy toolkit,[106] provided knowledge and insight to private sector counterparts so other companies can implement the toolkit, promoted and participated in several multi-institutional programs, and facilitated ongoing research working with academic institutions.

Conclusion

There are strong and mutually reinforcing links between improved population health and greater economic growth, productivity, and prosperity, as shown by decades of research. As expressed in the SDGs, the participation of women is key to each of these goals, as well as to maximizing the beneficial linkages between them. Women are consumers of healthcare and drivers of the health sector, as they produce the majority of paid and unpaid health services in most countries.[107] The "virtuous cycle" in which healthy women can invest more time and effort into their own economic pursuits—in the health sector and in other sectors and as caregivers—creates multiplicative positive effects.

Yet, women have been unable to realize their full potential as users and producers of health and healthcare due to the barriers and limitations they face. Gender continues to affect many aspects of life, including educational attainment, health status, personal safety, professional success, ability to exercise political power, and social standing.[108] This inequity of opportunities is unjust. It also stymies economic growth and efforts to improve well-being at all levels, whether individual, family, community, country, or global. In the health sector, these limitations are epitomized in both the challenges to the health of women and to their ability to contribute as providers of paid and unpaid healthcare.

Women face unique and often overlooked health risks that also affect their economic futures. Despite substantial progress in some aspects of women's health, and especially in reducing maternal mortality, women continue to face enormous barriers to access and a huge, unmet burden of ill health, especially in chronic diseases and NCDs.

The myriad contributions of women to health are an essential part of the foundation on which healthy lives are built, yet without support for this work, its full benefits cannot be realized.[109] To achieve UHC, society must recognize and fairly remunerate women's paid and unpaid healthcare work and seek gender equity and diversity in all spheres, both in the home and in the labor market. By creating and implementing gender-transformative policies that create economic and social support for the paid and unpaid healthcare and caregiving work that is concentrated among women—whether that be paid family leave, flexible working hours, legal protections, or equal pay for equal work—women will have greater ability not only to participate more fully in the economy but also to provide better care for themselves and their families. Equally important, men will be able and incentivized to more equitably and effectively participate in family life and caregiving.

While the policy-making and public financing aspects of gender-transformative health and economic development approaches to addressing the participation of women are primarily the role and responsibility of government, all-of-society approaches are required to most effectively evoke change. This is a point made clearly in SDG 17 and as part of UHC, which is embodied in SDG 3. The buy-in, participation, and partnership of the private, corporate sector—as employers and workplace managers, as well as leading institutional actors—is key to achieving the best outcomes and rapid change through innovation. The private sector can and should promote and implement policies that support women's health as well as be a partner in helping other sectors do the same, which highlights its distinctive role within the virtuous cycle of women's health that is central to UHC.

The case study of Healthy Women, Healthy Economies, a multi-institutional initiative originally conceived at APEC, speaks to these opportunities for the private sector to support gender-transformative policy making on health, the health sector, and female labor force participation. The Healthy Women, Healthy Economies initiative looks at access issues (women as consumers of healthcare), the interface between women and the production of healthcare through paid and unpaid work, and the impact on women's economic participation and success in the workplace. Merck KGaA, Darmstadt, Germany, is the private sector leader and partner of Healthy Women, Healthy Economies. The company has used its resources to implement programs that can shape policy, support research, and create better workplaces through Healthy Women, Healthy Economies, by partnering with both public and private stakeholders on issues of women's health and other issues such as the burden of unpaid work and the impact of NCDs. The Healthy Women, Healthy Economies policy toolkit provides a framework for other private and public sector entities to take up the opportunity and responsibility to become more gender-transformative internally and externally through, for example, advocacy, programs, and knowledge building.

Promoting gender diversity and equity is an essential strategy to both achieve UHC and strengthen economic performance. Empowering women, improving women's health, and addressing gender inequalities in health and other realms of life are moral imperatives as well as smart economic investments. A world in which neither health nor gender are barriers to an individual achieving his or her full potential in all spheres of life is a world of rising economic tide for all—for individuals and families, but also societies and the companies that do business with them. Everyone benefits from living in a nation and a world of healthy individuals who form empowered communities.

NOTES

1. United Nations, "Sustainable Development Knowledge Platform," accessed October 26, 2017, https://sustainabledevelopment.un.org/sdgs.
2. Ana Revenga and Sudhir Shetty, "Empowering Women Is Smart Economics," *Finance & Development* 49, no. 1 (March 2012): 40–43, http://www.imf.org/external/pubs/ft/fan dd/2012/03/pdf/revenga.pdf.
3. World Bank, "World Development Report 2012: Gender Equality and Development" (Washington, DC: The World Bank, 2012), https://siteresources.worldbank.org/INTW DR2012/Resources/7778105-1299699968583/7786210-1315936222006/Complete -Report.pdf.
4. Ana Langer, Afaf Meleis, Felicia M. Knaul, Rifat Atun, Meltem Aran, Héctor Arreola-Ornelas, Zulfiqar A. Bhutta, et al. "Women and Health: The Key for Sustainable Development," *The Lancet* 386, no. 9999 (2015), 1165–1210.
5. Revenga and Shetty, "Empowering Women Is Smart Economics."
6. World Bank, "World Development Report 2012: Gender Equality and Development."
7. Langer et al., "Women and Health."
8. Michelle Bachelet, "Towards Universal Health Coverage: Applying a Gender Lens," *The Lancet* 385, no. 9975 (April 2015): e25–e26, https://doi.org/10.1016/S0140-6736(14) 61781-5.

9. Women and Gender Equity Knowledge Network, "Unequal, Unfair, Ineffective and Inefficient, Gender Inequity in Health: Why It Exists and How We Can Change It," Final Report to the WHO Commission on Social Determinants of Health (Geneva: World Health Organization, 2007).

10. World Health Organization, "Glossary: Whole-of-Government, Whole-of-Society, Health in All Policies, and Multisectorial," accessed October 17, 2017, http://www .who.int/global-coordination-mechanism/dialogues/glossary-whole-of-govt -multisectoral.pdf?ua=1.

11. Langer et al., "Women and Health."

12. We refer to noncommunicable chronic diseases (NCDs) following the framework put forward in Felicia M. Knaul, Octavio Gómez-Dántes, Afsan Bhadelia, and Julio Frenk, "Beyond Divisive Dichotomies in Disease Classification," *The Lancet Global Health* 5, no. 11 (November 2017): e1073–e1074, https://doi.org/10.1016/S2214-109X(17) 30376-5.

13. There are several limitations to this chapter, as it was beyond the scope of work to provide a definitive treatment of any of the above topics. Further, this chapter does not provide a comprehensive overview of the myriad challenges to health that are faced by women and girls. While we include the health of young girls and older women in a life course approach to women's health, the discussion focuses on adult women who are caregivers and producers of healthcare.

14. Robert W. Fogel, "Health, Nutrition, and Economic Growth," *Economic Development and Cultural Change* 52, no. 3 (April 2004): 643–658, https://doi.org/10.1086/383450.

15. David E. Bloom and David Canning, "Policy Forum: Public Health, the Health and Wealth of Nations," *Science* 287, no. 5456 (February 2000): 1207–1209, https://doi.org /10.1126/science.287.5456.1207.

16. Dean T. Jamison, Lawrence H. Summers, George Alleyne, Kenneth J. Arrow, Seth Berkley, Agnes Binagwaho, Flavia Bustreo, et al., "Global health 2035: A World Converging within a Generation," *The Lancet* 382, no. 9908 (December 2013): 1898–1955, https://doi.org/10.1016/S0140-6736(13)62105-4.

17. David E. Bloom, David Canning, and Jaypee Sevilla, "The Effect of Health on Economic Growth: A Production Function Approach," *World Development* 32, no. 1 (January 2004): 1–13, https://doi.org/10.1016/j.worlddev.2003.07.002.

18. R. J. Mitchell and P. Bates, "Measuring Health-Related Productivity Loss," *Population Health Management* 14, no. 2 (2011), 93–98, http://doi.org/10.1089/pop.2010.0014.

19. Edward Miguel and Michael Kremer, "Worms: Identifying Impacts on Education and Health in the Presence of Treatment Externalities," *Econometrica* 72, no. 1 (January 2004): 159–217, http://cega.berkeley.edu/assets/cega_research_projects/1/.

20. Langer et al., "Women and Health."

21. Kristine Onarheim, Johanne H. Iversen, and David E. Bloom. "Economic Benefits of Investing in Women's Health: A Systematic Review," *PLoS ONE* 11, no. 3 (March 2016): 1–23, https://doi.org/10.1371/journal.pone.0150120.

22. David E. Bloom, Michael Kuhn, and Klaus Prettner, "The Contribution of Female Health to Economic Development," National Bureau of Economic Research Working Paper, no. 21411 (July 2015): 1–39, http://www.nber.org/papers/w21411.pdf.

23. Langer et al., "Women and Health."

24. Christian Gonzales, Sonali Jain-Chandra, Kalpana Kochhar, and Monique Newiak, "Fair Play: More Equal Laws Boost Female Labor Force Participation," IMF Staff Discussion Note, no. 15/2 (February 2015): 1–33, https://www.imf.org/external/pubs/ft/sdn/2015/sdn1502.pdf.

25. Revenga and Shetty, "Empowering Women Is Smart Economics."

26. Mayra Buvinic, Trine Lunde, and Nistha Sinha, "Investing in Gender Equality: Looking Ahead," *Economic Premise* 22 (July 2010): 1–10, http://siteresources.worldbank.org/INTPREMNET/Resources/EP22.pdf.

27. World Bank, "World Development Report 2012: Gender Equality and Development."

28. Jonathan Woetzel, Anu Madgavkar, Kweilin Ellingrud, Eric Labaye, Sandrine Devillard, Eric Kutcher, James Manyika, et al., "The Power of Parity: How Advancing Women's Equality Can Add $12 Trillion to Global Growth" (Shanghai: McKinsey Global Institute, 2015), http://www.mckinsey.com/insights/growth/.

29. World Bank, "World Development Report 2012: Gender Equality and Development."

30. World Bank, "World Development Report 2012: Gender Equality and Development."

31. Department of Economic and Social Affairs Population Division, "World Population Ageing" (New York: United Nations, 2015), http://www.un.org/en/development/desa/population/publications/pdf/ageing/WPA2015_Report.pdf.

32. Department of Economic and Social Affairs Population Division, "World Population Ageing."

33. Julio Frenk, José L. Bobadilla, Jaime Sepúlveda, and Malaquias López Cervantes, "Health Transition in Middle-Income Countries: New Challenges for Health Care," *Health Policy and Planning* 4, no. 1 (1989): 29–39.

34. Institute for Health Metrics and Evaluation, "GBD Compare Data Visualization," accessed October 17, 2017, http://www.healthdata.org/data-visualization/gbd-compare.

35. GBD 2016 SDG Collaborators, "Measuring Progress and Projecting Attainment on the Basis of Past Trends of the Health-Related Sustainable Development Goals in 188 Countries: An Analysis from the Global Burden of Disease Study 2016," *The Lancet* 390, no. 10100 (2017): 1423–59, https://doi.org/10.1016/S0140-6736(17)32336-X.

36. World Economic Forum, "The Global Risks Report 2018" (Geneva: World Economic Forum, 2018), http://www3.weforum.org/docs/WEF_GRR18_Report.pdf.

37. World Economic Forum, "The Global Risks Report 2018."

38. GBD 2016 Disease and Injury Incidence and Prevalence Collaborators, "Global, Regional, and National Incidence, Prevalence, and Years Lived with Disability for 328 Diseases and Injuries for 195 Countries, 1990–2016: A Systematic Analysis for the Global Burden of Disease Study 2016," *The Lancet* 390, no. 10100 (2017): 1211–59.

39. NCD Alliance, "Non-communicable Diseases: A Priority for Women's Health and Development" (Geneva: NCD Alliance, 2011), http://www.who.int/pmnch/topics/maternal/2011_women_ncd_report.pdf.pdf.

40. Felicia M. Knaul, Ana Langer, Rifat Atun, Daniel Rodin, Julio Frenk, and Ruth Bonita, "Rethinking Maternal Health," *The Lancet Global Health* 4, no. 4 (2016): e227–e228.

41. Langer et al., "Women and Health."

42. Melinda Gates, "Valuing the Health and Contribution of Women Is Central to Global Development," *The Lancet* 386, no. 9999 (September 2015): e11–e12, https://doi.org/10.1016/S0140-6736(15)60940-0.

43. Jim Yong Kim and Timothy Evans, "Promoting Women's Health for Sustainable Development," *The Lancet* 386, no. 9999 (2015): e9–e10, https://doi.org/10.1016/S0140-6736(15)60942-4.

44. NCD Alliance, "Non-communicable Diseases."

45. NCD Alliance, "Non-communicable Diseases."

46. NCD Alliance, "Non-communicable Diseases."

47. Knaul et al., "Rethinking Maternal Health."

48. Institute for Health Metrics and Evaluation, "GBD Compare Data Visualization."

49. Institute for Health Metrics and Evaluation, "GBD Compare Data Visualization."

50. Institute for Health Metrics and Evaluation, "GBD Compare Data Visualization."

51. Institute for Health Metrics and Evaluation, "GBD Compare Data Visualization."

52. Marvin M. Goldenberg, "Multiple Sclerosis Review," *Pharmacy and Therapeutics* 37, no 3 (2012): 175–84, https://www.ncbi.nlm.nih.gov/pmc/articles/PMC3351877/.

53. World Heart Federation, "Press Backgrounder: Women and Cardiovascular Disease," accessed October 27, 2017, https://www.worldheartfederation.org/wpcontent/uploads/2017/05/PressBackgrounderApril2012WomenCVD-1.pdf.

54. International Diabetes Federation, *IDF Diabetes Atlas*, 8th edition (Brussels: International Diabetes Federation, 2017), https://www.idf.org/e-library/epidemiology-research/diabetes-atlas.html.

55. NCD Alliance, "Non-communicable Diseases."

56. NCD Alliance, "Non-communicable Diseases."

57. NCD Alliance, "Non-communicable Diseases."

58. NCD Alliance, "Non-communicable Diseases."

59. NCD Alliance, "A Call to Action: Women and Non-communicable Diseases," accessed November 30, 2017, https://ncdalliance.org/sites/default/files/resource_files/Women%20and%20NCDs%20infographic_WEB_fv.pdf.

60. Lancet, "Keeping Watch on Women's Cancers," *The Lancet* 385, no. 9980 (May 2015): 1804.

61. American Cancer Society, "The Global Burden of Cancer in Women," accessed October 20, 2017, http://www.cancer.org/acs/groups/content/@research/documents/document/acspc-048547.pdf.

62. International Agency for Research on Cancer, World Health Organization, "Cancer Fact Sheets: Breast Cancer," accessed October 20, 2017. https://gco.iarc.fr/today/data/pdf/fact-sheets/cancers/cancer-fact-sheets-15.pdf.

63. American Cancer Society, "Global Cancer Facts and Figures," accessed October 20, 2017, https://www.cancer.org/research/cancer-facts-statistics/global.html.

64. NCD Alliance, "Non-communicable Diseases."

65. Langer et al., "Women and Health."

66. Felicia M. Knaul, Héctor Arreola-Ornelas, Julio Rosado, and Oscar Méndez, "Valuando lo invaluable: las contribuciones de las mujeres a la salud y a la economía en México" (Ciudad de México: Fundación Mexicana para la Salud, A.C., 2017), http://www.funsalud.org.mx/competitividad/Pdfs/Valuando_invaluable15112017.pdf.

67. Gaëlle Ferrant, Luca M. Pesando, and Keiko Nowacka, "Unpaid Care Work: The Missing Link in the Analysis of Gender Gaps in Labour Outcomes," OECD Develop-

ment Centre Issues Paper (2014): 1–12, https://www.oecd.org/dev/development-gender
/Unpaid_care_work.pdf.

68. World Health Organization, "WHO Sustainable Development Knowledge Platform:
Progress of goal 5 in 2017," accessed October 27, 2017, https://sustainabledevelopment
.un.org/sdg5.

69. World Health Organization, "Gender, Women and Primary Health Care Renewal: A
Discussion Paper" (Malta: World Health Organization, 2010), http://apps.who.int
/iris/bitstream/10665/44430/1/9789241564038_eng.pdf.

70. World Health Organization, "Gender, Women and Primary Health Care Renewal."

71. Langer et al., "Women and Health."

72. Woetzel et al., "The Power of Parity."

73. Langer et al., "Women and Health."

74. Langer et al., "Women and Health."

75. World Health Organization, "Universal Health Coverage (UHC)," last modified December 2017, http://www.who.int/mediacentre/factsheets/fs395/en/.

76. World Health Organization and International Bank for Reconstruction and Devel-
opment/The World Bank, "Tracking Universal Health Coverage: 2017 Global Monitoring Report," (Washington, DC: The World Bank, 2017), http://documents.worldbank
.org/curated/en/640121513095868125/.

77. World Economic Forum, "The Global Gender Gap Report 2017" (Geneva: World Economic Forum), http://www3.weforum.org/docs/WEF_GGGR_2017.pdf.

78. Inter-Parliamentary Union/United Nations Entity for Gender Equality and the
Empowerment of Women, "Women in Politics: 2015," last modified January 1, 2015,
http://archive.ipu.org/pdf/publications/wmnmap15_en.pdf.

79. Veronica Magar, Megan Gerecke, Ibadat Dhillon, and Jim Campbell, "Women's Contribution to Sustainable Development through Work in Health: Using a Gender Lens
to Advance a Transformative 2030 Agenda," in *Health Employment and Economic
Growth: An Evidence Base* (Geneva: World Health Organization, 2016), http://www
.who.int/hrh/com-heeg/Womens_work_health_online.pdf?ua=1&ua=1.

80. Knaul et al., "Valuando lo invaluable."

81. Langer et al., "Women and Health."

82. United Nations, "Goal 17: Revitalize the Global Partnership for Sustainable Development," accessed November 3, 2017, https://sustainabledevelopment.un.org/sdg17.

83. International Bank for Reconstruction and Development/World Bank, *Healthy
Partnerships: How Governments Can Engage the Private Sector to Improve Health in
Africa* (Washington, DC: World Bank, 2011), https://openknowledge.worldbank.org
/handle/10986/2304.

84. Kwame S. Jomo, Anis Chowdhury, Krishnan Sharma, and Daniel Platz, "Public-Private
Partnerships and the 2030 Agenda for Sustainable Development: Fit for Purpose?,"
Working Paper No. 148 ST/ESA/2016/DPW/148, UN Department of Economic & So-
cial Affairs, 2016, http://www.un.org/esa/desa/papers/2016/wp148_2016.pdf.

85. Norbert Hultenschmidt and Eva-Maria Hempe, "The Silent Pandemic That Threat-
ens the Global Economy," World Economic Forum, February 15, 2016, https://www
.weforum.org/agenda/2016/02/.

86. Merck KGaA, Darmstadt, Germany, is a 350-year-old global science and technology company with over 52,000 employees in 66 countries worldwide. It focuses on diseases that disproportionately affect women, such as thyroid disorders and multiple sclerosis. See https://www.emdgroup.com/en/company/who-we-are.html and http://reports.emdgroup.com/2016/cr-report/facts-figures.html ("Corporate Responsibility Report Facts and Figures").

87. Asia-Pacific Economic Cooperation (APEC) is a regional economic forum established in 1989 to leverage the growing interdependence of countries. APEC's 21 members aim to create greater prosperity for the people of the region by promoting balanced, inclusive, sustainable, innovative, and secure growth and by accelerating regional economic integration. See https://www.apec.org/About-Us/About-APEC.

88. Asia-Pacific Economic Cooperation, "About: Healthy Women, Healthy Economies," accessed November 5, 2017, http://healthywomen.apec.org.

89. Egon Zhender, "2016 Global Board Diversity Analysis," accessed October 28, 2017, https://www.egonzehnder.com/gbda.

90. Sylvia A. Hewlett, "More Women in the Workforce Could Raise GDP by 5%," *Harvard Business Review*, November 1, 2012, https://hbr.org/2012/11/.

91. Amanda Weinstein, "When More Women Join the Workforce, Wages Rise—Including for Men," *Harvard Business Review*, January 31, 2018, https://hbr.org/2018/01/.

92. Vivian Hunt, Dennis Layton, and Sara Prince, *Diversity Matters* (London: McKinsey & Company, 2015), https://assets.mckinsey.com/~/media/857F440109AA4D13A54D9C496D86ED58.ashx.

93. Susanne Dyrchs and Rainer Strack, "Shattering the Glass Ceiling: An Analytical Approach to Advancing Women into Leadership Roles," The Boston Consulting Group, August 14, 2012, https://www.bcgperspectives.com/content/articles/leadership_change_management_shattering_the_glass_ceiling/#chapter1.

94. CATALYST Information Center, *Why Diversity Matters* (New York: CATALYST, 2013), http://www.catalyst.org/system/files/why_diversity_matters_catalyst_0.pdf.

95. Julia Santucci and Ann Katsiak, "Healthy Women, Healthy Economies—2016 Updates for Policy Partnership on Women and the Economy," presentation 2016/PPWE1/004, Policy Partnership on Women and the Economy Meeting, 2016, http://mddb.apec.org/Documents/2016/PPWE/PPWE1/16_ppwe1_004.pdf.

96. Asia-Pacific Economic Cooperation, "Policy Toolkit," accessed November 5, 2017, http://healthywomen.apec.org/policy-toolkit/.

97. United States Agency for International Development (USAID)/Asia-Pacific Economic Cooperation (APEC), "'Healthy Women, Healthy Economies' Implementation Workshop: From Vision to Action" (Lima: USAID, 2016), http://healthywomen.apec.org/wp-content/uploads/HWHE-2016-Workshop-Outcomes-Report.pdf.

98. United States Agency for International Development/Asia-Pacific Economic Cooperation, "Healthy Women, Healthy Economies."

99. Merck, "Merck and the Royal Health Awareness Society Partner to Advance Women's Health in Jordan," CISION PR Newswire, September 22, 2016, http://www.prnewswire.co.uk/news-releases/merck-and-the-royal-health-awareness-society-partner-to-advance-womens-health-in-jordan-594460341.html.

100. Merck KGaA, "Merck KGaA, Darmstadt, Germany Launches Global Initiative to Recognize and Support the Pivotal Role of Unpaid Caregivers," Merck KGaA News Release, October 5, 2017.

101. Embracing Carers, "A Community Caring for Caregivers," accessed December 15, 2017, https://www.embracingcarers.com/en_US/home.html.

102. EMD Serono, Inc., "EMD Serono to Collaborate with March of Dimes to Improve Health of Mothers and Babies," EMD Serono, Inc., March 22, 2018, media.emdserono.com/2018-03-22.

103. Langer et al., "Women and Health."

104. Knaul et al.,"Valuando lo invaluable."

105. Women Deliver, http://womendeliver.org/.

106. Caroline Rubin, Ram Tamara, Zeynep Akalin, Austin Weatherholt, and Ann Katsiak, "Making the Business Case, Implementation of the APEC Healthy Women, Healthy Economies Policy Toolkit" (Lima: Asia-Pacific Economic Cooperation / United States Agency for International Development, 2016), http://healthywomen.apec.org/wp-content/uploads/.

107. Langer et al., "Women and Health."

108. B. Garijo, "Healthy Women Make for Healthy Economies," Women Deliver, 2018, http://womendeliver.org/2018/healthy-women-make-for-healthy-economies/.

109. Langer et al., "Women and Health."

6

Reframing the Pharmaceutical Sector Contribution to Access to Medicines and Universal Health Coverage

A Business Ethics Perspective

Michael Fürst

I have to say right at the beginning: I have not managed to figure out what I am supposed to speak about. The thing has a name: business ethics. And a secret: its rules. But my assumption is that it belongs to the sort of phenomena, as well as the reason of state or the English cuisine, which both occur in the form of a mystery because they must keep secret that they do not exist at all. (Luhmann, 1993b)[1] _____

In the 25 years since Luhmann began his lecture thus, optimism has grown that something like an academic discipline called "business ethics" can actually exist and that moral factors and ethical reasoning can and need to be an element of economic theory and business reality.[2] This is no small achievement considering that the dominant paradigm in mainstream economics for almost 150 years has been that ethical and political aspects of economic action were excluded from economic reasoning and theory.[3] At the level of management theory, a similar development has unfolded against the long-standing doctrine of shareholder capitalism, finally echoing the views of influential management thinkers like Peter Drucker (2001a, 2001b), who argued that business has to avoid unnecessary harm and look at societal challenges as business opportunities.[4]

The debates on business ethics and sustainability are no longer just noise but are relevant topics that have found a wide audience in academic and practitioner circles. At the same time, the growing number of examples that illustrate how systematically and innovatively companies can deal

This chapter solely represents the personal opinion and perspective of the author and not of the affiliated organization.

with their ethical and societal responsibilities is remarkable, though not sufficient considering the scale of the global challenges ahead of us. Once the province of a few academic seminars and perceived as detached from business reality, the business ethics debate and corporate philanthropy teams have exploded into a full business reality—a sometimes fierce and not easy to manage intersection of business, ethics, human rights, universal healthcare, and related roles and responsibilities.

The range of issues connected to the burgeoning conversation around business ethics reaches from general topics like bribery and corruption to industry- and even company-specific ones such as access to medicines. Issues such as human rights in business are unfolding in new ways that companies must pay close attention to (UN, 2011).[5] For the pharmaceutical sector, the UN High-Level Panel on Access to Medicines has even increased attention to sector-specific human rights issues such as the right to health.

This chapter will discuss calls for universal health coverage (UHC) in light of these debates. In particular, we will consider whether the focus on intellectual property rights, often seen as a barrier to accomplishing the right to healthcare and access to medicines (UN High-Level Panel on Access to Medicines, 2016), captures all the necessary ethical dimensions, economic implications, and challenges facing these rights. By applying different theoretical ethical lenses to this subject, we conclude that the ultimate justification and universalization of an ethical norm do not necessarily allow us to draw deductive conclusions about that norm's application and implementation (Wieland, 2008). This means that the discourse on applying ethical norms or principles, such as the right to health, needs to inform the discourse on the legitimization and justification of ethical norms or principles (Wieland, 2008). In other words, the debate about the practical implementation of UHC has something important to say about the broader question in business ethics of what normative principles actually mean in concrete terms and how they should be applied.

The push to introduce UHC is prompting healthcare companies to consider the ethical and social dimensions of issues such as the affordability of generics and patented drugs—issues that go beyond questions about the prices set by manufacturers for their medicines when just considering the huge difference between ex-factory and retail prices in access-constrained markets[6]—regulatory frameworks around intellectual property rights, health systems strengthening activities, and health systems financing. We will consider how the private sector can strategically respond to the debate on intellectual property rights in order to widen access to medicines and how pharmaceutical companies should contribute to solutions that will finally allow affordable access within UHC,[7] using instruments that are tailored to the needs and access constraints in specific patient segments in individual countries.

Access to Medicines in the Context of the Business and Human Rights Debate

The controversy over the human rights responsibilities of businesses signals a material change in the business ethics debate, in general, and in the access to medicines discussion, in particular. In terms of materiality, human rights belong to a category of topics that have gained considerable attention and importance. For a number of years, human rights discourse predominantly took place in academic circles or in the community of non-governmental organizations (NGOs) but not—at least not explicitly by using the term *human rights*—in the business community, even among the corporate responsibility (CR) community (Wettstein, 2012). This is not to say that human rights issues were not managed in companies, but they were cordoned off as individual issues. For example, the Declaration of Helsinki (originally passed in 1964) defines ethical principles for medical research involving human subjects; these principles refer to specific obligations to human rights such as the protection of life and health but do not use the term *human rights* even once. Accordingly, pharmaceutical companies often work from these ethical principles but do not do so under the heading of human rights. Broadly, corporate human rights work has been issue-based and occasional. This started to change with the official launch in 2000 of the UN Global Compact and its principles that are partially focused on human rights issues, with the aim that business contributes to globalization with a human face by adhering to standards related to human rights. In 2005 John Ruggie from the Harvard Kennedy School was appointed the UN secretary-general's special representative on business and human rights with the mandate to develop principles that define how companies should manage human rights issues. In 2011 the UN Human Rights Council endorsed the UN Guiding Principles on Business and Human Rights. This date marks an inflection point in the business and human rights debate that has a strong anchoring in the UN's SDGs. It underlies the goal to implement UHC by 2030.

For pharmaceutical companies, this development is relevant since the sector has a direct exposure to the right to health and to the roles and responsibilities related to this right. The right to health that originates from the international covenant on economic, social, and cultural rights does not have inherently moral implications just for the sector but has also attracted increasing political attention and importance as part of "rights-based rhetoric" (Leisinger, 2004, p. 1), specifically since it is increasingly clear that health is a crucial development issue and economic asset.[8] This is especially true for people living in poverty, since their livelihood depends on having good health and because illness can push the poor into a downward spiral of lost income and high healthcare costs. The magnitude of this problem is not to be underestimated, considering that approximately 400 million people do not have access to even basic levels of affordable care (WHO & World Bank, 2015). The concept of UHC is trying to respond practically to these problems and inequalities, because poor health is not just a risk for local communities but also for the international community (Sachs, 2012). Theoretically, UHC is rooted in the acknowledgment that every individual is entitled to receive some basic healthcare accorded on the right to health.[9]

Recognition on the international agenda that health has a considerable impact on societal and economic development was powerfully demonstrated by the inclusion of health in the Millennium Development Goals of the UN and even more strongly in the subsequent UN SDGs 2030, which place the right to health even higher on the agenda of public discourse. As J. Mann et al. wrote in 1994, "Health and human rights are complementary approaches for defining and advancing human well-being" (p. 6).

Recognizing this complementarity is a prerequisite for finding ways to address problems and challenges related to these facts; it also requires agreement on the duties, responsibilities, and rights connected to these facts. Practically, then, if it were correct that a) governments have the primary responsibility to protect and fulfill human rights and companies have the duty to respect human rights, what does b) linking human health and human rights mean in terms of access to medicines, or to healthcare at large?

The answer to this question seems to be straightforward for some critics of the pharmaceutical sector, who say that pharmaceutical companies are not living up to their accountability to the right to health. These critics accuse pharmaceutical companies of irresponsible policies and practices on pricing and intellectual property and of limited research on diseases of the poor (UN High-Level Panel on Access to Medicines, 2016).[10] We would argue instead that the problem of limited access to medicines and health services is more complicated than just questions of price or intellectual property.

Getting to the root of the problem requires that the response of the pharmaceutical industry to the undoubtedly huge problem needs to be more faceted and adjusted to the numerous complexities and barriers to access, and it requires that critics recognize these complexities (and vice versa on the other side of the discursive fence), including the responsibilities and performance of other actors such as governments, other private sector companies, and NGOs. It also requires that we understand the root causes of health disparities and their implications for the right to health. This will allow us at a later stage to elaborate on a proposal for how healthcare companies can respond to this multifaceted and knotty problem.

Drivers of Health and Ill Health: A Quick Reality Check

According to the World Health Organization's (WHO) *World Health Statistics 2016,* "dramatic gains in life expectancy have been made," specifically in Africa, "where life expectancy has increased by 9.4 years to 60 years." However, huge inequalities still persist. Life expectancy at birth for women in Europe is 80.2 years, whereas in Africa it is 61.8 years. And worldwide, on an annual basis, 303,000 women die from complications of pregnancy and childbirth, 5.9 million children die before their fifth birthday, 9.6 million people are newly infected with tuberculosis and 214 million with malaria, and 1.7 billion need treatments for neglected tropical diseases (WHO, 2016).

These problems are staggering. And to make it worse, many of the low- and middle-income countries are being hit by a double burden of disease, since noncommunicable diseases are on the rise at a time when many basic health needs have not been sufficiently addressed. In 2012, approximately 75% of all deaths globally that were related to noncommunicable disease—28 million people—occurred in low- and middle-income countries (WHO, 2015). Moreover, according to a 2015 WHO and World Bank report, 400 million people do not have access to essential health services. And depending on the poverty measure used, 17% of people in the 37 countries in focus are impoverished by health expenses, while 6% are pushed into extreme poverty because of health spending (WHO & World Bank, 2015). The extent to which access to healthcare and positive health outcomes are still a variable of income, a country's economic performance, and social context is striking.[11]

It is important to recognize that access challenges are not just related to low-income countries but rather to low-income strata; in other words, there are considerable health inequalities in high-income countries with high income inequality, which just confirms that health outcomes are dependent on social status and income. This in turn means that every actor in the health space needs to think about income strata rather than about country GDP (gross domestic product) classifications when developing strategies to improve access to healthcare or medicines.[12] In countries with an increasing gap in income or wealth distribution, high unemployment, or an increasingly limited provision of social services—problems present even in Europe[13]—access to healthcare becomes a prevalent issue. This implies that the social determinants of health (which include income and social status; exposure to health risks from nonpotable water, malnutrition, and fragile health systems; health literacy and education; the interaction of multiple diseases; social networks; and policies that enable access) are important components that have to be considered when trying to identify sustainable strategies to protect, respect, and fulfill the right to health and improve health outcomes.[14]

Considering these determinants makes it obvious that only a systems perspective, and not a perspective that isolates issues like price or intellectual property rights, is the right choice to solve existing health inequities and disparities, since gaps in health systems are central to the challenges and failures related to achieving the right to health and access to medicines (Leisinger, 2012). It should also be quite clear that these determinants are not within the direct control of pharmaceutical companies. In fact, governments have more direct control over these determinants, or at least an obvious responsibility for them. This means that only a holistic policy approach and well-functioning health governance will allow actors to confront the factors that negatively influence differences in health status. The right to health is in a government's bailiwick: governments are to be addressed first when trying to protect people from the causes that can infringe

the right to health and when taking proactive measures to respect and fulfill this right. The goal of improving health status and health outcomes
also requires that states have adequate policy and political institutions
that enact and enforce the economic institutions that ultimately determine the economic status of a country at large and its citizens (Acemoglu,
Daron, & Robinson, 2012, p. 43), which then eventually enables a country
to make the needed investments to positively influence the determinants
of health and ultimately protect and fulfill the right to health. However,
these complex issues still encompass the debate on the responsibility of
the pharmaceutical sector, specifically the pricing of medicines and the
use of intellectual property. It seems, though, that these factors are necessary but not sufficient to achieve sustainable improvements.

Pharmaceutical companies cannot directly control most of the social
determinants of health. However, some, such as the availability of medicines, health education, or some systems-strengthening activities, are
within their sphere of influence. This obliges them to take on responsibilities to respect the right to health and avoid harm that could infringe the
right to health of rights holders. Likewise, they have a responsibility to
contribute to the progressive realization of the right to health by addressing social determinants in their policies and actions. They are a secondary
bearer of responsibility, which is a crucial challenge to be fulfilled.

Perspectives on the Nexus between Property Rights and the Right to Health

The right to (intellectual) property—also a human right, according
to article 17 of the Universal Declaration of Human Rights—is one of the
most heated issues surrounding UHC, since some perceive it as a key barrier for access to medicines and the fulfillment of the right to health. A
well-functioning regulatory framework on intellectual property can incentivize innovation and create an ethical climate and legal framework
that promotes economic growth.[15] However, the majority of the most-needed
medicines worldwide are off-patent and have a generic status, which raises
a question: To what extent is the strong focus on intellectual property directed toward the main access barrier?

We can start unpacking this debate over intellectual property rights by
going all the way back to a Lockean perspective on property rights: that is,
intellectual property is the result of one's labor that increases the value of

the common good. In the case of a pharmaceutical company, it is intuitively logical that Locke's concept also applies to the development of novel medications since it is the result of mixed labor with a higher value than an idea or any previous good before.[16] Locke's position was adapted much later by libertarian philosophers such as Robert Nozick, who argued that intellectual property becomes an exclusive property only if states issue property rights that protect it (Nozick, 1974).

Before this legal guarantee is provided, a new idea from an innovator is intangible and difficult to protect, different from real, physical property. A patent is a practical expression of this guarantee; in economic terms it allows a monopoly for a limited period of time under the condition that the innovation is made transparent to society. The patent owner has full discretion over the usage of this patent that includes setting prices, issuing licenses, or selling the patent, which offers numerous economic opportunities. On the other hand, without legal protection (and enforcement), anyone could appropriate the innovation for his or her own use without having contributed anything to its creation: this presents a considerable dilemma in terms of the moral justification for appropriation. Arguably, only a granted and protected patent on intellectual property will result in academic and societal dialogue, since property owners otherwise would need to hide the intellectual and innovative core of a new product or service (Gewertz, 2012).

In Lockean terms, the appropriation of an idea requires that it is the result of its own labor; that the common is not substantially devalued by the exclusive use of the idea; and that the nonwaste condition is applied when ideas are appropriated. Nozick extends the proviso by stating that exclusive rights are only morally justifiable under the condition that the position of others is not worsened. Intellectual property rights are morally justifiable and permissible to Nozick since they do not disadvantage or deprive others; they would not have had access to this innovation because it did not exist prior to the innovator creating it.

The focus of his rationale is on situations in which property is acquired, not on the situation that results from the appropriation. He recognizes, however, that innovations are typically related to inventions or insights created by someone other than the owner of the patent (and well before patenting), which leads him to conclude that patents should be time limited. Finally, the distribution of goods is just as long as it results from a previously just distribution. This means that exclusivity linked to intellectual property is morally just as long as the acquisition of the intellectual property and the patent are just (Nozick, 1974).

These legitimate means are market-based mechanisms, which indicates that Nozick's position is rather well aligned with a laissez-faire economic model.[17] For pharmaceutical companies this implies that the exclusive use of patents is even then to be considered just and morally permissible, according to Nozick, if some might not have access to the products that are protected and purely traded along an economic market logic (Nozick, 1974).

The role of the state in this is primarily about protecting rights such as intellectual property rights. As shown by Nordhaus, though, the optimal patent life is finite since the returns on investments in innovations are decreasing over time, which means that governments should protect patents only for a limited period of time for economic reasons. This perspective has moral implications, of course, since this time limitation for the protection of an intellectual property right such as a patent is, in principle, a violation of property rights that just comes at a later point in time.[18]

Although Nozick's fundamentally laissez-faire rationale appeals to many market liberal economists[19] and is to a certain extent logically stringent, he overlooks some important ethical considerations and empirical effects of his theory.[20] His arguments do not sufficiently take into account that property rights can be in conflict with other rights. In the case of the pharmaceutical industry, his rationale does not account for the situation in which patients with a disease would have—from a human rights perspective—a right to access to medical treatments they could not afford. Nozick accepts that the acquisition of maximal possible market value from a patent derived from intellectual property overrides other rights such as the right to health.[21]

In principle, the main counterargument against the libertarian position is that the enjoyment of a property right must, at least, not conflict with other rights. And if rights are in conflict, there is a need to prioritize one over the other, which also means that the right to property can legitimately infringe other rights, and vice versa. Ownership and the right to property entails the obligation to respect the rights of others. "When those rights are violated," writes Donaldson (1982), "ownership carries liabilities instead of benefits" (p. 88). Property is an instrument for enhancing societal welfare and therefore deserves to be protected. But ownership "can properly serve the public interest" since "market failures and the physical characteristics of the resources at stake often require curtailing an owner's dominion" (Dagan, 2011, p. 44).[22]

As moral actors,[23] companies have the duty not to infringe others' rights by using and enjoying their property rights. This requirement derives from the concept of the right to property itself. Rights of others have to be respected by owners of property. According to John Rawls (1971, 2001), the use of property rights creates an obligation not to violate the rights of others: 1) Each person has the unalienable right to an adequate system of fundamental rights applicable to all, and government is primarily responsible for this system. 2) Social and economic inequalities can exist but only if they bring the biggest benefit to the least advantaged member of the society.

This second principle applies most specifically to economic institutions. Although both principles are directed toward different institutions, they are to be applied in a sequential order, which means that the infringement of basic liberties or rights is not morally justifiable even if economic gains could be realized. This implies that intellectual property is to be deprioritized in a case of conflicting rights since it is not a basic right or liberty (Rawls, 1971). The profits that are generated from intellectual property rights or patents through economic, market-based transactions have secondary order. As a consequence, both profits and intellectual property rights themselves can be redistributed by the state (Gewertz, 2012; Rawls, 1971). Ultimately such redistributions aim to provide a more just social distribution.

Therefore, according to such perspective, pharmaceutical companies need to accept that using their right to intellectual property must not infringe the rights of other rights holders. If such an infringement happened, by (for example) poorer patients being priced out of certain drugs, then the state has the right to redistribute the benefits of a patent. In other words, government could infringe on the intellectual property right, or use the profits to create benefits for the least advantaged patients, because it would lead to a more just and fairer distribution of economic benefits and social status.[24]

Is such an ethically justified infringement really just, and is it implementable? One obvious argument against redistribution or infringement of intellectual property rights in the pharmaceutical sector is obviously that the development of a medication is an expensive and risky endeavor. If profits were redistributed by the state and therefore considerably diminished, the allocation of financial resources for research and development might decrease, which could then lower the likelihood of further medical innovations in the future. At least it needs to be considered that the financial resources made available by shareholders or other stakeholders is dependent on a comparative analysis of the risk-benefit profile of investments in pharmaceutical research and development versus investments in other opportunities. A negative investment scenario could stifle research efforts and the development of next-generation treatments. From an ethical point of view, Rawls's position that property rights are not basic rights, and therefore are of second order, might be correct when considering current generations of patients—and thus ethically justifiable in the short term. However, future patient generations could benefit from a property rights system that has been shown to incentivize huge positive value and progress for society through its products and services,[25] a system that could be harmed by a lack of innovation that results from a weakened intellectual property rights framework negating those incentives. Rawls's framework might ultimately be an attractive shortcut that results in limited opportunities to provide basic rights in the long term.

When applying Rawls's principles to access challenges and intellectual property, pharmaceutical companies would only be entitled to enjoying the benefits of intellectual property as long as those do not infringe the basic liberties of patients. And in line with current thinking on human rights as basic rights (Shue, 1996), a just state must create, establish, and enforce policies that ultimately allow a more just social distribution. The problem is not what a just distribution means theoretically, but how a just distribution can practically be applied and managed in a real-world scenario, without prohibitively raising costs or creating too much of an administrative burden.[26] Combined with a set of negative incentives for innovation, this would result in lower investment in the next generation of treatments and in a policy landscape that undermines the original idea of a more just distribution.

Furthermore, consider that at the time when a Rawlsian appropriation of rights takes place—which is at an early stage of the research and development process—neither the clinical and financial benefits of the right, nor the potential harm, is fully known or understood. However, it requires continuous investments from the property owner to create a right that has an economic value and becomes an asset: again, this is the long-term perspective that considers future patient generations. It is ethically highly questionable whether access to treatment for current patients (i.e., fulfilling their right to health) should be traded off against the basic right of future generations of patients to have access to new, more effective treatments. A more just distribution of basic rights today might undermine the provision of basic rights and liberties tomorrow.

Overall, it appears that infringement of the rights of right holders typically happens at a stage when the property right is actually executed and applied in the marketplace through the use of the monopoly granted by a patent. If this is correct, then the intellectual property right in itself doesn't constitute the main problem for lack of access. The problem is instead an unenlightened enforcement of the right, which impedes access to affordable medicines and makes the goal of UHC at least problematic if not even unrealistic. Pharmaceutical companies should therefore make an ethical proviso when a property right is granted that its application needs to consider the rights of other right holders. However, this does not mean that the right to property should be slashed or substantially weakened. This could undermine a creative and productive institutional setting that drives economic development, creates healthcare innovation, and improves health[27] and is, to a considerable extent, stimulated by the incentives derived from property rights (North, 1981, 1990, 2005).[28]

However, the incentives provided by intellectual property rights do not stimulate economic and social welfare by default. They only do so if other socioeconomic factors such as appropriate levels of income, good political governance, drug reimbursement policies, and so forth exist in parallel in these settings (Lichtenberg, 2005). Since investing in well-working health systems and their underlying institutional settings has been shown to create considerable returns, where the benefits exceed the costs by an estimated 9 to 20 times (Jamison et al., 2013), a smoothly functioning access strategy requires stable protection of intellectual property rights and a parallel pricing model and enlightened use of patent filing and enforcement strategies that respond to various healthcare barriers within a given healthcare system or country.

Finally, when reminding ourselves that the primary duty bearer for protecting and fulfilling the right to health is the government, it is not necessarily the most just solution to prioritize certain basic rights over the rights of property holders. Rather, states should take care that these rights are not unnecessarily in conflict as a result of improper policy, insufficient systems financing, and weak governance. Having said this, companies also have a moral obligation tied to their intellectual property, which they must use in a manner that respects the rights of other rights holders.[29] Undermining the right to intellectual property or revoking property rights will erode the reciprocal nature of rights; that is, as much as rights must be respected by property owners, property must be respected by other rights holders for systematic reasons, especially given the importance that intellectual property has for incentivizing innovation and socioeconomic progress. These issues are difficult, sometimes convoluted, and largely ill served by easy and emotionally attractive "solutions" that may create some short-term wins in terms of widened access but that deal with the symptoms instead of the root causes of unequal access to medicines. Such solutions are not sustainable, either from a public health or an economic perspective.

Theoretically, it might sound like an appealing argument to prioritize basic rights over other rights. However, it leaves aside important considerations in regard to the *application* of such a principle and the resulting consequences (Wieland, 2008). Social categories such as property and its incentives operate alongside economic, moral, and legal codes, among others, all of which are needed to optimize the performance of each individual system, such as the economy, but also recursively to stabilize the order between the systems (Luhmann, 1993a, p. 453). As a result of this functional differentiation, a hierarchical order between ethical and economic logic is in principle thinkable but in practice not implementable. This, however, is a main pillar of the traditional philosophical program that persists in modern societies. A modern theory of business ethics has to describe how moral ambition can realistically be enabled in business and economy,[30] "beyond daydreams and educational aspirations" (Wieland, 2001, p. 25).

A starting point toward a solution follows John Rawls's argument that a society is best "interpreted as a cooperative venture for mutual advantage" (Rawls, 1971, p. 84); in other words, problems of cooperation and interaction are the defining element of modern societies. Issues (such as access to medicines) that arise at the intersection of business and ethics require differentiated functional reasoning, simultaneously applied in cooperative settings, instead of an automatic prioritization of basic rights such as the right to health. Instead of a purely normative understanding of ethics, contextual and descriptive ethical reasoning can help to develop a concept or theory of local justice.[31]

Put simply, we need a theory that has a distinct empirical orientation and practical implications. To get there, it makes sense to differentiate between a theoretical discourse and a "local" discourse on ethical norms, applied to economic, legal, or political systems. In regard to theoretical reasoning, ethics is autonomous. However, in regard to the application, it is not. Decoupling the theoretical discourse from practical applications allows us to develop implementable and sustainable solutions that also remain theoretically robust. As a precondition, both theoretical and philosophical reasoning need to accept that the ultimate justification and universalization of an ethical norm does not necessarily allow us to deduce conclusions about its ability to be applied and implemented (Wieland, 2008).[32] In turn, the applied discourse on ethical norms, linked as it is with real-world systems, needs to inform the theoretical discourse on the legitimization and justification of ethical norms or principles (Wieland, 2001). Ethical challenges emerge in a real socioeconomic context, and every line of argument should consequently inform appropriate choices in this real world.

Therefore, the question is whether the responsibility to respect the right to health can be properly balanced with the protection of intellectual property rights that bring innovative medicines to the market and are the pipeline of future generic medicines. Can corporations deploy access solutions that contribute to global health, without systematically undermining basic rights—whether the right to health or property rights? Market-based approaches that benefit from a strong patent regime need to recognize and respond to the legitimate requirement for and responsibility to each individual's right to health. Recognizing this, companies have to process not just economic signals but also ethical signals (such as polylingual collective actors). Put another way, they must operationalize ethical re-flections as part of an economic allocation problem.[33] Only this allows companies to maintain or gain a position of being a collaborative partner in societal discourse about ethical challenges that have economic conse-quences and about economic challenges that can have ethical implications. The debate needs to be shifted away from the predominant argument that property rights and patents are the main cause for endangering the right to health.

Implications for the Role of Companies in Society

The focus of pharmaceutical companies should be on solutions that rely on property rights but, at the same time, that respect the right to health by providing access to underserved patients at a scale that contributes to the goals of UHC. Such an approach takes into consideration the strong ethical arguments in favor of property rights but also considers the argu-ment that economic benefits should not be maximized at the expense of the basic right to health. This means that sometimes tough choices have to be made.

Ultimately, companies are a collaborative project of multiple stake-holders that have decided to cooperate in order to optimize their individual resources in a competitive market. This implies that economic cooperation is also societal cooperation: only this enables companies to mobilize and integrate the needed resources required for a success. This proposition ar-gues against the classical economic theory that conceptualizes social order as an exogenous element that sets boundaries for economic transactions. The social responsibility of companies—such as respecting the right to health—is not nonexistent, but it has been excluded by theory. The soci-etal character of a company needs to be conceptualized as endogenous, for economic reasons (Wieland, 2009, p. 282).

This does not, however, mean that the governance of a company has to be relocated to an external control mechanism such as governmental policy or societal discourse. Rather, companies should use stakeholder dialogues, deliberative discourse, and engagement as mechanisms to manage their re-sources in order to complete economic transactions that result in higher factor returns and cooperative rents. However, such social engagement will only generate these benefits if it is genuine. Companies have to truly want to contribute to solving societal and economic problems.

Nor is this just politics. A company can gain legitimacy by really engaging in a social, political, and economic discourse. It remains an economic actor in a political market (Wieland, 2009). A company is providing nothing other in a political discourse than it provides in its economic environment: distinct resources that have to be identified, prioritized, and incentivized in order to generate a cooperative rent. The distinct governance form of the firm simply enables the members of what is, in the end, a cooperative project to accomplish their needs and interests for mutual gain.

Thus, companies need to engage with resource owners in societal discourse on challenges that are surrounding the right to health and should share their resources for the mutual benefit of stakeholders involved.[34] For example, governments or policy makers are such stakeholders since they are providing a policy framework that allows companies to generate benefits from their property rights (which then, policy makers hope, turn into innovations that can create mutual benefits). In reality, this requires that both parties are willing to accept the "fuzzy logic"[35] of ethical values or norms such as the right to health and to find ways to apply it in difficult situations that are often defined by disagreements, dilemmas, and tough choices.

In a situation in which two ethical norms such as the right to health and the right to property are in conflict, the goal is to determine, through dialogue and debate, the best solution that doesn't undermine the central core of the principles at issue (that avoids, for example, suspending property rights). An example would be an innovative mechanism that situationally relinquished a company's patent claim (a nonexclusive voluntary licensing agreement, for example) without giving up the fundamental right to that property. The main goal here is to avoid access constraints that can develop through a stringent application of a monopoly arising from a patent without giving up the right to property or patent itself. However, this does not absolve governments from their responsibility for their citizens' health (by, for example, providing sufficient healthcare). The breach of other rights such as the right to property is a last resort.

Important in this context is to understand that thinking beyond traditional business indicators such as sales, profits, or margin requires pharmaceutical companies to consider two essential parameters. First, they need a values-based governance through which economic transactions can be ethically managed and successfully completed. This argument primarily refers to the policies and procedures by which a company meets its societal role (which is the provision of goods and services, not, notably, the maximization of shareholder value) by adhering to ethical standards (Drucker, 1973; Heracleous & Lan, 2010). Second, they have to be increasingly more visible and more involved in solving societal challenges that are outside—though connected to—the scope of traditional business models, which often emphasize short-term success and typically define a company's sphere of influence and responsibility narrowly.

Society demands, as a prerequisite for the allocation of legitimacy, that companies assume a greater degree of social responsibility in areas where market failure, lack of political governance, or weak infrastructure exists. These are places where crippling societal needs outweigh the purchasing power needed to make traditional business models work. These are, in fact, precisely those sorts of places where businesses have often avoided involvement and ignored any sense of obligation since they did not and could not see any relevant commercial opportunities. C. K. Prahalad (2004) has pointed out very lucidly that people in low-income segments of the global income pyramid have a certain level of purchasing power that indicates opportunities for companies, if they can learn how to develop catalytic business models that meet the needs of the poor and provide them with social opportunities (Prahalad & Hammond, 2002). The attempt to build business models for the underserved and poor recognizes and appreciates that any economic cooperation requires social cooperation, cooperation that companies can signal by their willingness to address societal problems. In effect, companies can recognize a responsibility (since no other entity can mobilize the needed resources) and receive a reward: legitimacy in the eyes of a society.

Classical economic theory defines institutional settings in the business environment as an exogenous behavioral restriction, and thus rejects the idea of the company as having a role as a responsible collective actor in society. We argue instead that the socially cooperative nature of the firm implies a linkage to the normative social legitimacy of corporate objectives and business activities, and thus embraces the desirability and necessity of corporate contributions to social welfare beyond the legal requirements. The social character of an enterprise and its nature are endogenous for economic reasons because, otherwise, transactions and cooperation cannot be managed successfully (Wieland, 2009).

From the perspective of social theory, this definition of the firm conceptualizes a company as a corporate citizen that bears rights and duties as a morally proactive citizen. The company as corporate citizen is not a legal status but, according to Wieland (2003b), is instead a "concept of citizenship as-a-desirable-activity" (p. 17), referring to Wood and Logsdon (2002, p. 68). In this sense, CR refers back to the values-driven allocation of corporate resources to pursue solutions to social problems (Wieland, 2003a, p. 18). In other words, the benefits of corporate activities must not only be directly allocated to the transaction partners within a legally binding contract, or consist of financial philanthropic contributions as a mode for wealth redistribution or to prevent negative external effects.

On the one hand, this implies that the successful realization and stabilization of economic transactions and cooperative relationships constitutively requires ethical behavior. On the other hand, the attempt to decouple economic action from its ethical consequences is doomed to failure, since companies represent a specific form of societal cooperation that has a normative nexus to the legitimacy of its goals and behavior (Wieland, 2009).

In practical terms this means that companies are held responsible for negative effects on society (and the avoidance of them) caused by their activities, even if legal. It also implies that companies should work together with other stakeholders in order to solve societal problems (such as, for example, the lack of healthcare for people living in the middle and at the base of the global income pyramid). Pharmaceutical companies are then tasked to reframe societal challenges such as UHC also as economic opportunities, and to transfer those into a socioeconomic model of cooperation—a model that is able simultaneously to generate economic benefit for a company and substantially and sustainably solve the targeted societal problem. In principle, it is in the enlightened self-interest of companies to accept this increased level of responsibility, but—and this needs to be pointed out very clearly—only if they define their specific spheres of responsibilities as precisely as possible. This is a process that needs to consider the individual core competencies and resources of each organization.

Managing Access to Medicines Strategically with a Portfolio Approach

Historically, many CR initiatives have concentrated too much on philanthropic initiatives that cannot be scaled or copied at the local level. In the pharmaceutical sector, many companies have invested considerable amounts of resources in such philanthropic and mostly donations-based access programs.[36] These initiatives reached many patients who had no chance to get the needed treatment without these efforts. Although this is genuinely a positive outcome—that is, deprived patients getting access to needed treatment for free—these attempts were often neither strategic nor really sustainable or even scalable, because they were not built on the basis of a sustainable and inclusive business model. Such an approach can't work for an effort such as UHC that, by definition, needs scalability and replicability. Instead, genuine entrepreneurial activity, in the form of new, sustainable business models that transform societal challenges into innovative and sustainable services, needs to be emphasized. Fortunately, corporations seem to be trending toward this sort of alignment of social and commercial ambition.

An effective strategic approach to access to medicines, one that is responsive to the needs of UHC, should therefore aim to operate with a portfolio of tailored activities,[37] including philanthropic initiatives, zero-profit, inclusive business models, and Shared Value[38] or lower-margin business models. These should all be closely linked to a company's strategy and core competencies and be operated with a strong ethical governance that encompasses values such as integrity, fairness, and respect for human rights, so that the company conducts business transactions in line with ethical standards and avoids or minimizes negative external effects (Fürst & Schotter, 2013). Society demands that legitimate companies take responsibility in areas where market failure, lack of political governance, or weak infrastructure exist, and where social needs outstrip the purchasing power required to make traditional business models work.

Figure 6.1 explores this rationale and typology by showing that specific CR and access intervention types should be differentiated along the different income segments of the global income pyramid.[39] This segmentation is, in principle, country-agnostic but is specific in terms of income and types of health expenditures; in other words, the strategy should consider whether expenditures for healthcare services and medicines are covered by insurance, are reimbursed, or need to be financed out-of-pocket, since this will obviously have an impact on the instruments chosen to provide access to medicines. There are many more instruments that companies can use and deploy besides those pictured; the point is that companies strategically need to use a suite of different instruments as part of an access strategy that contributes to the goal of UHC.

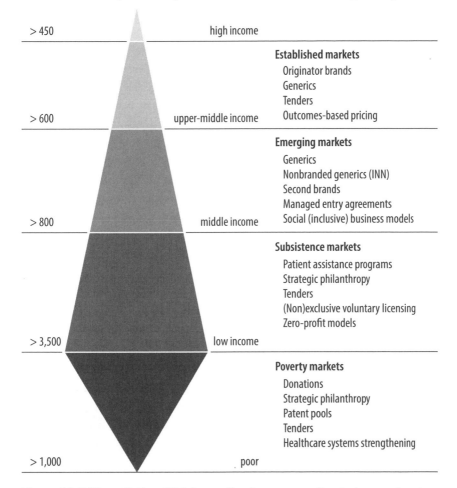

POPULATION SIZE
in millions per income segment

MARKET ARCHETYPES
Intervention type (examples)

> 450   high income

Established markets
Originator brands
Generics
Tenders

> 600   upper-middle income   Outcomes-based pricing

Emerging markets
Generics
Nonbranded generics (INN)
Second brands
Managed entry agreements

> 800   middle income   Social (inclusive) business models

Subsistence markets
Patient assistance programs
Strategic philanthropy
Tenders
(Non)exclusive voluntary licensing
Zero-profit models

> 3,500   low income

Poverty markets
Donations
Strategic philanthropy
Patent pools
Tenders
Healthcare systems strengthening

> 1,000   poor

Figure 6.1. Differentiating CR intervention types according to income levels, needs, and market types. This is a conceptual illustration for a strategic portfolio approach that would need further specifying to fit the strategic needs and capabilities of a particular company. Source: Data on income distribution from Kochhar (2015) with reference to the World Bank's PovcalNet and the Luxembourg Income Study database.

Established Markets

Typically, the business models of global pharmaceutical companies—similar to the business models of most other global commercial businesses—are tailored to serve the needs of consumers at the top or the upper-middle segment of the global income distribution. Companies can work here with the full spectrum of products and services they have in their portfolio, typically with a focus on highly innovative offerings. Originator brands and (branded) generics are portfolio assets that would be typically deployed for this customer base and covered either through public or private health insurance or through sufficient private income or wealth in the case of out-of-pocket payment. Intellectual property rights are typically guaranteed and can be enforced, and the pricing of medicines follows not necessarily a cost-based approach but is calculated according to the socioeconomic value that the product provides from a clinical, patient, and healthcare systems perspective. Access to medicines is not a typical challenge in this income stratum since patients are mostly covered by insurance or can even afford to pay out of pocket.[40] We will therefore not further elaborate on this but will mention that pharmaceutical companies are operating in high and higher income segments with innovative instruments such as outcome guarantees, price-volume agreements, or other elements that fall under the category of managed entry agreements. Other innovative pricing models should be developed and deployed in order to respond to pricing pressures and fiscal constraints in healthcare budgets in these market segments. For highly expensive treatments where the price is calculated based on benefits for the patient, the healthcare system, and the socioeconomic environment over a certain time period, a pricing model might also consider payment terms that are reflecting this same time period in order to avoid a budget impact just at the time when the product is prescribed, dispensed, and used.

Emerging Markets

The next level of the global income pyramid comprises two different income segments that represent emerging markets, with a medium to low-medium level of income and unmet needs at the upper end and subsistence markets with a high level of unmet needs at the lower end.

The segment of emerging markets with many middle- to low-middle-income customers is a somewhat different story. Here, companies can approach existing needs with market-based solutions at lower prices, therefore offering treatment for more patients with lower purchasing power. We could refer to these interventions as social (inclusive) business models that allow a business-oriented scale-up approach, since they generate an appropriate level of profitability or business value and simultaneously add social value by tapping into new patient segments.

Companies need to differentiate very carefully the specific income segments within this income bracket and understand different factors influencing buying decisions. These factors include the willingness to pay, the ability to pay, prices (the prices for basic goods and services are sometimes higher in these market segments than in established markets, likewise in even lower income segments), the rural versus urban distribution of population, cultural determinants, educational and awareness levels, infrastructure gaps, supply chain constraints, and more. A thorough understanding and careful assessment of such factors will allow the company to develop a holistic and successful intervention. Typically, social business models are built as volume models: they operate according to the principle of economies of scale, in order to keep the margin levels of the unit low and therefore the product affordable. This can be problematic during the starting phase of such a model, as it needs a certain level of up-front investment in order to quickly achieve scale and pass break-even.

The portfolio of access instruments in emerging markets can further offer "new-market disruptions,"[41] such as second-brand models that respond to affordability challenges by understanding the willingness and ability to pay of certain income groups, or the development of a specific product brand, different from the originator brand and distributed and sold through specific channels that are separated and protected from the channels used by the originator brand. This second-brand model can be used for products protected as intellectual property and for generic medicines, for example. With such brand differentiation strategies, it is important to note that the products need to have equivalent quality, since patients in lower-income segments cannot waste scarce resources on low-quality products.

In addition, inclusive business models support the buildup of local, sustainable health systems, next to the distribution of medicines at price points that are affordable to the local patient base and are chosen based on the local disease burden. Such inclusive business models can be effective in geographic areas beyond the usual reach of pharmaceutical companies, where fragile health systems can be most ameliorated through improved health literacy and education, healthcare provision through mobile services, and the improved availability of affordable treatments—not to mention activities that address broader determinants of health. It is important to develop and manage such sustainable business models, even though they will likely have lower profit margin goals, since only this kind of business-model thinking will allow replication and scale-up. Programs from pharmaceutical companies such as Novartis Social Business and Novartis Access[42] that are trying to respond to distinct health needs with innovative models have actually achieved financial sustainability or are geared toward achieving it.[43] Crucially, they were developed and deployed as horizontal programs instead of vertical access programs; they cover not just one disease vertically but a group of diseases or therapeutic areas that are prevalent in the targeted communities.

Patient assistance programs can be interesting portfolio assets in emerging markets, especially with specialty services and chronic condition treatment. These programs share the cost of medicines with private or public institutional payers, or directly with individual patients who lack the purchasing power to fully afford these medicines out of pocket. This requires that such a model be able to assess the income or wealth of individual patients to then decide how much of the costs can be borne by the patient and how much should be covered by the pharmaceutical company (co-pay). As opposed to classical donation-based programs, companies can expand access on a more sustainable basis by generating at least a limited income stream, whereas donation-based programs by definition do not generate any income. In these shared contribution models, public payers and the pharmaceutical companies share the costs of the treatment, although they typically require a well-functioning network of physicians and healthcare centers to allow patients to access the system and receive treatments. This is a challenge, but one that can be met through multi-company partnerships.

In a competitive market for generic medicines, companies can participate in national or international tenders, which allow governments to reduce and contain costs for a specified tender item. This can be effective if the underlying pricing model is able to respond to market conditions in the public sector, which often might require allowing different margin models for different channels and sectors. It also requires an appropriate desire, incentive structure, and dedicated resources that allow companies to offer competitive tender prices at potentially lower margin levels than the ones that can be achieved and obtained in private market segments. For patented products, exclusive or nonexclusive volunteer licensing is yet another access instrument, in which licensees produce or import the licensed drug in an area with a different brand for a lower price than the originator product. The incentive for the licensor is the royalty for every unit sold. Although such licensed products are typically priced too high for the lowest-income segments and instead target the middle- to lower-middle-income segment, they are a practical demonstration of how the right to property can be upheld and protected, but with enough flexibility to honor the right to health and make drugs available for many more patients in lower-income segments.

Subsistence and Poverty Markets

Further down the pyramid in the subsistence market, where significant unmet needs exist and where many people are working in an informal economy, access interventions can consider inclusive business models operating with low prices or zero-profit models that offer a more limited but still existent potential for scale, and can still definitively improve the frame conditions for (social) business in the long run.[44] Such zero-profit models can either be operated in public channels through appropriate reimbursement agreements with governments or international donor organizations, or they can be managed in private, out-of-pocket markets. Companies can also provide treatments at cost in subsistence markets through participation in tenders from governments or NGOs.

At the poverty level, access should instead focus predominantly on philanthropic interventions that have a strong strategic rationale for the company and therefore unfold an appropriate level of impact. These interventions are still linked to the core competencies and assets of a pharmaceutical company, are patient-centric, and aim to improve the frame conditions in the healthcare system. At a programmatic level, donation-based assistance programs with individual patients, or collaborative donation agreements with governments or NGOs, fall into this category, as do interventions at the systems level with catalytic effects, such as capability and capacity building. Providing molecules to a patent pool is a reasonable option if a company does not have or want to build a commercial presence in a country in which the disease is specifically prevalent and if no capabilities exist to develop and manage an access model that is able to bring the medication to patients. Local companies or international organizations might be much better suited to license the molecule for local distribution.

Since healthcare systems in lower-income settings are typically weak or barely existing, companies can engage in activities of healthcare systems strengthening in areas in which they have capabilities and expertise. But companies should not claim accountability or create long-lasting dependencies while doing this; instead they should conduct systems strengthening with the intention to seed-fund activities and catalyze positive developments. They should always have an exit option, which is, ironically, a signal of a sustainable solution.

By focusing on trying to solve challenges where a company has competencies and resources, a well-designed access strategy can legitimately generate shared benefit with a society struggling with insufficient healthcare systems and poor outcomes. Thinking in terms of legitimacy ensures that the company only considers socially acceptable and desirable activities carried out in accordance with ethical principles. And when a pharmaceutical company connects both CR and access to their strategic value drivers and core competencies, they narrow the range of activities to the ones that will generate sustainable, replicable, scalable solutions. If they fail to integrate CR and their proposed access program with their strategic vision, the program, however interesting and morally motivated in theory, might very well die aborning—canceled because of priority changes or economic crisis. Corporate stakeholders see costs being generated, not value being added, in such misaligned programs.

Pharmaceutical companies need a portfolio of different intervention types to drive access to medicines across income bands, to contribute to the goal of health for all, and finally to be a solution partner for government in their journey to introduce UHC. This portfolio should encompass more established access instruments such as patient access programs or donations, but, more important, focus on innovative inclusive business models that have the potential for scale, replication, and sustainability. Crucially, removing or lowering protection for intellectual property would put up higher barriers against such programs. Pharmaceutical companies, thrust into struggles with further margin erosion by losing their intellectual property protection, would place less emphasis on plans to invest in lower-margin business models that are geared toward reaching lower income strata.[45]

The access strategy outlined here requires robust monitoring and evaluation of its social achievements.[46] These programs focus on vulnerable patient groups, with the principle of "do no harm," and it is important to ensure that access programs result in positive outcomes and impacts for those patients. And from a company perspective, these access programs are often considerable investments; it is simply good management practice to ensure that the money is well spent. Therefore, monitoring and evaluative data complement the standard economic and business metrics that allow companies to correct their course when results don't match expectations. Meaningful metrics should then also be the backbone for setting appropriate objectives regarding access to medicines and for the alignment of these objectives with a meaningful and targeted approach to internal incentives. If there is a discrepancy between the proclaimed goal of reaching patients in lower-income settings and the existing reality in terms of incentivizing other activities, the likelihood of achieving this goal is rather limited because of misaligned incentives.

All these different instruments are relevant and much-needed pieces in the global puzzle of UHC; they help to minimize negative impacts while creating opportunities out of societal challenges (such as access to medicine), with the final goal of protecting and fulfilling the right to health.

What we need is an ethical approach to access that goes beyond a moral plea, that is more than a "means against moral itchiness"[47] because it deals with the real structural problems of modern societies that can't be successfully addressed with the traditional concept of an ethical primacy. What we also need in the private sector are virtuous leaders who are willing to put their hands on the wheel of history, as Max Weber had it, and dedicate the organizations they manage toward the real purpose of business: not maximizing profits but fulfilling a social purpose. Fortunately, they can fulfill such a purpose (like developing medicines and making them available to the underserved) while still succeeding financially. In the final analysis, truly entrepreneurial companies that are willing to accept a wider societal responsibility recognize that taking smart risks can allow them to develop an access strategy that not only contributes to the common good but also allows them to get a jump on future, as yet untapped, growth markets.

NOTES

1. Luhmann, "Business Ethics—As Ethics?" (author's translation). Luhmann continued in this ironic vein, saying that he was already looking for the car key in his pocket at the beginning of the debate, since he could not really expect a relevant answer from the lecture's attendees.
2. See also Sandel (2013).
3. For a reconstruction of the emergence of economic thinking, we highly recommend the oeuvre of Josef Wieland, specifically Wieland (2012).
4. For a further analysis, see Fürst (2017).
5. This is especially true since the UN Guiding Principles on Business and Human Rights were endorsed by the Human Rights Council in 2011 (UN, 2011).
6. According to a Health Action International/WHO study, in extreme cases, retail markups can account for up to 90% of the final price (Ball, 2011).
7. We will not elaborate on the key elements and requirements of UHC but rather refer readers to articles and reports—including the chapters in this volume—that can do this in a much more detailed and appropriate fashion than we can, given that our chapter has a different focus. For exemplary literature on UHC, please see Sachs (2012) or O'Connell, Rasanathan, and Chopra (2014).
8. See, for instance, an instructive article from Bloom and Fink (2014).
9. More specifically, UHC can be described as "access to key promotive, preventive, curative and rehabilitative health interventions for all at an affordable cost, thereby achieving equity in access." From a World Health Assembly 2005 resolution, quoted in O'Connell et al. (2014).
10. The report from the UN High-Level Panel on Access to Medicines provides an overview of many arguments used in this debate, albeit the report focuses mostly on intellectual property (UN High-Level Panel on Access to Medicines, 2016). The Access Campaign from Médecins Sans Frontières (MSF, 2017) is another platform that conveys these arguments.
11. We do not address factors such as malnutrition, lack of clean water and proper sanitation, exposure to toxics, and others in this paper.
12. We explain in this chapter what this could mean for a pharmaceutical company to have an access to medicines strategy.
13. For details, see the instructive report *Understanding the Socio-economic Divide in Europe* from the OECD (OECD Centre for Opportunity and Equality, 2017).
14. For the social determinants of health see Carr (2004).
15. As an example for this view, see the recent report from the UN High-Level Panel on Access to Medicines (2016).
16. As briefly mentioned before, property rights are a human right and therefore deserve to be protected, respected, and fulfilled. In philosophical literature, one of the best known lines of reasoning in defense of property rights links back to the work of John Locke in his second of *Two Treatises of Government*, in which he argues that every free being owns his body and therefore should own the products resulting from the activity of his body (Locke, 1690). Locke derives physical property rights from one's labor mixed with so-far-unclaimed property, resulting in a higher value. Locke makes a proviso that appropriation is defendable but just as long as

there is enough of the commons left for others and as long as the new owner will not take out more of the commons than he can use to his own advantage. Although there is a considerable difference between physical property rights and intellectual property rights in terms of their form, Locke's concept can still be applied since intellectual property is, in principle, nonexclusive. For a discussion on rights such as property rights from a business ethics perspective, see Donaldson (1982).

17. To exemplify the libertarian view of Nozick, it might be interesting to point to the fact that, for him, taxes are an infringement of each individual's right to enjoy the results of his or her own labor. In this sense, a tax can be understood similar to forced labor. For this rationale, see Nozick (1974).

18. See Nordhaus (1969) and Hu and Jaffe (2007).

19. An obvious example is Milton Friedman.

20. See Donaldson (1982).

21. The protection of intellectual property by law typically takes place through patents, copyrights, or trademarks. For an overview in the context of regulatory developments in the United States, see Besen and Raskind (1991).

22. For an economic position on this, see, for example, Demsetz (1967).

23. For this figure of a corporation as a moral actor, see Wieland (2003b) or French (1979).

24. One can see the Doha Declaration on Trips and Public Health as a practical expression of this thought.

25. See Jamison et al. (2013).

26. For this argument, see Gewertz (2012).

27. In regard to the improvement of health through pharmaceuticals, see, for example, Kremer (2002).

28. See also Acemoglu and Robinson (2012). Lichtenberg (2005, p. 17) also references Schmookler (1966) and his empirical work that illustrates that the "expected profitability of inventive activities determines the pace and direction of industrial innovation."

29. This social-obligation norm of property can be found, for instance, in German constitutional law and has many historical references: in article 17 of the Déclaration des Droits de l'Homme et du Citoyen from 1789 or in German philosophy of law.

30. For the following, see Wieland (2001).

31. For this argument see the work from Josef Wieland (2008) on the ethics of governance.

32. As Richard Rorty (2006) has written, "It is the ability to come up with new ideas, rather than the ability to get in touch with unchanging essences, that is the engine of moral progress" (p. 372).

33. See previously made references (French, 1979; Wieland, 2003b) on the figure of the collective actor and its moral responsibility.

34. For the following, see Wieland (2008).

35. We borrow this term from Josef Wieland (2014b), who also provides a broader background on the relevant literature.

36. For an interesting article counting the number of initiatives, see Rockers et al. (2017) or Boston University School of Public Health (2018).

37. For some of the basic arguments, see Fürst (2014).

38. We will not elaborate on the concept of shared value in detail but rather refer readers to the original paper published in 2011 in the *Harvard Business Review* (Porter & Kramer, 2012). A critical but positive discussion of the shared value model can also be found in Fürst (2016).

39. A similar model is used by Novartis for its access to medicines strategy. See Novartis CR report, July 15, 2018, p. 18, https://www.novartis.com/sites/www.novartis.com/files/novartis-cr-performance-report-2017.pdf. For the conceptual thinking behind this model, see Fürst (2014).

40. Pricing of medicines has, however, become an increasingly heated topic even there, because of stretched healthcare budgets, new and expensive treatments, the growing expectation of patients to receive the latest technology, and the change in demographics toward an aging population. For example, a hepatitis C treatment from Gilead was launched in the United States at a list price of more than US$ 80,000.00.

41. For the distinction, see Christensen (2006, 2011).

42. See the chapter from H. Nusser in this volume.

43. A program that responds to healthcare needs in rural communities as part of UHC—as pointed out in Reddy's chapter in this volume—is the Novartis program Healthy Families that originally started in India 2007 and is now operational in Kenya and Vietnam; see Fürst (2014) and Porter and Kramer (2014).

44. For an instructive article on segmenting different income levels in the lower range of the global income pyramid, we recommend Rangan (2011).

45. From a pure financial perspective, such dual business models with different margin potentials and goals are already difficult to maintain simultaneously. The reason is that a volume business with lower margin is a challenge for the higher-margin business because of margin dilution at an aggregate level when the volume created does not result in a considerable lower cost base for the manufactured products. Without an appropriate alignment of objectives—for example, different hurdle rates for different access models that are allowing and even incentivizing an effective and results-oriented management of such different models—it will not be possible to remove the barriers that are otherwise impeding growth, scale, and replication.

46. For monitoring and evaluation in the pharmaceutical sector, See Rockers et al. (2017), and as a concrete example, see Boston University School of Public Health (2018).

47. This we borrow from Niklas Luhmann.

REFERENCES

Acemoglu, D., & Robinson, J. (2012). *Why nations fail. The origins of power, prosperity and poverty.* London: Crown Publishers.

Ball, D. (2011). *WHO/HAI project on medicine prices and availability.* Review series on pharmaceutical pricing policies and interventions (working paper). Retrieved from http://www.haiweb.org/medicineprices/24072012/CompetitionFinalMay2011.pdf.

Besen, S. M., & Raskind, L. J. (1991). An introduction to the law and economics of intellectual property. *Journal of Economic Perspectives, 5*(1), 3–27.

Bloom, D. E., & Fink, G. (2014). The economic case for devoting public resources to health. In J. Farrar et al. (Eds.), *Manson's tropical diseases* (23rd ed.) (pp. 23–30). New York, NY: Elsevier.

Boston University School of Public Health. (n.d.). *Evaluation of Novartis Access: An (NCD) medicine access initiative.* Retrieved February 11, 2018, from http://sites.bu.edu/evalua tingaccess-novartisaccess/.

Carr, D. (2004). Improving the health of the world's poorest people. *Health Bulletin: A Publication of the Population Reference Bureau, 1*(1), 1–39.

Christensen, C. M. (2011). *The innovators dilemma.* New York, NY: HarperCollins.

Christensen, C. M., Baumann, H., Ruggles, R., & Sadtler, T. M. (2006). Disruptive innovation for social change. *Harvard Business Review, 84*(12), 94–101.

Dagan, H. (2011). *Property: values and institutions.* Oxford, UK: Oxford University Press.

Demsetz, H. (1967). Toward a theory of property rights. *American Economic Review, 57*(2), 347–359.

Donaldson, T. (1982). *Corporations and morality.* Englewood Cliffs, NJ: Prentice-Hall.

Drucker, P. (1973). *Management: Tasks, responsibilities and practices.* New York: Harper Paperbacks.

Drucker, P. (2001a). Social impacts and social problems. In *The essential Drucker* (pp. 51–68). New York, NY: Springer.

Drucker, P. (2001b). The purpose and objectives of a business. In *The essential Drucker* (pp. 18–38). New York: Springer.

French, P. (1979). The corporation as a moral person. *American Philosophical Quarterly, 16*(3), 207–215.

Fürst, M., & Schotter, A. (2013). Strategic integrity management as a dynamic capability. In *Strategic Management in the 21st Century* (pp. 1–35). Santa Barbara, CA: Praeger.

Fürst, M. (2014). Opening the door to opportunities: How to design CR strategies that optimize impact for business and society. In C. Weidinger et al. (Eds.), *Sustainable entrepreneurship* (pp. 265–268). Cham, Switzerland: Springer.

Fürst, M. (2017). Just when you thought it couldn't get worse, you hear: "The business of business is business"—some reflections on a self-fulfilling prophecy and alternative perspectives on the purpose of companies. In J. Wieland (Ed.), *Creating shared value— Concepts, experience, criticism* (pp. 55–77). Cham: Springer International Publishing.

Gewertz, N. M. (2012). Intellectual property and the pharmaceutical industry. *Journal of Business Ethics, 55*, 295–308.

Heracleous, L., & Lan, L. L. (2010). The myth of shareholder capitalism. *Harvard Business Review, 88*(4), 24.

Hu, A. G. Z., & Jaffe, A. B. (2007). *IPR, innovation, economic growth and development.* Unpublished manuscript.

Jamison, D. T., et al. (2013). Global health 2035: A world converging within a generation. *The Lancet, 382*, 1898–1955.

Kochhar, R. (2015). *A global middle class is more promise than reality: From 2001 to 2011, nearly 700 million step out of poverty, but most only barely.* Pew Research Center. Retrieved from http://www.pewglobal.org/files/2015/07/Global-Middle-Class-Report_FINAL_7-8-15 .pdf.

Kremer, M. (2002). Pharmaceuticals and the developing world. *Journal of Economic Perspectives, 16*(4), 67–90.

Leisinger, K. M. (2004). *The right to health: what corporate duties?* Unpublished paper.

Leisinger, K. M. (2012). Poverty, disease, and medicines in low- and middle-income countries. *Business and Professional Ethics Journal, 31*(1), 135–185.

Lichtenberg, F. R. (2005). Pharmaceutical innovation and the burden of disease in developing and developed countries. *Journal of Medicine and Philosophy, 30*(6), 663–690.

Locke, J. (1690). *Two Treatises of Government.* Retrieved from http://socserv2.socsci.mcmaster.ca/econ/ugcm/3ll3/locke/government.pdf.

Luhmann, N. (1993a). *Das Recht der Gesellschaft.* Frankfurt am Main: Suhrkamp.

Luhmann, N. (1993b). Wirtschaftsethik—als Ethik? In J. Wieland (Ed.), *Wirtschaftsethik und Theorie der Gesellschaft* (pp. 134–147). Frankfurt am Main: Suhrkamp.

Mann, J. M., Gostin, L., Gruskin, S., Brennan, T., Lazzarini, Z., & Fineberg, H. V. (1993). Health and human rights. *Health and Human Rights, 1*(1), 6–23.

Médecins Sans Frontières (MSF). (2017). Access Campaign. Retrieved from https://msfaccess.org/.

Nordhaus, W. D. (1969). *Invention, growth and welfare: A theoretical treatment of technological change.* Cambridge, MA: MIT Press.

North, D. C. (1981). *Structure and change in economic history.* New York, NY: W. W. Norton.

North, D. C. (1990). *Institutions, institutional change and economic performance.* Cambridge, UK: Cambridge University Press.

North, D. C. (2005). *Understanding the process of economic change.* Princeton, NJ: Princeton.

Nozick, R. (1974). *Anarchy, state, and utopia.* New York, NY: Basic Book.

O'Connell, T., Rasanathan, K., & Chopra, M. (2014). What does universal health coverage mean? *The Lancet, 383*(9913), 277–279.

OECD Centre for Opportunity and Equality (COPE). (2017). *Understanding the socio-economic divide in Europe.* Retrieved from https://www.oecd.org/els/soc/cope-divide-europe-2017-background-report.pdf.

Porter, M., & Kramer, M. (2012). Creating shared value. *Harvard Business Review, 89*(1–2), 62–77.

Porter, M. E., & Kramer, M. R., & Lane, D. (2014). *Social business at Novartis: Arogya Parivar.* Harvard Business School Case 715-411. Retrieved from https://www.hbs.edu/faculty/Pages/item.aspx?num=48341.

Prahalad, C. K., & Hammon, A. (2002). Serving the world's poor. *Harvard Business Review, 80*(9), 48–58.

Prahalad, C. K. (2004). *Fortune at the bottom of the pyramid: Eradicating poverty through profits.* Upper Saddle River, NJ: W. S. Publishing.

Rangan, V. K. (2011). Segmenting the base of the pyramid. *Harvard Business Review, 89*(6), 113–117.

Rawls, J. (1971). *Theory of justice.* Cambridge, MA: Harvard University Press.

Rawls, J. (2001). *Justice as fairness.* Cambridge, MA: Harvard University Press.

Rockers, P. C., Wirtz, V. J., Chukwuemeka, U. A., Swamy, P. M., & Laing, R. O. (2017). Industry-led access-to-medicines initiatives in low- and middle-income countries: Strategies and evidence. *Health Affairs, 36*(4), doi:10.1377/hlthaff.2016.1213.

Rorty, R. (2006). Is philosophy relevant to applied ethics? *Business Ethics Quarterly, 16*(3), 369–389.

Sachs, J. D. (2012). Achieving universal health coverage in low-income settings. *The Lancet, 380*(9845), 944–947.

Sandel, M. J. (2013). Market reasoning as moral reasoning: Why economists should re-engage with political philosophy. *Journal of Economic Perspectives, 27*(4), 121–140.

Schmookler, J. (1966). *Invention and economic growth.* Cambridge, MA: Harvard University Press.

Shue, H. (1996). *Basic rights: Subsistence, affluence, and U.S. foreign policy.* (2nd ed.). Princeton, NJ: Princeton University Press.

UN Human Rights. (2011). *Guiding principles on business and human rights: Implementing the United Nations "Protect, respect and remedy" framework.* Retrieved from https://doi.org/U.N. Doc. E/CN.4/2006/97.

UN High-Level Panel on Access to Medicines. (2016). *Promoting innovation and access to health technologies.* Retrieved from http://www.unsgaccessmeds.org/final-report/.

Wettstein, F. (2012). CSR and the debate on business and human rights: Bridging the great divide. *Business Ethics Quarterly, 22*(4), 739–770.

WHO. (2015). Noncommunicable disease factsheet. Retrieved from http://www.who.int/news-room/fact-sheets/detail/noncommunicable-diseases.

WHO. (2016). *World Health Statistics 2016.* Retrieved from http://www.who.int/gho/publications/world_health_statistics/2016/en/.

WHO & World Bank. (2015). *Tracking universal health coverage: First global monitoring report.* Retrieved from http://www.who.int/healthinfo/universal_health_coverage/report/2015/en/.

Wieland, J. (2001). Eine Theorie der Governanceethik. *Zeitschrift für Wirtschafts- und Unternehmensethik, 2*(1), 8–49.

Wieland, J. (2003a). Corporate citizenship und strategische Unternehmenskommunikation in der Praxis. In *Corporate citizenship und strategische Unternehmenskommunikation in der Praxis.* München: Hampp.

Wieland, J. (2003b). Die Tugend kollektiver Akteure. In J. Wieland (Ed.), *Die moralische Verantwortung kollektiver Akteure* (pp. 22–40). Heidelberg: Physica.

Wieland, J. (2008). Governanceethik als anwendungsorientierte Ethik. In M. Zichy & H. Grimm (Eds.), *Praxis in der Ethik. Zur Methodenreflexion in der anwendungsorientierten Moralphilosophie* (pp. 303–324). Berlin: De Gruyter.

Wieland, J. (2009). Die Firma als Kooperationsprojekt der Gesellschaft. In *CSR als Netzwerkgovernance—Theoretische Herausforderungen und praktische Antworten.* Marburg: Metropolis.

Wieland, J. (2012). *Die Entdeckung der Ökonomie. Kategorien, Gegenstandsbereiche und Rationalitätstypen* (2nd ed.). Marburg: Metropolis.

Wieland, J. (2014). *Governance ethics: Global value creation, economic organization and creativity.* Heidelberg: Springer.

Wood, D. J., & Logsdon, J. M. (2002). Business citizenship. From individuals to organizations. *Business Ethics Quarterly 2*(3), 59–94.

7

The Private Sector Joins the Trek on India's Meandering Path to Universal Health Coverage

K. Srinath Reddy

Despite starting with the vision of public-sector-provided free health-care to all its citizens at the time of her independence 70 years ago, India has evolved a mixed health system that has many barriers to access to essential health services and high levels of personal expenditure on healthcare. Attempts to improve access and affordability began with the launch of the National Rural Health Mission (NRHM) and national health insurance program Rashtriya Swasthya Bima Yojana (RSBY) during 2005–7, paralleled by some state governments also launching pro-poor social insurance programs. However, these schemes have not provided the expected levels of access, comprehensive care, or financial protection. Low levels of public financing and weak regulatory systems have detracted from efforts to advance the agenda of universal health coverage (UHC). A freshly articulated National Health Policy (NHP 2017) aims to double public spending by 2025, with strategic purchasing of health services from both public and private sectors, accompanied by much needed regulatory reform.

While the private sector has emerged as the dominant provider of healthcare, it is neither well distributed nor well regulated enough to assure universal access or uniform quality. Several successful models of private sector contribution have emerged in recent decades but have still not reached the scale needed for supporting UHC across India. Public-private partnerships are part of the planned path to UHC, as charted in NHP 2017, but their role needs to be clearly defined. A major new initiative, Ayushman Bharat, announced in the union budget of 2018, opens up further opportunities for private support to UHC but awaits evolution of system architecture.

India's Health Lags behind Its Economy

Despite the sharp and well-sustained growth of India's economy over the past 25 years, performance in the health sector has lagged. This is evident from several key indicators of health system performance. Life expectancy at birth has risen from 32 years at the time of India's independence to 68.5 years in 2016; however, the nation is still second from the bottom in South Asia. Nepal has a life expectancy of 70 years and Sri Lanka is far ahead, with a life expectancy of 75 years.[1] The differences in life expectancy among states within India is stark. Assam and Uttar Pradesh are 11 years behind Kerala in life expectancy. Under-five mortality in India has dropped by 65% in the last 25 years. However, in 2016, it was still six times higher than the child mortality rate in Sri Lanka. Similarly, the maternal mortality ratio in India is four to six times higher than in China and Sri Lanka.[2] Child immunization rates are around 64% in India, while many sub-Saharan countries have rates over 90% and Sri Lanka has close to 100% coverage.[3]

India can be proud of the successes achieved in polio eradication and reduction in the incidence of HIV/AIDS. Deaths due to tuberculosis (TB) have decreased, but drug-resistant TB is, alarmingly, on the rise. Vector-borne diseases like malaria, dengue, Chikungunya, and Japanese encephalitis continue to pose serious challenges to public health. Even as India is achieving some success in the control of infectious diseases and is striving to bring down infant and maternal mortality, cardiovascular diseases, diabetes, cancers, and chronic respiratory diseases are now the dominant causes of death. These diseases account for 63% of all deaths. Over the past 25 years, all states of India have experienced a sharp rise in these disorders, which claim many lives below the age of 70 years. Indeed, over a third of the cardiovascular deaths occur below the age of 65. Even conservative estimates indicate that 63 million Indians presently have diabetes.[4] These avoidable early deaths, often occurring in the productive prime of midlife, impose huge economic burdens on families and pose a threat to the nation's development.[5] A study by the Harvard School of Public Health and the World Economic Forum estimated that noncommunicable diseases would cost India 4.3 trillion dollars between 2011 and 2030.[6] Mental health disorders are also disabling many Indians and burdening their families. If we also add the lost lives and severe disabilities caused by road traffic injuries, the level of preventable disease is disastrously large. Taking all diseases into account, per capita disease burden (expressed as disability-adjusted life years) dropped by 36% in India between 1990 and 2016. However, even in 2016, per capita disease burden was 72% higher than in China or Sri Lanka in 2016.[7]

One of the reasons for the poor performance of the health sector is the low level of public financing of health, resulting in high levels of out-of-pocket and catastrophic health expenditures and healthcare-related impoverishment. It is estimated that over 63 million Indians are pushed below the poverty line each year by healthcare-related expenditure.[8] A recent study by Brookings India shows that the many social health insurance schemes introduced by central and state governments between 2004 and 2014 have improved access to advanced healthcare but have not reduced out-of-pocket health expenditure or catastrophic health expenditure.[9] Healthcare-induced poverty levels remained at 7% of the population over this decade. With public financing for health stuck between 0.9% and 1.2% of our GDP for several decades, India figures at the bottom rung of international rankings in terms of per capita public financing of health.[10] As India sets out to achieve UHC by 2030, there is a great need to strengthen the health system performance by supplementing public sector investments and service provision with contributions from the private sector.

Indian Healthcare: A Complex System

India has a federal structure, with 29 states and 7 union territories. The constitution places the main responsibility for the delivery of health services on the state governments, while the national government assumes the responsibility for the design and provides partial funding of national health programs, regulation of health professional education, pharmaceutical policy, and international regulation and cooperation in health.

India's mixed health system has evolved, mostly by default and not by design, to feature shared healthcare provision by an unevenly distributed and highly heterogeneous composite of public and private providers. At the time of independence, healthcare was envisioned principally as a freely provided public sector service. Private sector presence was mostly confined to individual general practitioners providing outpatient care, small family-owned nursing homes, and a few charitable or missionary hospitals. The public sector offered a three-tier structure of care stretching from primary health centers to large medical college–linked hospitals. Underfinancing of the public sector health services led to progressive decline in their availability and quality, even as population growth and changing demographic profiles expanded healthcare needs. The private sector expanded to fill the space unoccupied by the public sector and is now competing with it across all levels of care. The rapid growth of large metropolitan corporate hospitals and their later branching to smaller cities has been a feature of the past three decades, spurred by domestic economic liberalization and foreign investments brought in by globalization.

Presently, the private sector is the primary source of care for 44% of rural and 52% of urban households. For hospitalized care, the private sector is the port of call for 58% of rural and 68% of urban patients.[11] The private sector represents both charitable (not-for-profit) and commercial (for-profit) entities, with the latter forming the larger segment, both among small and large healthcare facilities.

The Private Sector in Healthcare: A Scattered Spectrum of Providers

The recognized health systems in India include the allopathic (modern) system, as well as four indigenous or alternate systems. The latter include Ayurveda, Unani, Siddha, and Homeopathy and are collectively known as AYUSH. Practitioners of these systems form part of the public sector health services, apart from being a component of the variegated private sector. A large number of unqualified practitioners also provide health services of myriad unscientific varieties to rural and urban poor.

The allopathic system itself has a composite profile of medical, dental, and nursing professionals, with qualifications ranging from basic degree or certification to highly specialized postgraduate and doctoral degrees. A wide variety of allied health professionals also form a vital part of the health services. There is a severe shortage of health professionals across most of these categories, as a consequence of underproduction and migration. Those available are poorly distributed across states. The problem is compounded by their urban aggregation, leaving rural areas grossly underserved. In the initial decades after independence, government service was the most attractive option for health professionals due to the dominant stature of the public sector and the career security offered by government jobs. This has changed in recent decades not only because of low salary scales and poor governance practices in areas such as postings and trans-fers, but also due to the private sector expansion, offering higher pay scales and better-equipped work environments.

In the case of doctors formally engaged in government service but per-mitted private practice alongside, the distinction between the public sec-tor and private sector employment is fuzzy. Very few states in India have banned private practice by government doctors. Central government institu-tions do not permit private practice. In the rest, the dual identity of the public plus private care provider creates complementarity as well as conflict.

A large number of active but under-resourced nongovernmental organ-izations deliver health services ranging from health education to community-based primary care. Many of them have been active in the area of maternal and child health, adolescent health, HIV/AIDS, and tuberculosis.[12,13,14,15] Jan Swasthya Sahyog (JSS) has been providing dedicated health services in the predominantly tribal district of Bilaspur in the state of Chattis-garh.[16] Similarly, the Society for Education, Action and Research in Com-munity Health (SEARCH) has developed innovative models of community-based child and maternal healthcare in the very backward area of Gadchiroli in Maharashtra.[17] It is now extending these models to other health problems, especially noncommunicable diseases. An excellent model of community-supported palliative care for cancer has been developed in Kerala and ten other states and union territories of India.[18] Arogya World has been part-nering with Indian industries to promote worksite wellness programs.[19] There are also many women who are driving India's efforts to improve the demand and delivery of health services at the frontline. Nearly a million Accredited Social Health Activists are functioning as social mobilizers at the village level as part of the National Health Mission.[20] Self-help groups of women have also been actively promoting better maternal and child health practices in the state of Uttar Pradesh.

Private Healthcare in India: Successes and Scars

The growth of the private sector has seen many successes, both for the organized private sector institutions and for public-private partner-ships. Chains of corporate hospitals now extend across India and have ex-panded to other countries. Starting with the Apollo Group that emerged in 1983, several large corporate hospitals now dot Indian cities and second-tier towns. Some of them have also diversified into medical education, medical insurance, and large-scale laboratory services. Medical tourism offered by India's private hospitals is growing in volume and is enthusiastically supported by the government.

Low cost–high quality models of healthcare by the private sector first emerged visibly in the area of eye health, where Aravind Eye Care, LV Prasad Eye Institute, and Shankar Nethralaya have set globally applauded benchmarks. They also practice pro-poor models of cross-subsidization by the more affluent patients. Their innovations in community outreach, low-cost lens production, and task shifting to well-trained allied health professionals have won acclaim and awards.

Low-cost cardiac surgery has been popularized by Narayana Hrudayalaya. In other areas, such as obstetric and general surgical services, models of focused low-cost care centers have emerged over the past decade. "Health Spring" is now offering organized primary care services across several states.[21] 'Vaatsalya' Hospitals are providing low-cost care in rural and semi-urban areas of Karnataka and Andhra Pradesh. However, these models have not reached the scale needed to meet national needs.[22]

Public-private partnerships in health came into the limelight over the past two decades with the success of emergency transport services, which were started experimentally in Andhra Pradesh and were rapidly adopted across the country. The Chiranjeevi program in Gujarat saw the government incentivizing private obstetricians to supplement government services.[23] Recently, renal dialysis centers are being operated in government facilities by the private sector, with government funding. In Karnataka, Arunachal Pradesh, and Rajasthan, some primary healthcare centers set up by the government have been handed over to private (mostly not-for-profit) providers for management. The organized private sector has also been actively partnering with major national health programs for control of blindness, tuberculosis, and HIV/AIDS.

Private sector engagement in government-funded health insurance programs began in a big way in the past two decades with the advent of health insurance programs for economically weaker sections, which were funded or mostly subsidized by state and central governments. Even earlier, these governments purchased some services from private hospitals for their employees. However, the large government programs, which were initiated to provide the poor and other vulnerable sections with access to secondary and tertiary care through financially supported hospitalization, opened the gates for private healthcare providers to participate in a big way in the public-funded programs. The government schemes engaged both public and private healthcare providers, but the latter were better positioned to provide advanced medical care. The Aarogyasri scheme of Andhra Pradesh was copied by many other states, while the centrally funded Rashtriya Swasthya Bima Yojana (RSBY, which translates as the National Health Insurance Program) has grown to be the largest health insurance program in the world, covering over 300 million beneficiaries.[9,24,25]

The recent union budget, presented to parliament on February 1, 2018, announced a major new initiative under the name Ayushman Bharat (which translates as "Long Life to India"). Ayushman Bharat combines two programs. The first proposes delivery of comprehensive primary health services through 150,000 Health and Wellness Centers, which will be frontline health posts close to the community. The government has invited private sector support through corporate social responsibility funding. The other proposal seeks to expand RSBY into an all-encompassing National Health Protection Scheme (NHPS) whereby 100 million poor and vulnerable families will receive financial coverage for secondary and tertiary hospital care (with coverage up to US$ 8,000 per family per annum, a huge increase from the RSBY cap of US$ 500).[26]

The private sector has a more direct role to play here, as a service provider from whom the government will procure services through strategic purchasing. Though disconnected, these two initiatives are beginning to lay the road for UHC.

Despite the growing role of the private sector as a leading healthcare provider, it has also attracted much criticism. Its concentration in urban areas deprives the rural population of easy access in many parts of India. With both cost and quality unregulated, there is a tendency among many private care providers to prescribe unnecessary tests and treatments, resulting in inappropriate and expensive care. The corrupt practice of kickbacks for referrals escalates costs. Participation in government-funded health insurance programs initially led to a surge in induced care, which cashed in on patient entitlements. High costs of care in corporate hospitals are seen as exploitative in the Indian context, even though they compare favorably with costs in high-income countries. Despite benefiting from heavily subsidized land allocation and tax concessions, some of these hospitals have failed to honor their commitment to provide free care to persons from economically weaker sections in a small fraction of their bed capacity. All of these have added to public skepticism of the role corporate hospitals can play in UHC. Thus, the paradox of dependence and suspicion continues, in the absence of a well-defined UHC framework and weak regulatory processes.

Other Areas of Private Sector Participation: Drugs, Diagnostics, and Education

India's pre-eminence as a generic drug manufacturer has earned it the title of "pharmacy of the world," particularly because of its potential to provide essential drugs to low- and middle-income countries. The private pharmaceutical sector replaced the public sector long ago in the manufacture of drugs and vaccines. While the prices are much lower than global market prices, multiple markups make many branded generics high priced in the Indian context. Pooled public procurement practiced by some state governments, together with centrally determined price control measures, is attempting to counter this challenge and contain drug prices. Availability of quality-assured generics at low prices can certainly be a valuable private sector contribution to UHC in India.

Availability of good diagnostic facilities varies across India. Private laboratories have grown in profusion in urban areas, but rural penetration is poor. Some of the larger laboratory chains cover several cities and towns. Private laboratories have been contracted by some state governments to provide free or subsidized service for a set of essential diagnostic tests. Since the government-funded health insurance schemes do not presently cover outpatient care, barriers of access and high cost exist presently. These will have to be addressed in a UHC framework that incorporates outpatient care and creates a network of laboratories that perform the tests covered in the essential package. The private sector has a large role to play in such a network, but it must be prepared to expand to underserved areas, enhance quality, and control costs to be of value to UHC.

The private sector has rapidly expanded its footprint in health professional education in the past 25 years. The number of private medical, dental, and nursing colleges now far exceeds the government colleges, in a dramatic reversal of the ratios that existed in 1990. However, the quality is highly variable, ranging from stellar to abysmal. The commercial motive of investing in these colleges as a profit-making business, often fed by large amounts of "capitation fees" collected on admission, has detracted from attention to quality and adherence to standards in many of the more recently established institutions. Many institutions that train allied health professionals, where certification does not attest to competency, are in a similar situation. The large gaps in India's health workforce, as well as the demographic opportunity to export health workers to other countries in need, make private sector participation in health professional education necessary for the success of UHC in India and elsewhere. However, it calls for a commitment to standards and quality that goes beyond the laissez faire attitude that currently dominates private sector engagement in this area.

India's Journey toward UHC: Late Start in Race to 2030

India voted in favor of the World Health Resolution on UHC in 2005. The same year, the central government set in motion two major national programs: the National Rural Health Mission (NRHM) and the RSBY. The NRHM focused on increasing access by the rural population to health services aimed at improving maternal and child health and controlling major infectious diseases, with emphasis on primary healthcare. It has now been transformed into the National Health Mission (NHM) with the addition of an urban component. The platform of NHM has also been expanded to include noncommunicable diseases and mental health.[20]

The RSBY started as a program of government-subsidized health insurance for the informal workforce and evolved from coverage of people below the poverty line to include many other categories who were deemed vulnerable. The limited financial coverage improved access to hospitalized secondary care but did not provide the anticipated financial protection, as measured through the three indicators of out-of-pocket expenditure, catastrophic health expenditure, and healthcare induced impoverishment. Even the state government schemes, which had higher levels of financial coverage for tertiary care, showed similar results.

In late 2010, the Planning Commission of India created a High-Level Expert Group (HLEG) to develop a framework for UHC in India. The HLEG report of 2011 recommended an increase in public financing from 1.2% of GDP to 2.5% of GDP over five years, with strong emphasis on primary health services. A merger of all state and central health insurance schemes and employer-provided insurance into a single payer system was proposed, with taxes as the major source of UHC funding. The role of private insurance, relatively small so far, was seen as supplementary. Strengthened public sector health services and contracted private healthcare providers were to be networked to provide an essential health package, which would progressively expand with accrual of more resources.[27] Several of these recommendations were reflected in the Twelfth Five Year Plan of 2012–17.[28] However, the slowing down of economic growth in India and prioritization of other welfare programs saw the level of public financing static at 1.2% of GDP, and UHC remained stuck at the starting line.

National Health Policy (2017): The Vision Resurfaces

A change of government in 2014 saw the slogan of Universal Health Assurance come forth, without a clear articulation of what it meant in terms of policy. A draft National Health Policy (NHP) developed in late 2014 remained wrapped in governmental deliberations for over two years and was finally unveiled in March 2017.[8,29,30] This policy now provides a direction toward UHC, which India embraced as part of the Sustainable Development Goals (SDGs) in 2015. Indeed, the NITI Aayog, the government's policy think tank, which replaced the Planning Commission in 2014, has tagged India's developmental milestones to the SDG targets for 2030.

NHP (2017) proposes an increase in public financing to 2.5% of GDP by 2025, with prioritization of primary healthcare. It articulates a vision for UHC that includes "collaboration with the nongovernment sector and engagement with the private sector." It also calls for gap-filling in primary care services through collaboration with not-for-profit organizations and incentivized participation of private primary care providers in underserviced communities. It also calls for strategic purchasing of secondary and tertiary care services from public, voluntary, and private healthcare institutions. In addition, it sees a role for the private sector in a variety of areas, such as the following: skill development programs for allied health professionals; disaster management; immunization; disease surveillance; mental healthcare programs; and health information systems. Finally, it proposes several regulatory measures and institutions, with particular emphasis on the Clinical Establishments Act for registration and regulation of healthcare facilities.

The NITI Aayog later adopted a three-year action plan (2017–20) that further defined the targets to be achieved by 2020 and the pathways to reach them. Notably, it called for reduction of out-of-pocket expenditure to 50% by 2020, from the present level of 63%, while addressing the need to provide "assurance of health care," as stated in the plan.

The overlapping role of the government in financing, providing, and regulating healthcare has reached its limitations of accountability and quality of service delivery. There is a large capacity within the private sector for delivery of health services. However, in the absence of the stewardship role of the government, services delivered in the private health sector are now at varying levels of quality and cost.

Having recognized the potential value of the private sector in serving the assurance function of UHC, the plan declares, "The government must therefore adopt the function of strategic purchasing. They should leverage this purchasing power to obtain the desired services from service providers, both private and public, through autonomous structures created for this purpose."[31]

It is in the mode of payment that the NHP and the Action Plan tread slippery terrain. They propose a "capitation" mode of bundled payment for purchase of primary health services and a "fee-for-service model" for strategic purchase of secondary and tertiary care services. By disconnecting the primary services from secondary and tertiary care, the provider incentive for improving primary care to save on the cost of advanced care is lost. There may be a perverse incentive for the primary care provider to refer early and more often to secondary and tertiary care to gain savings from the capitation fee paid for primary health services. A fee-for-service model at the higher levels of care will still be fraught with the danger of inappropriate and unwarranted care, replete with unnecessary visits and procedures. The high healthcare costs of a fee-for-service model are only too evident in the US health system. The evolving UHC framework has to address this challenge to strategic purchasing with an improved capitation fee model that links all levels of care.

Continuing its enthusiasm for engaging the private sector, the NITI Aayog has recently proposed that the private sector be permitted to invest in infrastructure, equipment, and human resources within existing government-owned district hospitals to provide technology-intensive clinical services for noncommunicable diseases like cardiovascular disorders and cancer. The private partner would do so on a renewable 30-year lease and share some of the common facilities with the hosting government hospital. The proposal has been hotly debated in the media, since the terms of engagement are unclear at present. Since the district hospitals fall within the jurisdiction of state governments, it remains to be seen how many of them will opt for this model.

The Ayushman Bharat initiative announced by the central government in February 2018 carries forward some of the proposals of the National Health Policy. The scope of the programs within that plan, as well as the resources allocated so far, fall short of the funding needed to make it the platform for UHC. The state governments are expected to contribute 40% of the funding required for the National Health Protection Scheme and to merge whatever state health insurance plans they have been running with this large national scheme.[26] How this cooperative federalism will evolve to create the countrywide consensus and coordination needed for UHC remains to be seen. Nevertheless, many areas of private sector collaboration with the public sector will emerge as the program unfolds.

Molding the Mixed (Up) Health System: Is the Private Sector Ready to Deliver UHC?

There is now an unprecedented openness on the part of the central government to engage with the private sector and provide it with opportunities to partner in delivering UHC. Most state governments, too, are ready to partner, but the needs assessment and framework of strategic purchasing are still works in progress. Regulatory structures need to be strengthened to secure quality and control costs. While the Clinical Establishments Act provides an important regulatory pathway, private healthcare providers have been protesting what they see as unreasonable restrictions and disproportionate penalties. As the health system proceeds from a lax regulatory state to one of tighter controls, such clashes are inevitable but will not create insurmountable barriers, since there is eagerness on both sides to cooperate. While voluntary accreditation systems exist for hospitals and laboratories, the advent of large publicly funded health programs, which propose to use strategic purchasing, should catalyze credible and transparent accreditation systems as a precondition for empanelment.

The private sector does see a major opportunity in UHC, which helps it to access public funding through the strategic purchase gateway. With private insurance likely to remain a small player and the paying capacity of large sections of the population being low, the expanding private sector has a growing appetite for tapping government funding. It can do so by partnering with the government in providing healthcare, performing diagnostic tests in empaneled laboratories, supplying drugs, and training health professionals. The private sector, however, has to look beyond urban-centered secondary and tertiary care if it wants to contribute meaningfully to UHC. The government, too, must engage with the different components of the private sector to identify how best they can be engaged in the public interest. From the individual practitioner who can be engaged for primary care to the multispeciality hospitals that dominate the tertiary care arena, the specific nature of contributions have to be carefully identified and incorporated into the UHC framework.

The private sector must also recognize that UHC involves health beyond healthcare and includes health promotion and disease prevention as important components. It must help in the implementation of health-friendly nutrition and environmental policies while extending support for multisectoral measures that aim to minimize harm from tobacco, alcohol, and substance abuse. Whether it is enhancement of childhood immunization coverage or prevention of childhood obesity, the private sector has a useful contribution to make. While supporting the goal of accessible, affordable, and appropriate healthcare for all, the private sector should also endorse and advance the public health objectives of UHC. This is of utmost importance in India, where health promotion and disease prevention have long been neglected, to the huge and highly avoidable detriment of health.

Health beyond Healthcare

UHC in India has to evolve through active engagement and optimal utilization of the public, voluntary, and private sectors in the provision of health services. Often, public-private partnerships (PPPs) have been seen as marriages of convenience with ill-defined contractual arrangements and have failed to achieve expected outcomes because of a culture clash. It is time to redefine PPP as "partnership for public purpose," based on common commitment to a mutually agreed-upon goal that is wedded to societal good and fosters trust and cooperation.[32] Clearly defined deliverables and processes for ensuring mutual accountability will spring from that common commitment. While this poses a great challenge in a hitherto disorganized health system, it is urgent that this healthcare Rubik's cube become aligned by 2030. With both the public and private sectors ready to engage, both hands may now move the pieces of the puzzle quickly, with coordinated purpose.

NOTES

1. World Bank. 2016. "South Asia." https://data.worldbank.org/region/south-asia.
2. GBD 2016 Mortality Collaborators. 2017. "Global, Regional, and National Under-5 Mortality, Adult Mortality, Age-Specific Mortality, and Life Expectancy, 1970–2016: A Systematic Analysis for the Global Burden of Disease Study 2016." *Lancet* 390 (10100): 1084–115.
3. "Global Vaccine Action Plan: Regional Vaccine Action Plans 2016 Progress Reports." Geneva. http://www.who.int/immunization/sage/meetings/2016/october/3_Regional _vaccine_action_plans_2016_progress_reports.pdf.
4. Patel, Vikram, Somnath Chatterji, Dan Chisholm, Shah Ebrahim, Gururaj Gopal-akrishna, Colin Mathers, Viswanathan Mohan, Dorairaj Prabhakaran, Ravilla D. Ra-vindran, and K. Srinath Reddy. 2011. "Chronic Diseases and Injuries in India." *Lancet* 377 (9763): 413–2.
5. Mohan, S., K. S. Reddy, and D. Prabhakaran. 2011. "Chronic Non-Communicable Diseases in India: Reversing the Tide." New Delhi. http://www.indiaenvironment-portal.org.in/files/file/PHFI_NCD_Report_Sep_2011.pdf.
6. Bloom, D. E., V. Candeias, E. T. Cafiero-Fonseca, E. Adashi, L. Bloom, L. Gurfein, E. Jané-Llopis, A. Saxena, A. Lubet, E. Mitgang, and J. Carroll O'Brien. 2014. "Econom-ics of Non-Communicable Diseases in India: The Costs and Returns on Investment of Interventions." http://www3.weforum.org/docs/WEF_EconomicNonCommunica bleDiseasesIndia_Report_2014.pdf.
7. Dandona, Lalit, Rakhi Dandona, G. Anil Kumar, D. K. Shukla, Vinod K. Paul, Kalpana Balakrishnan, Dorairaj Prabhakaran, et al. 2017. "Nations within a Nation: Variations in Epidemiological Transition across the States of India, 1990–2016 in the Global Burden of Disease Study." *Lancet* 390 (10111): 2437–60. doi: 10.1016/ S0140-6736(17)32804-0.
8. Ministry of Health & Family Welfare. 2017. "National Health Policy 2017." New Delhi. http://cdsco.nic.in/writereaddata/National-Health-Policy.pdf.
9. Ravi, S., R. Ahluwalia, and S. Bergkevist. 2016. "Health and Morbidity In India (2004–2014)." New Delhi. https://www.brookings.edu/wp-content/uploads/2016/12/201612 _health-and-morbidity.pdf.
10. World Health Organization. 2014. "Global Health Expenditure Database." Geneva. http://apps.who.int/nha/database.
11. International Institute of Population Sciences. 2017. "National Family Health Survey 4: India Fact Sheet." Ministry of Health and Family Welfare. http://rchiips.org/NFHS /pdf/NFHS4/India.pdf.
12. "Child In Need Institute." 2018. http://www.cini-india.org/.
13. "India HIV/AIDS Alliance." 2018. http://www.allianceindia.org/.
14. "Janani." http://www.janani.org/News.aspx?ID=SC0005.
15. "Operation ASHA." 2018. http://www.opasha.org/.

16. Jan Swasthya Sahyog. http://www.jssbilaspur.org/.
17. Society for Education, Action and Research in Community Health (SEARCH), http://searchforhealth.ngo/who-we-are/.
18. Pallium India, https://palliumindia.org/about/about-pallium-india/.
19. "Arogya World." 2018. http://arogyaworld.org/.
20. NHM. 2012. "Framework for Implementation National Health Mission, 2012–2017," 1–68. https://nrhm.gujarat.gov.in/Images/pdf/nhm_framework_for_implementation .pdf.
21. "Health Spring." 2018. https://www.healthspring.in/vision-and-mission.
22. "'Vaatsalya' Hospitals." 2018. https://www.vaatsalya.info/.
23. Bhat, Ramesh, Dileep V. Mavalankar, Prabal V. Singh, and Neelu Singh. 2009. "Maternal Healthcare Financing: Gujarat's Chiranjeevi Scheme and Its Beneficiaries." *Journal of Health, Population and Nutrition* 27 (2): 249–58. doi:10.3329/jhpn.v27i2.3367.
24. Selvaraj, S., and A. K. Karan. 2012. "Why Publicly-Financed Health Insurance Schemes Are Ineffective in Providing Financial Risk Protection." *Economic and Political Weekly* XLVII (11).
25. Srivatsan, R., R. Shukla, and V. Shatrugna. 2011. "Aarogyasri Healthcare Model: Advantage Private Sector." *Economic and Political Weekly* 46 (49).
26. Ministry of Finance, Government of India. 2018. "National Health Protection Scheme to Provide Hospitalisation Cover to Over 10 Crore Poor and Vulnerable Families." Press Information Bureau, February 1. http://pib.nic.in/newsite/PrintRelease .aspx?relid=17.
27. "High Level Expert Group Report on Universal Health Coverage for India." 2011. New Delhi. https://docs.google.com/viewer?url=http://planningcommission.nic.in /reports/genrep/rep_uhc0812.pdf.
28. Planning Commission of India. 2013. "Twelfth Five Year Plan (2012–2017): Social Sectors." New Delhi. http://planningcommission.gov.in/plans/planrel/12thplan/welcome .html.
29. Mathur, Manu Raj, K. Srinath Reddy, and Christopher Millett. 2015. "Will India's National Health Policy Deliver Universal Health Coverage?" *BMJ* (Clinical Research Ed.) 350: h2912. http://www.ncbi.nlm.nih.gov/pubmed/26033390.
30. Ministry of Health and Family Welfare. 2014. "National Health Policy 2015 Draft." New Delhi, India. https://www.nhp.gov.in/sites/default/files/pdf/draft_national _health_policy_2015.pdf.
31. NITI Aayog. 2017. "India: Three Year Action Agenda 2017–18 to 2019–20." New Delhi. http://niti.gov.in/writereaddata/files/coop/IndiaActionPlan.pdf.
32. Reddy, K. How to Define Public Purpose for a PPP to Move Beyond Marriage of Convenience; Here Is What Is Critically Crucial. *Financial Express*. July 13, 2017. http:// www.financialexpress.com/opinion/how-to-define-public-purpose-for-a-ppp-to -move-beyond-marriage-of-convenience-here-is-what-is-critically-crucial/761151/.

8

A Reality Check

Sierra Leone, the Private Sector, Sustainable
Development Goal 3, and Universal Health Coverage

Sowmya Kadandale and Robert Marten

The aspiration of Sustainable Development Goal 3 (SDG 3, introduced at the 2015 UN General Assembly) to improve the health and well-being of populations is staggering, and this ambitious initiative brings with it both opportunities and challenges. Nowhere are these issues more complex than in a country like Sierra Leone, which illustrates the path countries need to take as they navigate an intricate environment of government, development partners, civil society, and the private sector to attain the SDG 3 targets. Using Sierra Leone as a case study, this chapter seeks to draw out the key political, economic, structural, and systems issues linked to the attainment of SDG 3, including the potential role of the private sector in making progress toward universal health coverage and the implications for other countries as they move toward an ambitious 2030 agenda.

Drawing from the Sierra Leone case study, to ensure success in the SDG era countries need to focus on prioritizing key actions, such as

- *Ensuring political commitment, in order to integrate and align the key actions with national development efforts.* Improving health and well-being is as much a political process as it is a technical one. Multi-sectoral actions, including stronger private sector engagement where appropriate, require high level and *sustained* political commitment.
- *Tempering ambitious targets with realistic prioritization.* In low-resource settings, it might not be feasible to address *all* targets at the same time. Countries should prioritize realistically and strategically, taking into account sequencing and phasing of interventions. Development partners, civil society, academia, and the private sector can support governments in their efforts.

- *Adapting and contextualizing the SDGs to the local setting.* Further work might be needed to contextualize SDGs to each individual setting and operationalize strategies to make progress toward targets.
- *Securing the necessary national and global financial resources.* International institutions, including those from the private sector and academia, should work with the government to facilitate greater investments.
- *Focusing on data, data, data!* Countries should strengthen routine health information systems (including aligning, integrating, and consolidating vertical platforms in both public and private sectors), improve data reliability, and, most important, ensure that data generated through the different systems and surveys are used for informed decision making.

The SDGs provide a tremendous opportunity for countries to move beyond the aspiration of high-quality, affordable, accessible healthcare toward the reality of improving health and well-being for all. This challenges governments, development partners, and the private sector to work together not only to address issues aimed at ensuring universal health coverage but also fundamental problems of health security and resilient societies. On the eve of the new SDG era, nowhere are these realities more evident than in Sierra Leone as the country emerges from the shadows of a devastating Ebola Virus Disease (EVD) outbreak. Using the experiences of Sierra Leone as a case study, we first examine Sierra Leone's experience with the Millennium Development Goals (MDGs) and the transition to the SDGs. Second, we consider and contextualize the realities of Sierra Leone's health system and health sector within the new SDG framework. Third, we reflect upon the implications of Sierra Leone's situation for the SDGs and suggest potential ways to accelerate progress. Finally, we consider the opportunities afforded by the sustainable development agenda and what this could signify for similar countries seeking to implement the SDGs.

Sierra Leone's Experience with the Millennium Development Goals

To understand Sierra Leone's future work to achieve the SDGs, it is useful to review the country's past experience with the MDGs. Numerous indicators, such as poverty reduction and under-five stunting, improved.[1] However, for a number of reasons, Sierra Leone did not meet the health

MDGs. When the MDGs were launched in the early 2000s, Sierra Leone was still embroiled in a bloody civil war, an 11-year conflict that ended as recently as 2002. In the early MDG period, Sierra Leone was still recovering from this devastating conflict, which left much of the health system in shambles: numerous health facilities were destroyed, qualified health workers left the country, and the overall health and economic infrastructure was completely decimated.[2] As the 2005 National MDG report noted, "while there is demonstrated political will and favourable support from development partners, achievement of the MDGs poses enormous challenges."[3]

In advance of the 2010 Global MDG Review, Sierra Leone's government, with support from UN agencies, expanded the use of the MDG framework to assess progress and inform the country's national development strategies.[4] However, serious challenges persisted with each of the three MDG health goals (reducing child mortality, improving maternal health, and combating HIV/AIDS, malaria, and other diseases), despite notable progress against HIV/AIDS, malaria, and tuberculosis (TB). For example, child and maternal mortality rates remained among the highest in the world (table 8.1).[5] The 2010 MDG review concluded that the HIV/AIDS, malaria, and TB goal would likely be met, but the goals for maternal and child health would only be met with sustained effort, including increased political commitment, greater attention to vulnerable groups, and a clearer focus on addressing inequities.[6] Civil society believed that

Table 8.1. Health-related MDG targets in Sierra Leone

Indicator	Baseline year	Baseline estimate	2015 target	2015 status	% achieved
Infant mortality rate	2000	170/1,000	50/1,000	92/1,000	65%
Under-5 mortality rate	2000	286/1,000	95/1,000	156/1,000	68%
Maternal mortality ratio	2000	1,800/100,000	450/100,000	1,165/100,000	47%
No. of malaria deaths	2013	4,326	1,082	2,848	48%
Under-5 children with bednets	2000	2%	100%	49.2%	48%
HIV prevalence	2005	1.5%	0%	0.12%	58%

Note: These figures are self-reported by the Government of Sierra Leone, but some of the numbers vary from other data sources, such as those from the Demographic and Health Survey, the WHO Global Health Observatory, and the Global Burden of Disease.

"significant progress" was made on child and maternal mortality, with "mixed progress" on HIV/AIDS, TB, and malaria.[7]

More specifically, between 2008 and 2013, Sierra Leone made progress on several key coverage indicators, including measles immunization coverage (from 60% to 79%) and pregnant women receiving at least four antenatal visits (from approximately 56% to 76%).[8] However, despite these gains in coverage, health outcomes remained poor, with the country grappling with one of the world's smallest health workforces per capita in an extremely weak health system.[9] And this was before Ebola.

Between May 2014 and February 2016, close to 9,000 Sierra Leoneans were infected with Ebola, with close to 4,000 dying in the world's largest outbreak of the disease. Ebola's impact in Sierra Leone was profound. The health system was severely weakened by the deaths of healthcare workers, initially limited resource allocations toward Ebola, and the closure of health facilities. Trust in the system declined, and access to care was limited. Substantial reductions in healthcare utilization were reported, including over 80% reductions in maternal delivery care in Ebola-affected areas, 40% national reductions in malaria admissions among children younger than five years, and substantial reductions in vaccination coverage.[10]

One of the reasons for the Ebola outbreak as well as such weak outcomes was that prior attention to and investments in the health system were insufficient.[11] This issue was well highlighted during and in the aftermath of the outbreak.[12,13,14] The reasons for this inadequate investment in the health system were multifold and complex, including lack of political will and weak local capacities. For example, the government's sectoral allocation to health as a percentage of the overall budget was between 8.2% and 11.2% from 2008 to 2013, while the roads sector saw an increase from 19.5% to 29.2% during that same timeframe.[15] Similarly, as the country struggles to meet WHO-recommended staffing norms, approximately 50% of the health workers are outside of the government payroll system.[16] Additionally, as highlighted in Sierra Leone's 2017 health sector strategy, much of the governance of the health sector requires significant strengthening.[17] It could also be that some of the MDG priorities distorted national priorities and investments. For example, despite a national HIV/AIDS prevalence rate of only 1.5%, $8 million out of $14 million spent in 2004 on health prevention in Sierra Leone focused on HIV, only one of the MDGs.[18] Sierra Leone's experience also aligned with an in-depth commission reviewing global progress, which, while recognizing the country's progress, highlighted the fact that MDGs disregarded and fragmented health systems, ignored changing demographics, and overlooked emerging health challenges such as noncommunicable diseases,[19] mental health, or road traffic injuries.[20]

Additionally, a lack of consistently reliable national data provided an inaccurate picture of service coverage in Sierra Leone, thereby hindering efforts to design and implement needed interventions as well as track progress. This national experience was similar to that of other countries and helped contribute to the much more consultative and inclusive process to develop and create the SDG framework.[21] Starting in 2012, the United Nations facilitated a complex, multisectoral, and multilevel process building on the MDG experience to develop a post-2015 development framework to follow the MDGs. Sierra Leone participated and engaged in these discussions. Indeed, Sierra Leone's Ebola experience, coming near the end of the negotiations, helped influence and shape the final outcome in SDG 3. A shift toward a focus on health systems was affirmed, but the Ebola experience also pushed policy makers to consider issues of global health security and resilience. After what was likely one of the most inclusive and consultative processes in the history of the UN, states agreed upon the seventeen Sustainable Development Goals and their accompanying 169 indicators, including 1 health goal (SDG 3) with 9 health outcome indicators and 3 process indicators.[22]

To consider the transition from the MDGs to SDGs, it is important to understand Sierra Leone's socioeconomic situation. Following the dual shock of the EVD outbreak and a drop in global iron ore prices, Sierra Leone's GDP decreased by 21.5% in 2015, with slow recovery to 4.3% in 2016. However, the economic forecast as of early 2017 was positive, with GDP growth expected to increase to around 6.5% by 2020. Within this context, the government launched a series of initiatives aimed at adapting SDGs to the Sierra Leone situation, with the Office of the President actively leading the effort. The national development plan and the 2016 national budget incorporate the SDGs.

For SDG 3, comprehensive initiatives such as the President's Recovery Priorities (PRPs) are aimed at not only maintaining zero new cases of Ebola infections but also tackling the daunting task of drastically reducing maternal and child mortality. This effort addresses key elements, such as an insufficient skilled workforce, unreliable data systems, and a weak procurement and supply chain.[23] Partners such as the Department for International Development (DFID), the Global Fund, Gavi, the African Development Bank, and the US government—as well as UN agencies—committed to supporting these initiatives and aligned their support with the government's priorities. Furthermore, the first Sierra Leone Development Finance Forum, hosted by the government and the World Bank in 2017, recognized the vital role the private sector can play in making a positive impact on people's lives.

New health policy strategies developed in 2016–17, such as those for human resources targeted toward reproductive, maternal, newborn, child, and adolescent health, ensure that the SDG targets and indicators are reflected in the plans. The development of an overarching sector-wide health strategic plan was completed, with the SDGs forming the foundational basis for this document. Additionally, data systems are being strengthened to ensure routine information is collected and analyzed with a view to monitoring indicators and taking remedial actions to meet the targets and achieve better health outcomes.

However, in terms of the private sector, significant gaps in knowledge and data persist. It is estimated that approximately 50% of the hospitals in the country are privately owned, along with networks of private pharmacies and informal drug peddlers. The exact utilization and expenditure figures are difficult to obtain, and there are no significant organized trade associations.[24] However, it is anticipated that a recently concluded census of service availability and readiness assessment of all the health facilities in the country will yield much-needed information on private facilities and will aid in better informing policy. These sorts of data could help the government to explore and steward potential partnerships with private sector actors; however, at this point, understanding about the extent of the private sector's engagement in the health sector is limited.

The country's recently developed National Health Sector Strategic Plan 2017–2021 attempts to bridge some of these gaps, recognizing the need to map private sector stakeholders in the country, determining the types of engagement that might be needed, and having more structures in place for private sector involvement in health. One example of this is the Ministry of Health's effort to create a clear framework on the opening and closure of health facilities. Using the development of a master facility list as the start-

ing point, the government hopes to identify the most appropriate locations of existing health facilities as well as mechanisms to guide public
and private providers on where services should be provided (based on population needs). This will afford an opportunity to further engage the private sector in areas where they might have a comparative advantage (near
mines, for example).

Furthermore, progress has been made to ensure that Sierra Leone is
prepared and ready to respond to future outbreaks or shocks to the system. A recently concluded Joint External Evaluation of the International
Health Regulations and the Global Health Security Agenda in the country
identified a series of remedial actions and corrective measures that need to
be undertaken to improve health security and build the resiliency of the
system.[25] This includes strengthening legislation, tackling antimicrobial
resistance, improving emergency surveillance, preparedness, and response
for human and animal health, and ensuring that there is an adequate health
workforce capable of identifying and responding to outbreaks and other
disasters.

Sierra Leone was able to make some progress on the MDGs despite just
emerging from a civil war. Then, just before the dawn of the SDG era, the
country experienced Ebola. The virus was, thankfully, not as destructive
as the civil war, but the SDGs are a significantly broader agenda. While
there were 3 health goals in the 8 MDGs, there is now only 1 health goal in
the 17 SDGs. Despite this, the single health SDG agenda is broader and more
ambitious than the previous three health MDGs and encompasses key elements across the systems as well as different health programs and diseases.

Sierra Leone: Moving from Crisis to Resilience

It is important to have a clear understanding of Sierra Leone's economic situation. Prior to Ebola, following the discovery of iron ore in 2011,
Sierra Leone achieved a growth of 21% in 2013. Following the outbreak, the
economy significantly contracted in 2015, with signs of recovery in 2016
and 2017.[26] However, Sierra Leone today still ranks near the bottom of the
Human Development Index (179 out of 185 countries) and performs poorly
by most development and socioeconomic indicators.[27] Maternal and under-
five mortality are among the highest in the world (maternal mortality ratio
of 1,360 per 100,000 live births[28] and under-five mortality rate of 156 per

100,000).[29] Applying the World Health Organization's classification to identify countries in various stages of health system development, the Foundation Institution and Transformation (FIT) strategy, Sierra Leone clearly falls in the area of "F":

> Strategy 1: "F": Strengthening health systems *foundations* in least-developed and fragile countries with poor health system performance and negligible fiscal space to increase public spending on health.
> Strategy 2: "I": Strengthening health systems *institutions* in least-developed countries where the health system foundations are in place.
> Strategy 3: "T": Supporting health systems *transformation* in countries with mature health systems where reaching UHC and health security is still challenging.[30]

For Sierra Leone to achieve better health for its citizens, the government needs to ensure structural and systems elements are in place, including basic infrastructure and amenities such as water and electricity in health facilities. How would this affect the country's progress toward SDG 3?

Table 8.2 highlights the steep challenges facing Sierra Leone in the SDG era. In a country with fundamental challenges of infrastructure, personnel, and resources, the current situation compared to these targets offers a sobering reality. Perhaps one of the best illustrations of this can be observed in targets 3.1, 3.2, and 3.7—reduction of maternal and child mortality and access to reproductive health services. With the country being among the worst performers in the world for these indicators, a massive effort is required to meet the targets or, at the very least, make substantial progress in the coming years.

Combating communicable diseases and reducing the incidence of tuberculosis (target 3.3) is an equally pronounced challenge. In order to meet relevant targets, Sierra Leone would need to achieve a reduction in TB incidence of 4% to 5% per year, which, while not impossible, is extremely difficult for a country facing such severe challenges in the TB program, including a significant decrease in TB case notification rates in recent years (table 8.3).[31]

SDG targets 3.4, 3.5, 3.6, 3.9 and 3.a (noncommunicable diseases; substance abuse; road traffic injuries; hazardous materials, pollution, and contaminants; and tobacco use, respectively) all involve similarly daunting challenges. For example, at the time of writing, to promote mental health, the country has only one retired psychiatrist and one practicing clinical

Table 8.2. Key SDG 3 targets and current status in Sierra Leone

Target	Indicator	Value	Year
3.1. By 2030, reduce the global maternal mortality ratio to less than 70 per 100,000 live births.	Maternal mortality ratio (per 100,000 live births)	1,360	2015
	Proportion of births attended by skilled health personnel (%)	60	2006–14
3.2. By 2030, end preventable deaths of newborns and children under 5 years of age, with all countries aiming to reduce neonatal mortality to at least as low as 12 per 1,000 live births and under-5 mortality to at least as low as 25 per 1,000 live births.	Under-five mortality rate (per 1,000 live births)	120.4	2015
	Neonatal mortality rate (per 1,000 live births)	34.9	2015
3.3. By 2030, end the epidemics of AIDS, tuberculosis, malaria, and neglected tropical diseases and combat hepatitis, water-borne diseases, and other communicable diseases.	New HIV infections among adults 15–49 years old (per 1,000 uninfected population)	0.7	2014
	TB incidence (per 100,000 population)	310	2014
	Malaria incidence (per 1,000 population at risk)	406.0	2013
	Infants receiving three doses of hepatitis B vaccine (%)	83	2014
	Reported number of people requiring interventions against NTDs	7,564,272	2014
3.4. By 2030, reduce by one-third premature mortality from noncommunicable diseases through prevention and treatment and promote mental health and well-being.	Probability of dying from any of CVD, cancer, diabetes, CRD between age 30 and age 70 (%)	27.5	2012
	Suicide mortality rate (per 100,000 population)	5.6	2012
3.5. Strengthen the prevention and treatment of substance abuse, including narcotic drug abuse and harmful use of alcohol.	Total alcohol per capita (>15 years of age) consumption, in liters of pure alcohol, projected estimates	8.2	2015
3.6. By 2020, halve the number of global deaths and injuries from road traffic accidents.	Road traffic mortality rate (per 100,000 population)	27.3	2013

(continued)

Table 8.2. (*continued*)

Target	Indicator	Value	Year
3.7. By 2030, ensure universal access to sexual and reproductive healthcare services, including family planning, information and education, and the integration of reproductive health into national strategies and programs.	Proportion of married or in-union women of reproductive age who have their need for family planning satisfied with modern methods (%)	37.5	2005–15
	Adolescent birth rate (per 1,000 women aged 15–19 years)	125.0	2005–15
3.8. Achieve universal health coverage, including financial risk protection, access to quality essential healthcare services, and access to safe, effective, quality, and affordable essential medicines and vaccines for all.	N/A	N/A	N/A
3.9. By 2030, substantially reduce the number of deaths and illnesses from hazardous chemicals and air, water, and soil pollution and contamination.	Mortality rate attributed to household and ambient air pollution (per 100,000 population)	142.3	2012
	Mortality rate attributed to exposure to unsafe WASH services (per 100,000 population)	90.4	2012
	Mortality rate from unintentional poisoning (per 100,000 population)	5.7	2012
3.a. Strengthen the implementation of the WHO Framework Convention on Tobacco Control in all countries, as appropriate.	Age-standardized prevalence of tobacco smoking among persons 15 years and older (%, male)	60.0	2015
	Age-standardized prevalence of tobacco smoking among persons 15 years and older (%, female)	12.0	2015

3.b. Support the research and development of vaccines and medicines for the communicable and noncommunicable diseases that primarily affect developing countries and provide access to affordable essential medicines and vaccines, in accordance with the Doha Declaration on the TRIPS Agreement and Public Health, which affirms the right of developing countries to use to the full the provisions in the Agreement on Trade-Related Aspects of Intellectual Property Rights regarding flexibilities to protect public health, and, in particular, provide access to medicines for all.	N/A	N/A	N/A
3.c. Substantially increase health financing and the recruitment, development, training, and retention of the health workforce in developing countries, especially in least developed countries and small island developing states.	Skilled health professionals density (per 10,000 population)	1.9	2005–13
3.d. Strengthen the capacity of all countries, in particular developing countries, for early warning, risk reduction, and management of national and global health risks.	Average of 13 International Health Regulations core capacity scores	64	2010–15

Source: World Health Statistics 2016: Monitoring health for the SDGs, http://www.who.int/gho/publications/world_health_statistics/2016/en/

Table 8.3. SDG Target 3.3 (reducing the incidence of TB) and Sierra Leone

Baseline 2014	Milestone 2020	Milestone 2025	SDG 2030	End TB 2035
310	248 (20%)	155 (50%)	62 (80%)	31 (90%)

psychologist—for a population of over seven million. The country is served by only one psychiatric hospital (based in the capital Freetown), and until recent reform efforts, Sierra Leone's mental health legislation existed under the auspices of an archaic "Lunacy Act" developed in 1902.[32]

Other indicators aimed at strengthening health systems toward universal health coverage (SDG targets 3.8 and 3.c) provide additional insight into the challenges the country faces in the SDG era. Over 60% of health expenditure is through out-of-pocket (OOP) payments, and access to quality health services varies across districts, which severely limits progress. Furthermore, the country is heavily dependent on external sources of funding—net Official Development Assistance (ODA) in the country as a percentage of GNI (gross national income) was 21.1% in 2016.[33] The total health expenditure for 2013 was US$ 590 million, of which ODA accounted for 24.4%[34]—an increase of 295% from 2003 to 2013.[35] Following the recovery period post-Ebola, it remains to be seen to what extent this trend will continue. Hopefully, government investments in the sector will increase while efforts are made to tap into resources from the private sector (through, for example, effective public-private partnerships or stronger enforcement of tax collection).

Sierra Leone has initiated a dialogue around universal health coverage, but a series of political and technical challenges suggest that the country is a long way from making progress toward UHC. This includes the introduction of the Free Healthcare Initiative in 2010 to provide free services to all pregnant women, lactating mothers, and children under the age of five. However, the specific benefits package was not enshrined in any formal policy or legislation. While there has been evidence to suggest that the Free Healthcare Initiative did make some positive contributions, it is mostly financed by external donors (most notably DFID) with no clear long-term sustainability plans.[36] Furthermore, OOP payments remain high. The country also faces serious challenges in supply-side readiness, including quantity, quality, and access to human resources for health.[37]

More recently, attempts are being made at introducing the Sierra Leone Social Health Insurance Scheme (SLeSHI), a benefits package of primary health services to all citizens. The government of Sierra Leone indicated its intention to launch the scheme in 2017, but there were significant design and health systems challenges, including questions around actual reductions in OOP payments, an ambitious timeline for rollout, the viability of informal sector contributions, and a lack of available capacities to manage and administer such a complex and very limited supply-side readiness.[38]

There is a growing recognition in Sierra Leone that making progress on SDG 3.8 will require a significant collaborative effort between the government, development partners, civil society, and the private sector. This will entail mapping all service providers in the country, public and private, to determine the role and scope of health services along with the cost of service provision. Efforts will need to be made to ensure strong policy and regulatory frameworks are established and enforced. Additionally, the potential of public-private partnerships in the country's UHC space will need to be explored. Specific best practices can be identified and applied from neighboring countries and beyond. As illustrated by Srinath Reddy (see chapter 7), ensuring that the private sector is well organized is an important component in leveraging its potential. Since the private sector presence in Sierra Leone is currently scattered and lacks strong coherent structures, establishing and strengthening such bodies will take time and require strong government support and stewardship. But this process also offers valuable opportunities for improving service delivery.

Compounding the situation is the country's fragmented information systems and a dearth of reliable, high-quality data. A recent review found that many disease programs had their own information platforms, with little interoperability and no integration among the systems.[39] Due to problems with the routine data systems, much of the data used for decision making come from surveys such as the Demographic and Health Survey. Efforts are being made to address these challenges, but progress is slow, and many of these issues require significant investments in the long term to overcome the hurdles.

Looking beyond traditional health outcomes to recent developments around increased resiliency, progress has been made. The Integrated Disease Surveillance and Response (IDSR) system functions, reporting on priority health conditions every week.[40] There has been an increased understanding and implementation of infection prevention and control measures, and several efforts have been put in place to increase community engagement and ensure stronger linkages among different levels of care. This has included the establishment of a national coordination mechanism on social mobilization as well as expansion of partnerships on health promotion. However, two questions persist. First, as the memory of the EVD outbreak fades, will the country observe a decrease in resources and investments, thereby weakening the resiliency of the system? If there is indeed a decrease in investments for health, both externally and domestically, this will affect not only the post-recovery efforts in the country but could more broadly affect progress toward attaining SDG targets. Second, have too many parallel systems been set up during the Ebola epidemic to allow for any long-term gains toward the achievement of SDG targets?

In table 8.4, a sampling of other SDG targets that also affect health provides a more comprehensive view of the situation. While homicide rates are relatively low, much work needs to be done around improving nutrition and increasing access to safe water, sanitation, and clean, modern energy.

Table 8.4. Sampling of other SDG targets

Target	Global agreed indicator	Sierra Leone current status
2.2. End all forms of malnutrition.	Prevalence of stunting; prevalence of malnutrition (wasting and overweight)	37.9% of children under 5 years; SL has equal numbers for wasting and overweight; figures not provided)
6.1. Universal and equitable access to safe and affordable drinking water.	Proportion of population using safely managed drinking water services	63%
6.2. Access to adequate and equitable sanitation and hygiene.	Proportion of population using safely managed sanitation services	13%
7.1. Access to affordable, reliable and modern energy services.	Proportion of population with primary reliance on clean fuels and technology	<5%
16.1. Reduce all forms of violence and related deaths.	Victims of intentional homicide per 100,000 population	13 per 100,000

Source: World Bank World Development Indicators, http://datatopics.worldbank.org/sdgs/

This need signifies the importance of intersectoral action and the ongoing efforts by the government and partners to work closely across different systems and structures, using a holistic approach.

This brief overview of Sierra Leone's baseline situation provides a sobering reality check on the numerous challenges facing the country in the new SDG era. While the government is committed to progress, there are many financial and human resource constraints. Much of the physical infrastructure, in terms of roads, buildings, and electrical grids—not to mention the country's IT infrastructure—is extremely limited. Improving these basic services will need to be tackled at the same time Sierra Leone addresses a host of other issues needed to achieve the SDGs in the country. Extrapolating from Sierra Leone's experience with the MDGs, we provide some potential recommendations for maintaining and accelerating progress in this new SDG era.

SDG 3: What It Means for the Broader SDG Agenda and Era

Based on Sierra Leone's experience, to ensure success in the SDG era, countries need to focus on prioritizing a few key actions. We outline and illustrate these in the prioritized list below:

1. *Ensure political commitment to integrate and align the SDGs with national development efforts.* Improving health and well-being is as much a political process as it is a technical one. Multisectoral actions require sustained high-level political commitment. In response to the Ebola outbreak, Sierra Leone focused on health as a big part of the President's Recovery Priorities program following Ebola. At the time of writing, Sierra Leone's presidential elections were scheduled for March 2018. While it is hoped that the new president remains committed to achieving the SDG targets, competing interests and priorities could shift attention toward other pressing needs. In spite of this uncertainty, the government should continue its ongoing efforts to domesticate and integrate SDG goals into national plans and strategies. The Ministry of Health and Sanitation needs to ensure that the SDGs are integrated and aligned with its specific health strategies.

2. *Temper ambitious targets with realistic prioritization.* As illustrated, much of the SDG targets in Sierra Leone are ambitious. Other

low-income countries face similar challenges in overcoming obstacles towards achieving the SDGs. When SDG 3 was developed and agreed to at the global level, many of the targets were, rightly, ambitious— even aspirational. However, at the country level, particularly in low-resource settings, this means that difficult and at times unpopular choices need to be made. It might not be feasible to address all targets at the same time. Countries need to realistically and strategically prioritize, taking into account the sequencing and phasing of interventions. Strong leadership, lessons learned from similar countries, technical advice, and an inclusive policy dialogue are thus likely to determine priorities.

3. *Adapt and contextualize the SDGs to the local setting.* As they did in the MDG era, well-defined policy frameworks, strong political commitment, and realistic prioritization could help adapt the SDG 3 targets for Sierra Leone. Nevertheless, reaching consensus on feasible goals for a country can be difficult. Indeed, a 2016 review found that Sierra Leone was significantly behind on most goals: 15 out of the 17 SDGs were in the red, not on track to achieving the goals, with the remaining two in yellow.[41] Similarly, neighboring countries Guinea and Liberia have 15 out of 17 SDGs in red, with the two others in yellow.[42] While all countries have followed a rigorous process to domesticate the SDGs, further work might be needed to contextualize them to the individual settings and operationalize strategies toward progress.[43]

4. *Secure the necessary national and global financial resources.* While much of Sierra Leone's health spending is financed through domestic resources, even in low-income settings[44] or for countries in the "F" category of FIT, significant external financial and human resources are still needed in the short to medium term—again, linked to political will and commitment. This will be particularly important for investments in "hardware"—the structural elements that need to be in place in order to run the health system. For example, the World Bank and the African Development Bank provided support to the World Health Organization to facilitate the recruitment of faculty and provide infrastructural improvements to Sierra Leone's one and only medical school. This also implies technical advice from international institutions and agencies supporting countries in identifying and implementing efficiency gains and ensuring that the right interven-

tions are targeted for investments. International institutions, including those from the private sector and academia, should work with the government to enhance and improve their cooperation to facilitate greater investments. Furthermore, support should also be provided to the government in better understanding the private sector landscape in the country and potential opportunities for further engagement. Additionally, best practices from other countries and South-South collaboration can play a vital role in harnessing Sierra Leone's currently untapped potential with the private sector in health.

5. *Focus on data, data, data!* At the global level, significant investments have been made to monitor the SDGs by establishing relevant frameworks, technical bodies, databases, and systems. The Cape Town Global Action Plan for Sustainable Development Data[45] provides a clear way forward. At the country level, the situation remains more nuanced. In Sierra Leone, improvements have been made to strengthen routine health information systems (for example, as highlighted above, with IDSR). However, much work still remains, including aligning, integrating, and consolidating vertical platforms (including from the private sector), improving data reliability and, most importantly, ensuring that data generated through the different systems and surveys are used for informed decision making. As mentioned above, data and understandings of the private sector's role in Sierra Leone's health sector remain weak. However, there could be opportunities to consider partnerships with the private sector on improving data, particularly since current data are limited for some of the targets, thus inhibiting accountability and the ability to track and monitor progress.

Conclusion

While the MDGs were generally successful in generating political commitment, the SDGs aspire to provide a broader framework for enabling sustainable development. Health serves a critical role in this and is a key component of sustainable development.[46] The MDGs played an important role in helping to shape the field of global health, but the relationship between the SDGs and the future of global health remains unclear. This case study on Sierra Leone highlights three key elements: (1) the risk of global goals distorting national priorities; (2) the deep disparity across countries; and (3) the need to avoid distortion within/among SDG 3 targets.

1. *Global versus country priorities.* There is a risk that global efforts might undermine country-level priorities. This has been observed with the explosion of many well-intentioned and important global health initiatives—by some estimates standing at over 140,[47] with many of them bringing sufficient resources, attention, and influence to shift the dialogue at the country level. More recently, the discourse by the international community around "resilience" has led to a plethora of frameworks, concepts, and theories—all of which have implications for countries. Therefore, special attention needs to be paid to ensure that global goals do not skew efforts to address national needs.

2. *Universality of SDGs.* The SGDs are intended to be relevant for Sierra Leone as much as for Kenya or India or Australia. While this universality offers aspirations for improved development across all countries, it also brings with it certain limitations: for low-income countries like Sierra Leone, it could translate to very ambitious targets, while for high-income countries these targets might not be sufficiently ambitious. For health, the universality of SDGs provides countries of all income levels with a platform to share, collaborate, and build on each other's experiences. For example, tools such as the universal health coverage data portal allows countries to actively track key targets within SDG 3.

3. *Keeping sight of the overall goal, not just selected targets.* SDG 3 is aimed at ensuring healthy lives and promoting well-being at all ages. However, as seen with the MDGs, there is a risk that certain targets could become more visible, thereby creating a fragmented approach to achieving SDG 3. This is a risk not only in terms of disease outcomes but also for health systems–related targets. For example, UHC cannot and should not become a shorthand for SDG 3 but rather must remain as one of the key areas that countries need to focus on in order to improve health and well-being for their populations. Those making investments in SDGs should look at the totality of the structures and systems, instead of cherry-picking certain elements.

These constraints are not insurmountable. They simply suggest that the international community needs to be cognizant of the challenges and has to work with governments, local partners, and the private sector to adapt and contextualize the SDGs to local settings. Regional context and experience can also provide inspiration. For example, Ghana's experience could be instructive: it has focused efforts on strengthening data for sustainable development, including strengthening censuses and surveys, ensuring more disaggregated data, exploring geospatial data, improving data utilization and communication, and better harnessing big data, including through working with the private sector. With 2030 fast approaching, a concerted effort will be needed by governments, development partners, civil society, and the private sector to make progress toward the SDGs.

NOTES

1. Government of Sierra Leone. "Interim Millennium Development Goals Report 2015." Freetown, 2016.
2. Angel Desai. "Sierra Leone's Long Recovery from the Scars of War." *WHO Bulletin* 88, no. 10 (Oct 2010).
3. Government of the Republic of Sierra Leone. "Millennium Development Goals Report for Sierra Leone." Freetown, 2005.
4. "UNDP Sierra Leone Human Development Report 2007." *UNDP in Sierra Leone.* Accessed May 8, 2017. http://www.sl.undp.org/content/sierraleone/en/home/library /human-development-reports/undp-sierra-leone-2007-human-development -report.html.
5. Government of Sierra Leone. "Advanced Draft Report on Adaptation of the Goals in Sierra Leone." Ministry of Finance and Economic Development, July 2016.
6. United Nations Secretary General. "Millennium Development Goals Report," 2010.
7. Commonwealth Foundation and End Poverty 2015. "A Civil Society Review of Progress towards the Millennium Development Goals in Commonwealth Countries. National Report: Sierra Leone," 2013. Accessed May 8, 2017. http://commonwealthfoundation .com/wp-content/uploads/2013/10/MDG%20Reports%20Sierra_Leone_FINAL_2 .pdf.
8. Sierra Leone Demographic and Health Survey 2013.
9. Sierra Leone Ministry of Health and Sanitation. Human Resources for Health Profile 2012.
10. J. W. T. Elston, C. Cartwright, P. Ndumbi, J. Wright. "The Health Impact of the 2014–15 Ebola Outbreak." *Public Health* 143 (Feb 2017): 60–70. doi:10.1016/j.puhe.2016.10.020.
11. Phyllida Travis, Sara Bennett, Andy Haines, Tikki Pang, Zulfiqar Bhutta, Adnan A. Hyder, Nancy R. Pielemeier, Anne Mills, Timothy Evans. Overcoming Health-Systems Constraints to Achieve the Millennium Development Goals. *Lancet* 364, no. 9437 (Sept 2004): 900–906.
12. Lawrence O. Gostin, Eric A. Friedman. A Retrospective and Prospective Analysis of the West African Ebola Virus Disease Epidemic: Robust National Health Systems at

the Foundation and an Empowered WHO at the Apex. *Lancet* 385, no. 9980 (May 2015): 1902–9.

13. Marie-Paule Kieny, David B Evans, Gerard Schmets, Sowmya Kadandale. Health-System Resilience: Reflections on the Ebola Crisis in Western Africa. *Bulletin of the World Health Organization* 92, no. 12 (Dec 2014).

14. Margaret E. Kruk, Michael Myers, S. Tornorlah Varpilah, Bernice T. Dahn. What is a resilient health system? Lessons from Ebola. *Lancet* 385, no. 9980 (May 2015): 1910–12.

15. Sierra Leone Ministry of Health and Sanitation. "National Health Accounts 2013," 2014.

16. Sierra Leone Ministry of Health and Sanitation. "Human Resources for Health Profile 2016," 2017.

17. Sierra Leone Ministry of Health and Sanitation. "National Health Sector Strategic Plan 2017–2021," 2017.

18. Adia Benton. *HIV Exceptionalism: Development through Disease in Sierra Leone.* Minneapolis: University of Minnesota Press, 2015.

19. George Alleyne, Agnes Binagwaho, Andy Haines, Selim Jahan, Rachel Nugent, Ariella Rojhani, David Stuckler, on behalf of The Lancet NCD Action Group. "Embedding Non-Communicable Diseases in the Post-2015 Development Agenda." *Lancet* 381, no. 9866 (Feb 2013): 566–74.

20. Jeff Waage, Rukmini Banerji, Oona Campbell, Ephraim Chirwa, Guy Collender, Veerle Dieltiens, Andrew Dorward, Peter Godfrey-Faussett, Piya Hanvoravongchai, Geeta Kingdon, Angela Little, Anne Mills, Kim Mulholland, Alwyn Mwinga, Amy North, Walaiporn Patcharanarumol, Colin Poulton, Viroj Tangcharoensathien, Elaine Unterhalter. "The Millennium Development Goals: A Cross-Sectoral Analysis and Principles for Goal Setting after 2015." *Lancet* 376 no. 9745 (Sept. 2010): 991–1023.

21. Sustainable Development Knowledge Platform. "Sierra Leone National Voluntary Review 2016."

22. World Health Organization. Health In 2015: From MDGs to SDGs. WHO, 2015. Accessed June 12, 2017. http://apps.who.int/iris/bitstream/10665/200009/1/9789241565110_eng.pdf?ua=1.

23. The President of Sierra Leone. "The President's Recovery Priorities." Accessed May 8, 2017. http://www.presidentsrecoverypriorities.gov.sl/health.

24. Sierra Leone Ministry of Health and Sanitation. "National health sector strategic plan 2017–2021," 2017.

25. World Health Organization. Maximizing Positive Synergies Collaborative Group. "Joint External Evaluation of IHR Core Capacities of the Republic of Sierra Leone. Mission Report: 31 October–4 November 2016," 2017. http://apps.who.int/iris/bitstream/10665/254790/1/WHO-WHE-CPI-2017.16-eng.pdf?ua=1.

26. The African Development Bank Group. "Sierra Leone Economic Outlook." Accessed May 8, 2017. https://www.afdb.org/en/countries/west-africa/sierra-leone/.

27. United Nations Development Programme. "Human Development Report 2016: Human Development for Everyone."

28. World Health Organization Sierra Leone. "Statistics." Accessed May 8, 2017. http://www.who.int/countries/sle/en/.

29. Statistics Sierra Leone - SSL and ICF International. "Sierra Leone Demographic and Health Survey 2013." Freetown, Sierra Leone: SSL and ICF International, 2014. Accessed May 8, 2017. http://dhsprogram.com/pubs/pdf/FR297/FR297.pdf.

30. World Health Organization. "Strategizing National Health in the 21st Century: A Handbook." WHO, 2016.

31. Laura Anderson and Esther Hamblion. "Epidemiological review of TB disease in Sierra Leone." WHO, October 2015.

32. "Mental Health and Psychosocial Support—WHO | Regional Office for Africa." Accessed May 8, 2017. https://www.afro.who.int/.

33. Organisation for Economic Co-operation and Development. "ODA Data for Sierra Leone." Accessed May 8, 2017. https://public.tableau.com/views/OECDDACAidata-glancebyrecipient_new/Recipients?:embed=y&:display_count=yes&:showTabs=y&:toolbar=no?&:showVizHome=no.

34. Sierra Leone Ministry of Health and Sanitation. "National Health Accounts, 2013." Accessed May 8, 2017. https://mohs-portal.net/wp-content/uploads/2017/05/NHA-2013.pdf.

35. World Health Organization. "Country Planning Cycle Database: Sierra Leone." Accessed May 8, 2017. http://nationalplanningcycles.org/planning-cycle/SLE.

36. Oxford Policy Management. "Evaluation of Sierra Leone Free Healthcare Initiative, 2016."

37. World Health Organization. "Training and Managing the Health Workers of Tomorrow." Accessed May 8, 2017. http://www.afro.who.int/sierra-leone/press-materials/item/9574-training-and-managing-the-health-workers-of-tomorrow.html?lang=en.

38. "Joint position of Health Development Partners on the Sierra Leone Social Health Insurance Scheme (SLeSHI)," 2017.

39. Ministry of Health and Sanitation. "Detailed Meeting Report Sierra Leone Health Information Systems Interoperability Workshop, 2–4 August 2016, Bintumani Hotel, Freetown," 2016. https://www.healthdatacollaborative.org/fileadmin/uploads/hdc/Documents/SL_HIS_Interoperability_Meeting_Report_Final__2_.pdf.

40. Ministry of Health and Sanitation and WHO. "Weekly Epidemiological Bulletin—Week 13: 27 March–2 April, 2017." Vol. 10, Issue 13, n.d. http://www.afro.who.int/images/SiLReports/wk13.pdf?ua=1.

41. World Health Organization. "Sierra Leone Sustainable Development Goals." November 15, 2016. https://slsdg.org/how-are-we-doing/.

42. Issuu. "SDG Index & Dashboards - Country Profiles." Accessed May 8, 2017. https://issuu.com/unsdsn/docs/sdg_index_and_dashboards_country_pr.

43. Robert L. Cohen, David M. Bishai, Y. Natalia Alfonso, Shyama Kuruvilla, Julian Schweitzer. "Post-2015 health goals: Could country-specific targets supplement global ones?" *Lancet Global Health* 7 (July 2, 2014): e373–74.

44. World Health Organization. "Strategizing National Health in the 21st Century: A Handbook." WHO, 2016.

45. United Nations. "Cape Town Global Action Plan for Sustainable Development Data—SDG Indicators." Accessed May 8, 2017. https://unstats.un.org/sdgs/hlg/Cape-Town-Global-Action-Plan/.

46. David B. Evans, Robert Marten, Carissa Etienne. "Universal Health Coverage Is a Development Issue." *Lancet* 380, no. 9845 (Sept 8, 2012): 864–65. doi:10.1016/S0140-6736(12)61483-4.

47. H. Somanje et al. Optimizing Global Health Initiatives to Strengthen National Health Systems. *African Health Monitor* 16, 2013.

9

How Can the Private Sector Help Countries to Achieve Quality, Sustainable Universal Health Coverage?

Pfizer's Fight against Chronic Diseases

Justin McCarthy and Snow Yang

This chapter describes the role that the private sector—with a particular focus on the biopharmaceutical industry—can play in helping countries progress toward universal health coverage (UHC). We begin by setting out core objectives to be achieved through private sector engagement and then follow up by outlining a set of principles to guide these initiatives in the context of UHC. To illustrate, we highlight select programs and partnerships in which the private sector is engaged and conclude by providing more in-depth examples and a case study to model Pfizer's commitment as a private sector stakeholder toward achieving UHC as part of the United Nations Sustainable Development Goals (SDGs) by 2030. Our key conclusions are as follows: (1) the private sector and the biopharmaceutical industry both have an opportunity and a responsibility to support countries' move toward UHC by providing greater access to equitable, higher quality healthcare; (2) we can do this by sharing expertise and capabilities across a wide range of disciplines, such as research and development, capacity and infrastructure building, workforce training, supply chain management, education and outreach, improving access to supplies and services, and finance; and (3) our cross-sectoral partnerships should focus on the deployment of primary and secondary caregivers, use of off-patent drugs, application of regional and global mechanisms for financing and procurement, and inclusion of priority treatments in national health coverage to help countries achieve equitable, quality, sustainable UHC.

On September 25, 2015, world leaders adopted 17 SDGs at a historic United Nations Summit designed to end poverty, protect the planet, and ensure prosperity for all as part of a new sustainable development agenda. Each goal has specific targets to be achieved by 2030.[1] UHC was high on their list: in 2017, the WHO estimated that "as much as half the world's population lacks access to essential health services."[2] More than 1 billion people worldwide have uncontrolled hypertension, and nearly 20 million infants either fail to complete or never start DTP (diphtheria, tetanus, and pertussis) immunization.[3] An earlier WHO report estimated that as many as 2 billion people lacked access to essential medicines.[4,5] Such numbers are staggering. SDG 3.8 is part of the UN's response: its goal is to provide access to safe and effective medicines and vaccines for all without causing catastrophic financial hardship. Supporting research and development for vaccines is an essential part of this process.[6]

However, many lower- and middle-income countries (LMICs) lack the basic structural elements necessary to put UHC in place.[7] These countries commonly grapple with interlocking issues, including political agendas, policy formation, allocation of scarce resources, and high burdens of disease. Moreover, barriers including underinvestment in health in national budgets; poor supply chain integrity; lack of human capacity and expertise; trade and tariff barriers; regulatory obstacles; diversion of supply; and inadequate healthcare infrastructure hamper progress. To further complicate matters, many LMICs are in the midst of a surge in chronic disease that, combined with aging populations, will increasingly challenge already fragile healthcare ecosystems. In fact, four out of five deaths will be from chronic conditions in the next decade and expenditure on chronic diseases, the main driver of spending on healthcare, is expected to double from 2010 to 2030 globally.[8,9]

Role of the Private Sector

To achieve UHC, health systems strengthening (including creating resilience to health emergencies), capacity building, creation of innovative finance models, provision of integrated care and services, and a focus on prevention and efficient treatment of chronic conditions will all be required. The private sector has a critically important role to play by sharing expertise and experience in a wide range of disciplines, including research and development, workforce training, technology solutions, logistics and supply chain management, media and communications, strategic planning, and finance. However, no single actor is able to achieve these goals. The benefits the private sector can bring will be magnified and bolstered through participation in strategic partnerships with governments and various inter-governmental and nongovernmental organizations.

Such public-private partnerships in the health sector are by no means a new phenomenon. Objectives for partnerships in the context of sustainable health goals have been outlined in a report commissioned by the Business and Sustainable Development Commission.[10] They include: (a) strength-ening medical manufacturing, supply chain management, and delivery systems; (b) improving communications to increase the reach of public health promotions and behavior change initiatives; (c) building health workforce capacities, especially in resource-constrained settings; (d) im-proving humanitarian assistance and disaster relief; (e) increasing policy and practitioner focus on prevention and wellness; (f) tackling counter-feiting and improving product safety and efficacy; and (g) accelerating drug and vaccine discovery and development for key disease burdens. To achieve these goals, stakeholders in LMICs must pool their scarce re-sources in order to gain access to new sources of innovation and leverage economies of scale.

Perspective of the Biopharmaceutical Industry

SDG 3.8 brings a unique opportunity to recognize the role of health-care and medicines as a driver of global economic growth, while also build-ing on the experience and achievements of the Millennium Development Goals (MDGs),[11] where the biopharmaceutical industry helped achieve outcomes such as increased antiretroviral access for HIV patients and sig-nificant progress on decreasing child mortality.[12] Lessons learned and ap-plied since 2000 from the MDGs show the importance of partnerships in improving the architecture of health interventions. Moreover, to achieve UHC, the biopharmaceutical industry believes that health systems must focus on long-term sustainable frameworks to prevent and manage in-fectious, chronic, and injury-related conditions. This will require broader healthcare innovation across the public and private sectors, innovation that enables access and improves quality while at the same time being flex-ible enough to generate tailored and country-owned solutions. Industry associations have coalesced behind a set of broad core principles that in-form their efforts. These include: equitable access to essential services; efficiency of resources use; availability of quality healthcare; choice and inclusiveness of services for patients; availability of health services to all who need them; adaptable financing and delivery of health systems; and innovation in R&D.[13]

Biopharmaceutical Industry Partnerships and Engagement

Together with more than 1,000 partners, the biopharmaceutical industry is currently engaged in over 300 programs to improve health outcomes in LMICs: these include training and capacity building, strengthening the health system infrastructure, raising awareness, prevention and outreach, and improving availability of treatments.[14] Biopharmaceutical industry engagement can generally be categorized into the following types of activity:[15]

- *Aid-based initiatives.* These are fundamentally intended to be stop-gap relief measures to get medicines, supplies, services, volunteers, and education to populations in urgent need.
- *Inclusive business model development.* Such models incorporate a range of activities such as encouraging foreign direct investment or establishing a local presence in developing countries; technology transfer or licensing agreements; or incorporating local businesses into the company's value chain through sourcing of raw materials or outsourcing services such as information technology.
- *Capacity-building initiatives.* These have the potential for significant impact in developing countries, where educational and professional training opportunities are limited and local infrastructure systems are often weak. By helping to train workers and strengthen local institutions, these activities are precursors to stronger healthcare infrastructure.
- *Policy-shaping and value advocacy.* Companies can help shape policies that accelerate progress toward goals associated with UHC by influencing changes in public policy or regulation that foster better health system environments. These activities, while often longer term in nature, can lead to a large-scale impact on UHC in LMICs. Perhaps most salient to pharmaceuticals is raising awareness about the value that medicines can bring to society and the savings they can create for health systems.

These programs come together to improve the lives of people suffering from HIV/AIDS, malaria, tuberculosis, neglected tropical diseases (NTDs), and noncommunicable diseases (NCDs) and can improve the health of women, children, and aging populations.[16]

One of the newest, largest, and perhaps most significant collective initiatives was launched at the 2017 World Economic Forum in Davos, Switzerland, where twenty-two leading biopharmaceutical companies started Access Accelerated.[17] Access Accelerated is a first-of-its-kind collaboration focused on improving prevention, care, and treatment for NCDs, including cardiovascular diseases, cancer, chronic respiratory diseases, diabetes, and mental health conditions. The initiative includes partners such as the World Bank and the Union for International Cancer Control, and it attempts to help address the full spectrum of access barriers to NCD medicines in low-income and lower-middle-income countries. The initial stages of Access Accelerated focused around cancer, but it has since expanded to include other NCDs, such as cardiovascular disease and diabetes.[18] See table 9A.1 in the appendix for examples of other programs involving pharmaceutical corporations.

Pfizer's Response and Evolution of Our Approach

The UN has called for broad-based support of the SDGs, including active involvement by the private sector. To make a significant and sustainable impact, the public and private sectors, as well as civil society stakeholders, are seeking to align activities and work together. Pfizer is committed to helping facilitate this type of biopharmaceutical industry engagement by aligning our corporate objectives so as to increase the impact on healthy individuals and patients across the globe. As Pfizer CEO Ian Read has said, "we believe that access to quality healthcare and the opportunity to lead healthy lives is an extremely important social goal. The power and value of collaboration between public and private organizations in achieving that goal cannot be overstated." Read went on to say,

> At Pfizer, bringing patients innovative therapies that significantly improve their lives is the basis of our commitment to all 17 of the SDGs. The understanding that our business and societal missions are the same is fundamental to our approach in supporting UHC and global public health. We discover, develop, and bring to market life-saving medicines and

vaccines that improve people's lives while helping to ensure that individuals have access to these medicines.

To achieve global health goals, Pfizer has used traditional philanthropic approaches: large-scale financial and product donations. However, Pfizer has evolved our approach to philanthropy over time to go beyond traditional philanthropy. Against the backdrop of a dramatically changing world, private sector companies like Pfizer have to think and act differently about the global health challenges that affect the most vulnerable. We believe that addressing emerging global health challenges in this increasingly complex and technology-driven environment requires new and collaborative strategies that prioritize sustainability over short-term solutions. For example, we are prioritizing our R&D efforts in areas where the promise of science meets the greatest patient need: immunology and inflammation, oncology, cardiovascular and metabolic diseases, pain, and vaccines. We are using the latest manufacturing and packaging technologies to reduce our carbon footprint and increase energy efficiency. We are also exploring partnership opportunities with technology companies to advance innovations in healthcare delivery and health financing that benefit patients.

Whether we are helping to pioneer large-scale biopharmaceutical industry-wide collaborations such as Access Accelerated or engaging in smaller grassroots programs, Pfizer is continuously exploring ways to build commercially sustainable business models that address areas of significant public health need in developed, middle-income, and developing countries. By partnering with entrepreneurs and other stakeholders, we are working collectively to advance progress toward the health targets identified by the UN. In addition to working with partners directly, we work with various organizations based in Geneva and around the world to help inform governments and multilateral organizations and thus shape positive global health and policy environments.

Efforts under the umbrella of SDG 3 ("Ensuring Healthy Lives and Promoting Well-Being for All Ages") are inextricably linked to the pursuit of UHC. As such, Pfizer's efforts in pursuit of SDG 3 and their link to the biopharmaceutical industry's principles for advancing UHC warrant mention. For example, while the case study at the end of this chapter outlines specific ways that Pfizer is working toward SDG 3.8 (UHC), examples shown in table 9A.2 of the appendix illustrate how we are contributing toward specific targets under SDG 3—and how these relate to the UHC principles cited above.

For instance, as tied to the biopharmaceutical industry principle of "Choice and Inclusiveness" and in support of SDG 3 Target 2,[19] since 2014 the Pfizer Foundation has supported a program with Save the Children to improve access to childhood immunizations and family planning services for women in Malawi. The initiative provides vital newborn services like immunization, along with access to information and services in family planning for postpartum women. Through this program we have reached over 290,000 children with health and nutrition services while working with the local Ministry of Health to address barriers to family planning.[20]

Some of our other, more long-standing programs also have guiding principles that are related to the SDGs and other global initiatives (see table 9A.3 of the appendix). To promote skills-based employee investment and align with the biopharmaceutical industry principle of "Adaptability," the Global Health Fellows Program places Pfizer colleagues and teams in short-term assignments with leading international development organizations in key emerging markets. During assignments, these volunteer Fellows transfer their professional medical and business expertise in ways that promote access, quality, and efficiency of health services for people in greatest need. To date, 340 Pfizer colleagues have contributed approximately 340,000 hours of pro bono service across 44 countries.[21,22,23,24]

Quality, Sustainable UHC: Pfizer's Fight against Chronic Diseases

The chronic disease epidemic is a serious problem that is likely to grow worse, especially in LMICs but also in developed countries. Pfizer believes that chronic disease poses some of the biggest challenges in the design and implementation of UHC. Ensuring a core package of health services is available to the populations that need it is key. However, millions of people worldwide with chronic disease do not have access to lifesaving essential care because healthcare systems are not equipped to deliver these services equitably (or at all) and/or government funding is unavailable to pay for them. With "Efficiency" in mind, Pfizer believes that to reduce the burden of these conditions, all healthcare systems—not just those in LMICs—need to incorporate a holistic approach that addresses prevention, diagnosis, and treatment. This integrated approach includes multi-stakeholder partnerships, which are particularly important since many NCDs, including cancer, are caused by both genetic and environmental factors. Establishing partnerships with organizations aligned around a common goal of diminishing the impact of NCDs allows us to leverage resources and expertise in creative ways that speed progress to help patients.

With more than 30 programs in development to address chronic disease[25]—including some that focus on specific diseases like cancer and cardiovascular disease and others that address gaps in healthcare systems—Pfizer is working across a broad spectrum of programs and partnerships to achieve SDG 3.8. Two of the many important examples of how Pfizer is implementing this approach are (1) efforts to address oncology in LMICs and (2) programs to support China in addressing NCD risk factors and treat cardiovascular disease more effectively at scale.

Building Capacity and Improving Access for Cancer Patients in LMICs

Cancer is among the leading cause of morbidity and mortality in less-developed regions. Patients in poor countries often face significant barriers to quality care, including long travel distances to receive oncology care services, a shortage of trained professionals, poor equipment, and lack of information around screening and diagnosis. In stark contrast to the oncology-related resources available to patients in high-income countries, there has long been a widespread assumption that cancer will largely remain untreated in poor countries.

Groups such as the Global Task Force on Expanded Access to Cancer Care and Control in Developing Countries (GTF.CCC) are, however, challenging this notion, based on evidence that much can be done to prevent and treat cancer in poor countries by deploying primary and secondary caregivers, prescribing off-patent drugs, applying regional and global mechanisms for financing and procurement, and including cancer treatment in national health insurance coverage. Such strategies have been found to reduce costs, increase access to health services, and strengthen health systems to meet the challenge of cancer and other diseases.[26,27]

Pfizer concurs with this strategy; further, we believe that the private sector has an important role to play in advancing approaches through innovative partnerships and collaborations that catalyze innovation, advance policy, strengthen health infrastructure and financing mechanisms, and secure access to products and services. The following examples illustrate how Pfizer is helping countries achieve these goals and make progress toward UHC.

Leveraging Best Practices for Early Cancer Detection in Peru to Improve Early Diagnosis in Other LMICs

Since 2011, the international nonprofit PATH (formerly called the Program for Appropriate Technology in Health) has collaborated with Peruvian partners to implement a community-based breast cancer program in the northern region of La Libertad. The program has established a feasible, evidence-based approach to early detection at the community level and linked it to triage and diagnostic services at the network level.[28] With the Pfizer Foundation's support, PATH plans to scale up this program to reach 115,000 additional women and demonstrate that the model is replicable and sustainable. The Foundation's grant will help build healthcare worker capacity, train doctors and midwives in quality clinical breast exams, including ultrasound and fine-needle aspiration biopsy, and train volunteers as patient navigators. Pfizer-funded partnerships will explore opportunities to replicate and scale programs like these and expand access to quality oncology care services to thousands of individuals in Peru, Brazil, Rwanda, and Kenya.

Accelerating the Fight against Breast Cancer through Community Empowerment

Pfizer and the Union for International Cancer Control (UICC) joined forces to create the Seeding Progress and Resources for the Cancer Community (SPARC) Grants, an initiative aimed at empowering advocacy groups, hospital networks, support groups, and other organizations worldwide as they initiate projects to close the gap in information, support, awareness, and policy between metastatic breast cancer and early-stage breast cancer. This program will also help reduce the number of women diagnosed at the metastatic stage of breast cancer.[29]

In 2016, 20 competitively selected organizations were granted funding to implement novel and sustainable projects across 18 countries. Each organization is tailoring its activities to the needs of patients in specific countries or regions, creating diverse programming that takes a much-needed hyperlocal and grassroots approach to driving impact for breast cancer patients. To date, 3,000 patients have been reached, and 217 events have been held across 22 different countries.

Improving Access to Essential Cancer Medicines

An estimated 44% of all cancer cases in sub-Saharan Africa each year occur in Ethiopia, Nigeria, Kenya, Uganda, Rwanda, and Tanzania. Cancers such as breast and cervical cancer, which account for about 30% of cancers in the region, are highly treatable and preventable if patients are able to access the medicines and supports they need.[30,31] As part of our work with Access Accelerated[32] and in conjunction with the American Cancer Society (ACS) and the Clinton Health Access Initiative (CHAI) to improve the environment for cancer care in Africa and fortify the infrastructure, Pfizer is helping to expand access to essential medicines in cancer treatment.[33]

While the reach of this program launched in mid-2017 is not yet known, what is known is that deaths in sub-Saharan Africa remain high due to late diagnosis and lack of treatment, and deaths from cancer are expected to almost double by 2030.[34] Facilitating access to high-quality, affordable medicines is a critical step to improving cancer treatment, as are many other measures, including those facilitating access to treatment facilities and workforce shortages. Pfizer and partner organizations are committed to long-term strategies to address the many barriers to care facing cancer patients in sub-Saharan Africa.

Chronic Disease Risk Factors and Cardiovascular Treatment in China

Accelerated by rapid urbanization, industrialization, population aging, and changes in the ecological environment and lifestyles, chronic diseases in China account for 87% of all deaths and more than 70% of the total burden of disease.[35] In response to this epidemic, the Chinese government issued the "Medium-to-Long Term Plan of China for the Prevention and Treatment of Chronic Diseases (2017–2025)," which outlines strategic objectives to address chronic disease threats including, among others, control of risk factors, early diagnosis and treatment, and development of a healthy support environment.[36] One of the diseases with the highest and fastest growing incidence to be addressed by this plan is cardiovascular disease (CVD). With an estimated 8.1 million individuals in China affected by CVD in 2010, this number is predicted to nearly triple, to 22.6 million by 2030. Tobacco use, which kills more than 7 million people a year globally, is one of the leading causes of CVD (and other chronic disease). China is at the epicenter of the global tobacco health crisis, with approximately 300 million smokers and 1 million smoking-related deaths each year.[37] To address the challenges of CVD and its associated risk factors in China, Pfizer is working in cooperation with health authorities, medical communities, academics, and the media to build capacity, educate patients and providers, modernize policy, and scale successful pilot programs. Examples include:

Key Cardiovascular Risk Factor Education and Extension Program

Dyslipidemia is a major risk factor for cardiovascular disease. The dyslipidemia management initiative called KEEP (Key Cardiovascular Risk Factor Education and Extension Program) works to provide real-world evidence and advocacy for the enhancement of national policies that support comprehensive lipid screening and management in community clinics.[38] As part of KEEP, Pfizer provides grants to support widespread patient education and healthcare practitioner training across China. We are also working to encourage the government to support the incorporation of cholesterol management into national policy. By providing details of a study that underscores the disease burden, developing easy-to-implement tools, and conducting feasibility pilots, we are building a strong body of evidence to support this policy goal. To date, there have been three pilot initiatives in priority cities, including Beijing (an estimated 27,000 patients), Hangzhou (an estimated 27,000 patients), and Shenzhen (an estimated 15,000 patients). Each of these pilots implemented a program to train general practitioners on risk factors and guidelines for dyslipidemia management in cardiovascular and cerebrovascular disease to help speed diagnosis and guideline-based treatment to reduce disease progression.

The Beijing pilot program is just one example of a successful KEEP pilot: it has launched in 35 community centers and trained 500 health providers; evaluated and managed 28,000 high-cardiovascular-risk patients; and introduced comprehensive management approaches, including the Clinical

Decision Support System clinical pathway, key performance indicators, and customized training, which largely reduced repeated work for community doctors and increased standard treatment rates.[39]

China Tobacco Control Partnership

As just one of many programs to address tobacco use, Pfizer supports the China Tobacco Control Partnership (CTP), which aims to prevent the initiation of smoking, promote quitting, and eliminate exposure to secondhand smoke in five of China's largest and most influential cities (Chengdu, Chongqing, Xi'an, Xiamen, and Wuhan). The initiative also seeks to change social norms around tobacco use and to reduce its burden in these five large and influential cities, which have a combined population of almost 70 million.[40] Some of the activities include city-wide public legislation, indoor smoke-free policy implementation, training workshops, tobacco control–themed health events, large-scale World No Tobacco Day events, and cessation competitions.

Pfizer's grants build on tobacco control work conducted in China by a team of researchers from Georgia State University and Emory University that was previously funded by the Bill & Melinda Gates Foundation. The Gates-funded China Tobacco Control Partnership began in 2009 and has led to significant social norm changes and the development of extensive relationships with national and local public health leaders in both governmental and nongovernmental roles, especially through the CTP's Tobacco Free Cities initiative. To date, the partnership has resulted in (1) protection of more than 8.5 million people from secondhand smoke exposure where Smoke-Free Public Places policies were adopted; (2) delivery of health education to 6.72 million people via 1,237 health education events; and (3) adoption of 358 smoke-free policies in businesses.

Raising Public Awareness of Cholesterol Management

Since 2014, the China Public Health Media Education Program (CHEER), supported by Pfizer Independent Grants for Learning and Change (IGLC)[41] and jointly initiated by the China National Health and Family Planning Commission (NHFPC, the former Ministry of Health), the China Health Education Center, and the China Journalists Association, has built a bridge connecting government, healthcare professionals, media, people with cardiovascular diseases, and the public, in order to raise public awareness of cholesterol management. The CHEER program has been successfully conducted in 11 provinces, reaching nearly 300 million people.[42] Based on its success and contribution to public education and health, the CHEER program was recognized as a best practice of health education at the 9th Global Conference of Health Promotion in Shanghai.

Conclusion

The challenges that many countries face in achieving UHC should not be underestimated, and its promise can be seemingly elusive in countries where important gaps in health infrastructures and the health workforce, fragile economies, and high burdens of disease remain as obstacles. However, strategies including deployment of primary and secondary caregivers, use of off-patent drugs, application of regional and global mechanisms for financing and procurement, and inclusion of priority treatments in national health coverage have been found to be effective to reduce costs, increase access to health services, and strengthen health systems.[43]

Pfizer believes the private sector has both an opportunity and an obligation to support countries' move toward UHC by providing greater access to more equitable, higher quality healthcare. We can do this by sharing expertise and experience in a wide range of disciplines, such as research and development, capacity and infrastructure building, workforce training, supply chain management, education and outreach, improving access to supplies and services, and finance—all of which will improve access to healthcare supplies and services.[44]

The examples highlighted in this chapter, whether we are building capacity to improve access for cancer patients in LMICs or reducing health risks in China to effectively prevent and treat cardiovascular diseases, showcase just some of the many important ways cross-sectoral partnerships can adopt the guiding biopharmaceutical industry principles and help countries achieve equitable, quality, sustainable UHC.

APPENDIX

Table 9A.1. Biopharmaceutical industry initiatives align with Guiding Industry Principles

Industry Program*	Guiding Industry Principle
Global Alliance Vaccines and Immunization (GAVI). An international organization created to improve access to new and underused vaccines for children living in the world's poorest countries by bringing together the public and private sectors with the shared goal of creating equal access to vaccines for children. Key players include WHO, UNICEF, the World Bank, the Bill & Melinda Gates Foundation, and vaccine manufacturers such as Sanofi Pasteur, Pfizer, MSD, and GSK.	Equitable Access
Scientific Partnership for HER2 Testing Excellence. With partnership from Roche, aims to integrate testing of HER2 (an aggressive protein) of breast and gastric cancer patients at the point of disease diagnosis. Provides training in 12 Asia-Pacific countries to surgeons, lab technicians, pathologists, and oncologists on increasing reliability and reproducibility of HER2 testing.	Equitable Access
4 Healthy Habits. An innovative partnership between the International Federation of Pharmaceutical Manufacturers Associations and the International Federation of Red Cross and Red Crescent Societies, which provides information and tools to change behaviors and promotes healthy lifestyles in communities around the world to ultimately reduce the rise of NCDs. Tools have been deployed for use by the 98 Red Cross and Red Crescent National Societies worldwide, reaching more than 2.8 million beneficiaries all over the globe.	Efficiency
Global Pharma Health Fund (GPHF). A charitable organization maintained by Merck KGaA, set out to develop and supply at low cost the GPHF-Minilab, a mini-laboratory employing a set of chemical and physical tests for rapid drug quality verification and counterfeit medicines detection in low-income settings of developing countries. GPHF-Minilabs can instantly help boost medicine testing capacities in developing countries.	Quality
Young Health Program (YHP). AstraZeneca supports this program with global reach, working in partnership with over 30 expert organizations to deliver on-the-ground programs, research, and advocacy. All are focused on adolescents and preventing major noncommunicable diseases such as type 2 diabetes. Meaningful youth involvement is key to successful program delivery and achieving the desired improved health outcomes.	Choice and Inclusiveness

Industry Program*	Guiding Industry Principle
Multi-Drug Resistant Tuberculosis Technology Transfer. A long-standing initiative that has identified capable manufacturers in high-burden countries (China, India, Russia, and South Africa) and offered them, free of charge, access to know-how, technical manufacturing support, and trademarks. Lilly also identified and worked with companies in the US and Greece to provide additional capacity and supply to global markets, as well as funding to convert or upgrade facilities to meet international quality standards.	Availability
Next Billion Patients in Egypt. Sanofi supports this scheme that began in 2012, giving healthcare professionals continuous medical education to leverage skills in diagnosing and treating patients for diabetes. Access-to-medicine programs are provided to hard-to-reach patients in rural, disadvantaged areas, and a specific affordable therapeutic portfolio of low-cost chronic and acute medications is made available.	Adaptability
Global Health Innovation Technology Fund (GHIT). Five Japanese companies—Astellas, Daiichi Sankyo, Eisai, Shionogi, and Takeda—along with the Gates Foundation and the Government of Japan, established a product development fund in 2013 to facilitate R&D for neglected diseases, such as malaria, tuberculosis, and neglected tropical diseases. Grants are awarded to various projects that aim to advance the development of new health technologies such as drugs, vaccines, and diagnostics for low- and middle-income countries.	Innovation

* IFPMA Translating Principles into Practice: The Pharmaceutical Industry's Efforts toward Universal Health Coverage, 2016. https://www.ifpma.org/resource-centre/translating-principles-into-practice-the-pharmaceutical-industrys-efforts-to-work-towards-universal-health-coverage-uhc/.

Table 9A.2. Pfizer initiatives that address SDG 3 targets

Target by 2030	Pfizer Response and Progress*	Guiding Industry Principle
Target 3.1: By 2030, reduce the global maternal mortality ratio to less than 70 per 100,000 live births.	We support a program with the 2020 MicroClinic in Kenya to implement evidence-based interventions that decrease maternal and neonatal mortality and improve access to antenatal and postnatal services, including access to a skilled birth attendant.	Availability
Target 3.2: By 2030, end preventable deaths of newborns and children under five years of age, with all countries aiming to reduce neonatal mortality to at least as low as 12 per 1,000 live births and under-five mortality to at least as low as 25 per 1,000 live births.	Since 2014, the Pfizer Foundation has supported a program with Save the Children to improve access to childhood immunizations and family planning services for women in Malawi. The initiative provides vital newborn services like immunization, along with access to information and services in family planning for postpartum women. Through this program we have reached over 290,000 children with health and nutrition services while working with the local Ministry of Health to address barriers to integrating family planning services.	Choice and Inclusiveness
Target 3.5: By 2030, strengthen the prevention and treatment of substance abuse, including narcotic drug abuse and harmful use of alcohol.	We are working to help combat the opioid crisis and are committed to the manufacturing of naloxone, a prescription medicine indicated for complete or partial reversal of acute opioid over dosage. Pfizer has launched the Pfizer Naloxone Access Program, a multifaceted initiative that addresses the prevention, treatment, and effective response to the issue of opioid overdose. As part of the program, Pfizer will provide, free of charge, up to 1 million doses of naloxone between 2017 and 2020 to Direct Relief, a not-for-profit agency independent of Pfizer and licensed to distribute medicines to charitable and community clinics in all 50 states and the District of Columbia. Pfizer is also providing $1 million in charitable grants across five states to fund initiatives focused on increasing public awareness of the risks of opioid addiction.	Adaptability

Target by 2030	Pfizer Response and Progress*	Guiding Industry Principle
Target 3.7: By 2030, ensure universal access to sexual and reproductive healthcare services, including for family planning, information and education, and the integration of reproductive health into national strategies and programs.	Pfizer is engaged in a collaboration with the Bill & Melinda Gates Foundation and the Children's Investment Fund Foundation to help broaden access to Pfizer's long-acting injectable contraceptive, Sayana Press (medroxyprogesterone acetate), for women most in need in some of the world's poorest countries.	Equitable Access

* Pfizer Annual Report. https://www.pfizer.com/files/investors/financial_reports/annual_reports /2016/our-business/sustainable-development-goals-sdgs/index.html.

Table 9A.3. Select additional long-standing Pfizer initiatives that support UHC also link to Guiding Biopharmaceutical Industry Principles[a]

Engagement Type	Pfizer Program	Guiding Industry Principle
Skills-based employee investments	The Global Health Fellows Program is an international corporate volunteer program that places Pfizer colleagues and teams in short-term assignments with leading international development organizations in key emerging markets. During assignments Fellows transfer their professional medical and business expertise in ways that promote access, quality, and efficiency of health services for people in greatest need. To date, 340 Pfizer colleagues have contributed approximately 340,000 hours of pro bono service across 44 countries.[b,c,d,e]	Adaptability
Eliminating blinding trachoma	Pfizer cofounded the International Trachoma Initiative, which is a collaboration of partners, including governments, UN agencies, the Gates Foundation, World Vision, and many others, to eliminate trachoma. To date, ITI has coordinated the distribution of 650 million doses of Pfizer-donated antibiotics to help treat more than 100 million people across 33 countries globally.[f,g,h,i]	Availability
Humanitarian assistance	Pfizer colleagues around the world work collaboratively with governments, NGOs, civil service organizations, healthcare providers, and payers to enable prevention and treatment of disease by making medicines and vaccines available to as many people as possible.[j]	Availability

[a] http://www.who.int/mediacentre/news/releases/2017/ntd-report/en/.

[b] To learn more about Pfizer's Global Health Fellows, go to: https://www.pfizer.com/content/global-health-fellows-overview-0.

[c] Learning and Inspiration from 10 Years of Pfizer's Global Health Fellows Program, June 6, 2013. https://www.uschamberfoundation.org/blog/post/learning-and-inspiration-10-years-pfizer-s-global-health-fellows-program/31468.

[d] Vian, Taryn, Sarah C. Richards, Kelly McCoy, Patrick Connelly, and Frank Feeley. "Public-private partnerships to build human capacity in low income countries: findings from the Pfizer program." *Human Resources for Health* 5, no. 1 (2007): 8.

[e] Vian, Taryn, Sayaka Koseki, Frank G. Feeley, and Jennifer Beard. "Strengthening capacity for AIDS vaccine research: analysis of the Pfizer Global Health Fellows Program and the International AIDS Vaccine Initiative." *BMC Health Services Research* 13, no. 1 (2013): 378.

[f] To learn more about Pfizer's role in the International Trachoma Initiative, go to: https://www.pfizer.com/news/featured_stories/featured_stories_detail/we_refuse_to_turn_a_blind_eye_to_trachoma.

[g] Liese, Bernhard, Mark Rosenberg, and Alexander Schratz. "Programmes, partnerships, and governance for elimination and control of neglected tropical diseases." *Lancet* 375, no. 9708 (2010): 67–76.

[h] Barrett, Diana, James Austin, and Sheila McCarthy. "Cross-sector collaboration: lessons from the International Trachoma Initiative." In Michael Reich, ed., *Public-Private Partnership for Public Health* (2002): 41.

[i] Kumaresan, Jacob A., and Jeffrey W. Mecaskey. "The global elimination of blinding trachoma: progress and promise." *American Journal of Tropical Medicine and Hygiene* 69, no. 5–suppl_1 (2003): 24–28.

[j] To learn more about Pfizer's humanitarian assistance, go to: https://www.pfizer.com/purpose/medicine-access/humanitarian-aid.

NOTES

1. United Nations. http://www.un.org/sustainabledevelopment/development-agenda/.
2. Tracking universal health coverage: 2017 global monitoring report. World Health Organization and International Bank for Reconstruction and Development/World Bank, 2017.
3. Tracking universal health coverage: 2017 global monitoring report. World Health Organization and International Bank for Reconstruction and Development/The World Bank, 2017.
4. World Health Organization and World Bank. Tracking Universal Health Coverage: First Global Monitoring Report, 2015. Due to poor data, the WHO has since ceased estimating the number of people who lack access to essential medicines globally.
5. World Health Organization. Access to Medicines Index 2016. www.who.int.
6. United Nations. http://www.un.org/sustainabledevelopment/development-agenda/.
7. Tracking Universal Health Coverage: First Global Monitoring Report. World Health Organization, 2015. Ilona Kickbusch and Christian Franz have outlined these elements in chapter 1 of the present volume.
8. WHO Global Observatory. http://www.who.int/gho/ncd/mortality_morbidity/en/.
9. Global Status Report on Noncommunicable Disease. World Health Organization, 2014. www.who.int.
10. Nelson, J. Partnerships for Sustainable Development: Collective Action by Businesses, Governments, and Civil Societies to Achieve Scale and Transform Markets. Commissioned by the Business and Sustainable Development Commission, 2017. www.hks.harvard.edu/centers/mrcbg/programs/cri.
11. The United Nations Millennium Development Goals were 8 goals that all 189 UN Member States have agreed to try to achieve by the year 2015. The UN Millennium Declaration, signed in September 2000, committed world leaders to combat poverty, hunger, disease, illiteracy, environmental degradation, and discrimination against women. The MDGs were derived from this Declaration and had specific targets and indicators. The MDGs have been superseded by the Sustainable Development Goals, a set of 17 integrated and indivisible goals that build on the achievements of the MDGs but are broader, deeper, and far more ambitious in scope.
12. UNAIDS announced that the goal of 15 million people on life-saving HIV treatment by 2015 was met nine months ahead of schedule. http://www.unaids.org/en/resources/presscentre/pressreleaseandstatementarchive/2015/july/20150714_PR_MDG6report.
13. Innovative Biopharmaceutical Industry Perspectives on Universal Health Coverage: Joint Public Policy Principles Proposed by PhRMA, EFPIA, IFPMA, JPMA. March 2014. These principles were developed by biopharmaceutical industry associations including the Pharmaceutical Research and Manufacturers of America (PhRMA), European Federation of Pharmaceutical Industries and Associations (EFPIA), and Japan Pharmaceutical Manufacturers Association (JPMA), in coordination with the International Federation of Pharmaceutical Manufacturers Associations (IFPMA).
14. International Federation of Pharmaceutical Manufacturers Associations. Developing World Health Partnerships Directory. http://partnerships.ifpma.org.
15. Adapted from Mahmud, Adeeb, and Marcie Parkhurst. 2007. Expanding Economic Opportunity: The Role of Pharmaceutical Companies. Corporate Social Responsibility

Initiative Report No. 21. Cambridge, MA: Kennedy School of Government, Harvard University.

16. BSR. Working toward Transformational Health Partnerships in Low and Middle Income Countries (2012). https://www.bsr.org/reports/BSR_Working_Toward_Trans formational_Health_Partnerships.pdf.

17. https://accessaccelerated.org.

18. While initiatives such as Access Accelerated are new, engagement by biopharmaceutical companies certainly is not: select examples are highlighted in table 1 of the appendix.

19. Target 3.2: By 2030, end preventable deaths of newborns and children under five years of age, with all countries aiming to reduce neonatal mortality to at least as low as 12 per 1,000 live births and under-five mortality to at least as low as 25 per 1,000 live births.

20. Pfizer Annual Report. https://www.pfizer.com/files/investors/financial_reports/annual _reports/2016/our-business/sustainable-development-goals-sdgs/index.html.

21. To learn more about Pfizer's Global Health Fellows, see https://www.pfizer.com /content/global-health-fellows-overview-0.

22. Learning and Inspiration from 10 Years of Pfizer's Global Health Fellows Program, June 6, 2013. https://www.uschamberfoundation.org/blog/post/learning-and -inspiration-10-years-pfizer-s-global-health-fellows-program/31468.

23. Vian, Taryn, Sarah C. Richards, Kelly McCoy, Patrick Connelly, and Frank Feeley. "Public-Private Partnerships to Build Human Capacity in Low Income Countries: Findings from the Pfizer Program." *Human Resources for Health* 5, no. 1 (2007): 8.

24. Vian, Taryn, Sayaka Koseki, Frank G. Feeley, and Jennifer Beard. "Strengthening Capacity for AIDS Vaccine Research: Analysis of the Pfizer Global Health Fellows Program and the International AIDS Vaccine Initiative." *BMC Health Services Research* 13, no. 1 (2013): 378.

25. Partnering to Tackle Non-Communicable Diseases. https://www.pfizer.com/files /investors/financial_reports/annual_reports/2016/assets/pdfs/pfi2016ar -partnering-to-tackle.pdf.

26. For more information on the Global Task Force on Expanded Access to Cancer Care, see https://hgei.harvard.edu/materials/.

27. Farmer, P., et al. "Expansion of Cancer Care and Control in Countries of Low and Middle Income: A Call to Action." *Lancet*, volume 376, no. 9747 (2010): 1186–93, 2 October.

28. To learn more about the PATH program in Peru, see https://www.path.org/projects /breast-cancer.php.

29. To learn more about Pfizer's role to support women diagnosed at the metastatic stage of breast cancer, see https://www.uicc.org/what-we-do/capacity-building/grants/sparc -metastatic-breast-cancer-challenge.

30. World Health Organization. Global Health Estimates Summary Tables: Projection of Deaths by Cause, Age and Sex, by World Bank Regions. 2013. Geneva, World Health Organization.

31. International Agency for Research on Cancer. GLOBOCAN 2012: Estimated Cancer Incidence, Mortality and Prevalence Worldwide in 2012. 2014.

32. https://accessaccelerated.org/about/.
33. To learn more about Pfizer's role in collaborating to expand access to lifesaving cancer medicines in Africa, see https://www.pfizer.com/news/featured_stories/featured _stories_detail/collaborating_to_provide_lifesaving_cancer_treatments_to _patients_in_africa.
34. World Health Organization. Global Health Estimates Summary Tables: Projection of Deaths by Cause, Age and Sex, By World Bank Income Group and WHO Region. 2013. Geneva, World Health Organization. http://www.who.int/healthinfo/global_burden _disease/projections/en/.
35. China Rise Financial Holding Investment Co. (CRFH). Report on Chinese Residents' Chronic Diseases and Nutrition, updated June 2016. en.nhfpc.gov.cn.
36. Kong, Ling-Zhi. "China's Medium-to-Long Term Plan for the Prevention and Treatment of Chronic Diseases (2017–2025) under the Healthy China Initiative." *Chronic Diseases and Translational Medicine* 2017 Sep; 3(3): 135–37.
37. World Health Organization Report on Global Trends in Tobacco Smoking: 2000–2025. 2015.
38. To learn more about Pfizer's KEEP initiative, go to https://www.pfizer.com/files /investors/financial_reports/annual_reports/2016/public-health-impact/accelerating -patient-engagement/index.html.
39. KEEP is supported by the Pfizer Medical team in China through grants from Pfizer Independent Grants for Learning and Change (IGLC) and spearheaded by the International Health Exchange and Cooperating Committee of the China National Health and Family Planning Commission, formerly known as the Ministry of Health.
40. To learn more about the China Tobacco Control Partnership, go to http://ctp .publichealth.gsu.edu.
41. https://www.pfizer.com/purpose/medical-grants/independent-grants.
42. For more information on Pfizer's role in the CHEER program, go to https://www .pfizer.com/files/investors/financial_reports/annual_reports/2016/public-health -impact/accelerating-patient-engagement/index.html.
43. Farmer, Paul, et al. "Expansion of cancer care and control in countries of low and middle income: a call to action." *Lancet* 2010; 376: 1186–93.
44. IFPMA Developing World Health Partnerships Directory. http://partnerships.ifpma .org.

10

Novartis Social Business

A Novel Approach to Expanding Healthcare
in Developing Countries

Harald Nusser

Only with the full participation of the private, commercial sector can United Nations Member States achieve universal health coverage (UHC) by 2030 at the scale necessary to meet the commitments each state has made as part of the Sustainable Development Goals (SDGs) established by the UN General Assembly in 2015. Government and civil society (including nongovernmental organizations [NGOs], faith-based organizations, and community-based organizations) both have roles to play, but we cannot get over the finish line without the energy, innovation, and scale of the private sector.

The World Health Organization (WHO) states that UHC "means that all people and communities can use the promotive, preventive, curative, rehabilitative and palliative health services they need, of sufficient quality to be effective, while also ensuring that the use of these services does not expose the user to financial hardship."[1] Yet the reality looks different. An analysis by the World Bank shows that 400 million people still lacked access to essential health services in 2015.[2] The WHO estimated in July 2017 that low- and middle-income countries would require an additional $134 billion per year between now and 2025 to reach the health-related targets under the SDGs.[3] Few states can afford this spending solely from public funds.

The private sector is a major source of healthcare for the world's poor. For example, 50% of healthcare now comes from the private sector in sub-Saharan Africa (excluding South Africa), and 60% of healthcare is delivered by the private sector in low-income countries generally.[4] Of the 50% of healthcare that comes from the private sector in sub-Saharan Africa, around 65% comes from the for-profit sector.[5] It seems that most of the remaining 40% of care is provided by faith-based organizations (although these figures are controversial).[6] In some areas, such as family planning or control of parasitic infections, local and international NGOs provide services to large numbers of patients, but this contribution is not as big as some think it is.[7]

"When it comes to NCD [noncommunicable disease] care in many African countries, including Ethiopia, the private sector has a major role to play," said Ahmed Reja Goush, chair of the International Diabetes Federation, Africa Region, and president of the Ethiopian Red Cross Society. According to him, any solution must include the private health sector, since so many NCD patients in Ethiopia resort to it. "In Addis Ababa, with a population of 4 million, there are 12 government hospitals and 33 private hospitals, 30 public health centers and more than 700 private health centers," he said.[8]

The private sector needs to be a full partner with government, not an outsider. "The value and contribution that industry can bring to this process by delivering innovation, increasing access and helping to strengthen healthcare systems is being recognized more and more and the private sector must be ready to support governments in achieving UHC," a panel discussion at the UN High-Level Political Forum on the SDGs concluded in 2016.[9] It is clear that there is a major role for the private sector to help achieve UHC in low- and lower-middle-income countries (L-LMICs), but it needs innovative new models for doing so at scale and in a sustainable way over the medium and long term. A 2018 WHO High-Level Commission on NCDs called for governments to engage "with the private sector, academia, civil society and communities, building on a whole-of-society approach to NCDs."[10] This can allow them, together, to capitalize on existing and new opportunities to bring essential packages of healthcare products and services to all who need them, while minimizing financial risk.

Private sector health companies cannot operate in a vacuum. During the World Economic Forum 2018, Novartis, Philips, and others hosted a roundtable discussion on new blended financing partnerships to unlock investment in global health. These blended investments and business models can help ensure the availability of sustainable financing and resources while maintaining a focus on the world's poorest communities.

Novartis: Twenty-First-Century Approaches

It is taking time for solutions to emerge, but the concerns were clear at the turn of the century. This prompted Novartis executives to start thinking about novel approaches to tackle both infectious and chronic diseases and to start partnering with public and private stakeholders and building health-care capacity on the ground. That vision first came to fruition in 2001 with the advent of the Novartis Malaria Initiative, which has become one of the pharmaceutical industry's largest access-to-medicine (AtM) programs.

Novartis also began thinking about moving beyond philanthropy to a more commercial approach for making critical drugs accessible to people in L-LMICs in a sustainable way. In 2005, management thinker C. K. Prahalad challenged the Novartis Executive Committee to do more to reach large numbers of the poor living in developing countries and encouraged them to develop a profitable way of serving those at "the bottom of the pyramid."[11] Such outside evaluations are often disruptive; they require rethinking established approaches and often lead management to invest attention in meeting challenges that had been ignored. They can also lead to positive change.

It is becoming clear that there must be a shift from philanthropy to reach more people with health products and services at scale. We need partnerships that put the unique skills of the private sector to work for these large numbers of people with innovative models of prevention and treatment. Meeting the SDGs now calls for new kinds of programs, many of which are designed to work at large scale and to provide medicines for diseases that are usually lifelong. So Novartis has been thinking about how to evolve its access programs to meet both the continuing demands of communicable diseases and the new demands that arise from NCDs in a sustainable way. To that end, Novartis launched Healthy Family in 2007 as a way of meeting Prahalad's challenge. More than a decade of learning from both the Malaria Initiative and the Healthy Family initiative informed the creation of Novartis Access (NA) in 2015. All three programs are now part of Novartis Social Business.

Novartis Social Business

Today, Novartis offers a variety of models that reach patients at all levels of the income pyramid. It is working toward making social business a central component of its access approach in a way that is scalable and replicable. To be sustainable, a social business must be a business: it needs to generate profit, even if it is modest. Initiatives that require continuing philanthropy are vulnerable to future competition for limited corporate resources or to belt-tightening in times of business challenges; those that make a contribution to net revenues are far more likely to survive, whatever the economic climate or the shifts in charitable trends. Profits make businesses scalable, bringing benefits to more and more people.

Because Novartis is a business, much of the data on investment, costs, and return on investment will remain confidential, because it could be misused by competitors seeking to set prices and margins in relation to those of another company rather than competing in an open marketplace. Making business data publicly available could be seen as a way of Novartis "telegraphing" its costs and intentions to other companies in order to limit their future competition.

A 10-year report on Novartis Healthy Family[12] reported that "Arogya Parivar broke even in less than three years and has been sustainable ever since, meeting both its commercial and social targets." The Vietnam program, launched in 2012, "broke even in 2015 and has been profitable ever since." This three-year window to profitability may thus be seen as something of a benchmark.

Novartis is applying the following framework to reach more patients:

- High and upper-middle income: Original brands, generics, patient assistance programs, and supply in response to competitive tenders (invitations for bids) issued by large health providers
- Middle and low income: Generics, differential pricing, Novartis Social Business, tenders, patient assistance programs, and strategic philanthropy
- Poor: Donations, strategic philanthropy, and tenders

The most important access-to-medicines programs are within the social business unit.

Novartis Malaria Initiative

The first attempt by Novartis to provide sustainable access solutions was the Novartis Malaria Initiative (NMI) in 2001. Through an agreement with the WHO, Novartis was the first healthcare company to commit to the supply of antimalarial treatments to the public sector of malaria-endemic countries without profit.[13] The supply is important but, equally important, Novartis committed to help promote prevention and to work to understand disease pathways.

The NMI has become one of the healthcare industry's largest AtM programs. A Harvard Business School case study noted in 2008: "Across the developing world, malaria was not only spreading, but also mutating dangerously, with deadly new variants appearing in both South America and Thailand in the 1990s. By 2001, similar mutations—resistant to all of the commonly available malaria drugs—had spread into Africa as well, threatening to ignite a virtual epidemic."[14] The case study describes the Novartis agreement with the WHO and the challenges of scaling up production of the antimalarial drug Coartem, from fewer than 100,000 doses in 2001.

This scale-up was complicated, because the entire production cycle for Coartem starts with planting the seeds of *Artemisia annua* (wormwood), the raw material for an important component. From that point to packaging the drug typically took around 14 months. It takes several hundred kilograms of *Artemisia annua* to produce just 4 kilograms of artemisinin, so Novartis needed to develop expertise and relationships in the cultivation of vast numbers of wormwood plants. Novartis has now sold more than 850 million Coartem treatments at cost and devised innovative strategies for getting treatment to patients, contributing to a significant reduction in the malaria death toll. Coartem was the first fixed-dose artemisinin-based combination therapy (ACT) to be brought to market.

Many of those in malaria-affected communities rely on the private sector to supply fixed-dose ACT. However, sometimes the poorest found it unaffordable, and sometimes medicine sellers found it more profitable to supply potentially ineffective monotherapies. To tackle this, Novartis worked with the Global Fund to Fight AIDS, Tuberculosis and Malaria to expand access to ACTs through a form of innovative financing, the co-payment mechanism. According to the Global Fund, "The model leverages Global Fund–negotiated ACT prices and further reduces the price to pharmaceutical importers in participating countries through a co-payment made by the Global Fund directly to manufacturers on their behalf. Country-led supporting interventions, such as large-scale mass communications around treatment seeking for malaria, are instrumental in rapid and large changes in price, availability and market share of quality-assured ACTs."[15]

Stock-outs and bottlenecks in distribution are a long-standing problem in assuring access and preventing the emergence of resistance. In 2016, Novartis launched a technology-based healthcare program called SMS for Life 2.0 in Kaduna State, Nigeria (discussed in more detail below). This enhanced program uses smartphones and tablet computers to enable local healthcare workers to track stock levels of antimalarials, other medicines, and vaccines, and send notifications to district medical officers when stock levels are low. The program also allows health systems to monitor disease surveillance and to train healthcare workers using on-demand e-learning modules. This program became an important part of delivery of medicines to combat NCDs in Pakistan.

Novartis Healthy Family

In 2007, Novartis launched Arogya Parivar (AP; "Healthy Family" in Hindi) to provide access to healthcare for people living in India's rural and remote areas. Although it is coordinated with public sector provision, the program does not rely on it.

AP is a social business model that uses a market-based approach to deliver healthcare. It is organized into 239 cells, each of which covers 35–40 square kilometers and includes 60 to 75 villages and small towns with 180,000 to 200,000 in each jurisdiction. In 2017, about 7.4 million people attended at least one of almost 150,000 health education meetings held in India. The program operates across 11 states, covering some 16,000 villages and small towns with a total population of 70 million.[16,17]

The social arm of the program deploys a team of health educators in each cell. The health educators work closely with village leaders and the local accredited social health activists[18] and government Anganwadi health workers. Together they teach and host meetings. Doctors provide screening, diagnosis, and therapies at the health camps. This integrates prevention into daily life and creates awareness ripples of disease recognition and treatment. The AP health educators raise awareness about health conditions and promoting health-seeking behaviors. They receive regular training and use storytelling to get key messages across in a compelling way.

The commercial arm of the scheme assigns a sales supervisor to each cell. The sales supervisors interact with distributors, pharmacists, and doctors to ensure that medicines are available. They play an essential role in ensuring a sustainable supply of medicines, which will help build a viable future business for Novartis. The supervisors also persuade doctors to participate in AP screenings and workshops. On average, a sales supervisor travels 80–90 kilometers a day and meets 11 doctors and 7 pharmacists. The strategy relies on Novartis products being available in the same areas in which the health educators are working, but there is no attempt to promote Novartis medicines during AP activities.

AP is a program that has been built on learning by doing. A 2013 Harvard Business School case study detailed many of the changes that happened in just the pilot phase. The authors reported, "The pilot product portfolio . . . required alteration. The national disease burden data gathered to inform product selection proved irrelevant to local needs. The Indian government provided free TB [tuberculosis] medicine and care across India, for example, eliminating commercial demand for Novartis TB drugs. Product packaging also became problematic. For instance, antibiotic tablets might come packaged individually on a blister pack strip containing a full weeklong course of treatment (i.e., 14 tablets). For villagers without funds for the full course, pharmacists would slice off and sell a single day's dose at a time. This encouraged patients to take medicine only until they began to feel better, encouraging the emergence of drug-resistant pathogens."[19] The attitude of those running AP is to look for shortcomings in the program and to think of better ways of meeting Prahalad's challenge.

The AP model is based on the six "A's of access":

- Awareness: Do patients understand that they have a disease that can be treated/managed?
- Adaptability: Is the medicine relevant to the patient's needs and the healthcare system used by the patient?
- Availability: Is the medicine available in a place that is convenient for the patient?
- Affordability: Can the patient afford to pay for the medicine?
- Adherence: Is the patient willing and able to take the medicines as needed?
- Alliances: Are all the right partners engaged in delivering this solution for patients?

AP offers more than 100 effective, affordable medications against communicable and NCDs prevalent in rural India.[20] The program employs around 500 people and works with more than 60,000 doctors, pharmacists, and distributors. Plans are under way to add more NCD screening and care and to add the Novartis Access portfolio to AP because of the rising incidence of chronic conditions such as hypertension and diabetes in rural India.

In 2017, almost 7.4 million people attended more than 149,000 AP health education meetings; over 9,200 camps were attended by a total of 398,000 people, 102,000 of whom saw a doctor afterward. The program is expected to reach 44 million people through health education meetings and health camps by 2022.

To ensure the long-term sustainability of the social arm of the work, health educators are being trained in communication, self-administration, leadership, and fundraising, so they can continue providing health education independently of the Novartis program when their areas "graduate" from AP. This approach is being piloted in 11 cells in Andhra Pradesh. Novartis calls this its "social legacy transfer strategy" and hopes to use it to introduce AP to new areas with high unmet need for healthcare, once existing cells are securely in place.

To support the ongoing development of rural physicians who volunteer for the program, doctors are offered extra training and links to specialized physicians to provide mentorship. AP is also now piloting and expanding its model to urban factory workers in a partnership with apparel company Levi Strauss & Co. and its supplier Aquarelle Clothing Ltd. To bring healthcare services to remote communities, AP has worked with Tech Mahindra, an information technology (IT) provider, to develop an online platform linking villagers to physicians in primary healthcare facilities.

The AP program in India builds a solid base for healthcare and also contributes to Novartis's future in the growing Indian market. It is thus considered to be a classic win-win program. Thanks to strong economic growth and rising incomes, India's base of the pyramid is expected to shrink significantly, from 379 million adults in 2015 to 145 million adults in 2030, according to Euromonitor International, a leading independent provider of strategic market research.[21] Companies targeting the Indian base of the pyramid need a long-term strategy that focuses on building brand loyalty in order to retain these consumers after they have exited the base of the pyramid, according to Euromonitor.

Expansion of Healthy Family

In 2010, Novartis began to look beyond India for new places to initiate its social business model. It calculated that between 1 billion and 2 billion people in 67 countries occupied the same layer of the income pyramid that AP had begun to serve in India. Using a multistep process, it narrowed the list of possible future sites to Kenya, Vietnam, and Indonesia based on social need, market attractiveness, and Novartis's existing capabilities. Novartis decided to give each new program a name corresponding to "healthy family" in each country's local language.

In Vietnam, Cùng Sông Khòe (CSK) was launched in 2012 as a public-private partnership in 23 provinces of the northern and Mekong regions. Together with doctors in community health centers, CSK educates rural people about prevention of several prevalent conditions including diabetes, hypertension, respiratory infections, malaria, and diarrhea, as well as hand, food, and mouth diseases. In 2016, CSK collaborated with the Vietnam Cardiology Foundation to address chronic diseases with diagnostic camps and training of doctors. In 2017 alone, 772 physicians from district and community health centers were trained in the diagnosis and treatment of hypertension and diabetes. Since the launch of CSK, more than 1 million people have either received health education or health screening. The program became self-sustaining in 2015.

In Kenya, Familia Nawiri (FN) was launched in 2012 to improve accessibility and availability of medicines and doctors across nine counties. FN collaborates with the Ministry of Health and invites government community health workers to its events to conduct their own outreach efforts. In the 3 years up to the end of 2017, about 473,000 people attended health education meetings. To cater to the needs of the urban poor, FN is conducting pilot programs with World Friends in four informal urban settlements around Nairobi. Nestlé is partnering with FN to bring health information and care to coffee farmers, in a system that allows farmers to access healthcare services when they need them, even if they have no cash on hand. Finally, FN teamed up with Novartis Access (NA) (see below) to raise disease awareness and diagnose chronic diseases. FN became self-sustaining in 2017.

In contrast, the effort in Indonesia never took off, partly because the program only had one product to offer and also because Novartis operations on the ground were lacking.

Novartis Access

The four main types of NCDs—cardiovascular diseases, diabetes, respiratory diseases, and cancers—are among the leading causes of death in L-LMICs. NCDs kill 40 million people each year, equivalent to 70% of all deaths globally. Each year, 15 million people between the ages of 30 and 69 die from an NCD; over 80% of these "premature" deaths occur in low- and middle-income countries.[22] From 2011 to 2025, cumulative economic losses due to NCDs under a "business as usual" scenario in low- and middle-income countries have been estimated at US$ 7 trillion.[23] Mental illness and substance abuse disorders also contribute substantially to the loss of healthy life, affecting all countries regardless of their socioeconomic status.[24] NCDs typically strike people in poor countries at a younger age than in wealthy countries; as a result, the effect on productive capacity is even higher than it is in Europe or North America, according to a 2010 report.[25] This impact should be an important part of the rationale for more investment in health services by L-LMICs.

In response, NA was launched in Kenya in 2015. It offers a portfolio of 15 on- and off-patent medicines[26] to provide better care for patients living with one or more of four kinds of NCD. The portfolio of medicines is offered as a basket to governments, NGOs, and other institutional customers at a price of US $1 per treatment per month. NA also works with faith-based health providers such as the Christian Health Association of Kenya (CHAK) and the Kenya Conference of Catholic Bishops (KCCB) to improve prevention and diagnostic capability. In a separate program to improve cancer treatment, Novartis is working with the American Society for Clinical Pathology to upgrade cancer diagnostic capacity in a number of East African countries.

The NA portfolio includes products selected for medical relevance: they are either on the WHO's Model List of Essential Medicines or belong to the most frequently prescribed medicines in these disease areas. For each disease, the aim is to offer various treatment options, including proven and standard first-line treatments, as well as some of the latest treatment options. From the list of the 107 countries in the scope of the *Access to Medicine Index*,[27] Novartis identified 30 countries where NA could have the greatest impact; all of these countries lack AtM programs and suffer from a high NCD burden.

In Kenya, NA coordinates its activities with the Ministry of Health. NA products are currently available through the networks of health facilities of the CHAK and the KCCB. The Mission for Essential Drugs and Supplies provides a reliable stock of essential medicines and medical supplies of good quality at affordable prices to over 1,800 public and private health facilities in Kenya and acts as the distributor for NA. A total of 10 counties (of 47 counties in Kenya) and 249 faith-based facilities were distributing the products at the end of 2017. NA also works with the Kenya Red Cross Society to deliver NCD care for 80,000 refugees in two refugee camps.

NA is working in a number of other countries as well, in Africa and in other parts of the world. Rwanda was one of the first countries to sign a memorandum of understanding to implement NA (a portfolio tender was awarded in 2017). There are partners in that country—including faith-based organizations and NGOs—that can carry out screening programs. NA workshops support capacity building in the area of clinical research. Also in 2017, NA was launched in Cameroon, and the first treatments were delivered in June of that year. The country has one of the highest rates of NCDs in sub-Saharan Africa, and chronic diseases cause 31% of deaths.[28] Initially, NA drugs were available through the 88 hospitals and clinics of the Cameroon Baptist Convention Health Services (CBCHS), spread across 6 of the country's 10 regions. The program will be extended to other faith-based organizations and eventually the whole country through public facilities.

Novartis signed a memorandum of understanding with the Ugandan Ministry of Health, complementing the government's efforts to improve NCD care. The country has already established dedicated NCD units with heart, lung, and cancer institutes. The ministry also provides funding to the private not-for-profit sector, through the Joint Medical Store (JMS), to improve healthcare provision (NA medicines are to be distributed through JMS). Novartis has also entered into a partnership with the Uganda Protestant Medical Bureau—one of the largest faith-based organizations in the country—to carry out capacity-building and screening programs in 2018. Village health committees can raise awareness about and screen for basic NCDs such as high blood pressure, providing an early warning and referral system to appropriate levels of care.

Finally, NA was also launched in Pakistan in 2017. It has signed an agreement with the federal government to provide medicines under the

Prime Minister's National Health Insurance Program, in which 1 million families are already enrolled. Patients will receive the medicines at no charge, while the government has agreed on a purchase price with Novartis that includes both the medicines and tracking and support services. NA has also contracted with the government of Punjab, the most populous province in Pakistan. In Punjab, medicines will be provided free of charge to poor patients through the public health system. The program aims to serve over 3 million people within a few years. These medicines will be purchased by the provincial government. Again, tracking and support services are part of the agreement.

NA needs to ensure that the Pakistan program reaches the right patients and that impact can be measured using key indicators. To address these challenges, NA has entered into a partnership with a technology company to develop an IT system to register patients and track medicines dispensed. This will provide essential, anonymized data to enable accurate stock management from warehouse to dispensing pharmacies. The system will be implemented first in Punjab province, using biometric information to ensure medicines reach eligible patients.

Beyond access to medicines, NA also has activities to strengthen healthcare systems. For example, it trains healthcare professionals on diabetes and hypertension management and provides community education and awareness raising. This ensures patients are referred into the formal healthcare sector appropriately.

In Cameroon, Novartis and the CBCHS have kicked off a Know Your Numbers campaign (expected to eventually reach 1 million persons) to encourage people to know their critical health numbers, while in Kenya, Novartis has formed a partnership with health authorities to develop NCD training curricula and treatment guidelines. In the field of cancer care, the company has started collaborating with two organizations—the American Society for Clinical Pathology and the American Cancer Society—across Ethiopia, Tanzania, Uganda, and Rwanda to strengthen the continuum of care for cancer patients.

When it launched Novartis Access in Kenya, the company commissioned Boston University (BU) to conduct an extensive baseline study, which was to be followed by an assessment of impact (detailed below). The baseline data, available about 18 months after the program was launched, gave important guidance on how the program should be developed. For example, the BU team found that half of those studied who knew they had asthma did not have medicines at home. This was perhaps unsurprising, but the details suggested needs that had not been identified before. Of those who did have medicine, many had tablets, not the inhalers recommended by international treatment guidelines. Although most had had their asthma diagnosed in the public sector, most were now obtaining treatment through private sector pharmacies.[29] In looking at overall access to medicines for a group of chronic diseases, the BU authors stated, "households in the poorest wealth quintile reported spending US$7.65 per month on medicines, while households in the least poor wealth quintile reported spending more than twice that amount (US$15.93)." Most surprising of all was that "among patients who had . . . [a] salbutamol inhaler (100 μg) in their home, those in the poorest quintile were least likely to have received the medicine free of charge."[30]

The BU impact data for NA are not yet available, but we do have some indications about reach and uptake. By the end of 2017, NA had reached 398,330 patients with NA products and provided 809,666 monthly treatments. Drug submissions to regulatory authorities for special NA packs are ongoing, with 221 already approved and 502 submitted in 24 countries. NA is losing money right now, but its low margins are offset by increasingly high volumes, which should enable it to become a contributor to net earnings in the coming years. This will ensure the continuity of its programs.

Measuring Health Outcomes

Health companies have had long experience in measuring inputs (how many dollars they invest) and outputs (how many treatments they ship or how many doctors they train, for example). Yet companies have not demonstrated the same agility in measuring health outcomes and impact, even though this is the most meaningful way to evaluate public health programs. Companies have to try to isolate the impact of their efforts from new prevention programs, service strengthening initiatives, care pilots, and other interventions, which may change the baseline against which company efforts are measured. This is particularly true of AtM programs.[31] Past measurement efforts have almost always occurred after the event, when a program decides to evaluate its efforts at the end of the project. The problem with this is that you do not know what the situation was at the beginning and how it has changed. There is also usually no control group, so the evaluations tend to be weak even when the best interventions have taken place, in part because the improvements might be due to existing factors that can't be separated from the impact of the intervention itself.

Good prospective research would enable policy makers to decide whether to continue or expand support for programs; it would enable healthcare providers to assess how well they are fulfilling their mandates, and it would allow healthcare professionals to assess the impact of their work. It has also allowed Novartis to adapt programs as they are expanded (see above). Perhaps most of all, it would give opinion leaders and voters evidence that they can use in holding governments and private firms to account.

An agreement with Novartis led to Boston University (BU) researchers publishing a study in *Health Affairs*[32] that found that the number of AtM initiatives had grown from 17 in 2000 to 102 in 2015, yet published evaluations existed for only 7 of them. From those 7 evaluations, the researchers found 47 articles that met their inclusion criteria for evidence and had been published in peer-reviewed journals. However, they found that 6% of those evaluations were of moderate quality, 62% were low quality, and 32% were very low quality. None of them were found to be of high quality.[33] The bottom line of the *Health Affairs* report was: "Overall, our findings suggest that current efforts to evaluate the impact of industry-led access-to-medicines initiatives are inadequate." Under their agreement, Novartis decided to fund a new kind of transparent, double-blind research by BU. Although it is paying for the evaluation, Novartis has no control over the evaluation process; BU publishes protocols, agreements, and all the results (positive or negative) on a website for all to see.[34]

The study protocol, published on *BMJ Open*,[35] states that the study will be a cluster-randomized controlled trial in eight randomly selected counties in Kenya. In intervention counties, public and private nonprofit health facilities will be able to order NA NCD medicines. Data will be collected from a random sample of 384 health facilities and 800 households for a baseline, after a year's intervention (the "midline" report), and after two years (the "endline"). Quarterly surveillance data will also be collected from health facilities and a subsample of households through phone-based interviews. The primary outcomes will be availability and price of NCD medicines at health facilities and availability, price, and expenditures on NCD medicines at households.

BU has posted the baseline data for the evaluation of NA online.[36] The BU team will provide insights into how heart disease, diabetes, cancer, and asthma affect Kenyans and whether NA has improved the situation. However, other researchers can query the entire database in any way they wish, to conduct their own analyses or as a contribution to future work.

Novartis has commissioned the evaluation for six reasons:

1. To develop and share methodology
2. To provide additional market and epidemiological data to help guide the program
3. To establish a monitoring and surveillance framework
4. To measure the change in availability of medicines at facility and household levels
5. To measure the change in price at outlets
6. To collect information about knowledge and opinions

According to Richard Laing (a professor at the BU School of Public Health who is working on the evaluation), programs offering low-priced products—not just medicines but also food or fuel—tend to benefit middle-income people, who know how to access the medicines and appropriate treatment, instead of the poorest people the programs are trying to reach. For this reason, Novartis is keen to find out what happens to the 15 medicines at the household level, especially with low-income families. The insights are expected to be so comprehensive that Novartis plans to use this research model as a basis for future evaluations in other places where it introduces NA. Novartis expects future evaluations to be simpler and more affordable because the results of the evaluation will show where to focus.

Novartis believes this evaluation methodology has the potential to be used by other pharmaceutical companies to measure their AtM programs. Since BU is posting all of the protocols and methodologies on its website, anyone can easily adapt the model to their own needs. It has already informed the development of a measurement and evaluation model being developed by the Access Accelerated initiative, a collaborative effort by 23 member companies of the International Federation of Pharmaceutical Manufacturers.[37] Furthermore, Novartis aims to apply the framework it developed with BU for NA to monitor and evaluate Healthy Family's impact on health, starting with India.

Challenges to Overcome

Throughout the expansion of each program, Novartis has come to believe that it has tended to underestimate the importance of the private sector in providing care and has committed to integrating it into many new and existing programs at a faster pace. For example, the decision to distribute NA medicines through public and faith-based channels was made early on to ensure that treatment reached the intended populations at prices they could afford. However, results from the BU baseline study conducted in Kenya revealed certain flaws in that logic: While more than 50% of chronic diseases are diagnosed in the public sector, over 40% of the patients actually buy their medicine in the private, for-profit sector.[38]

In addition, Novartis underestimated the paradigm shift its portfolio approach in NA would require in countries' medicines procurement systems and regulations. Moving from itemized sourcing to portfolio procurement continues to be the biggest hurdle for countries in adopting NA. Decentralization of procurement in many countries causes delays; there may be a memorandum of understanding with the central government, but it is local authorities that decide what to buy and how. Central government may need to develop new ways of issuing tenders for a basket of medicines instead of for individual products; this has been an extended process in both Ethiopia and Rwanda.

Access to medicines is necessary for better health services, but it is not sufficient: other frameworks need to be in place as well for such a program to succeed. These include up-to-date essential medicines lists and treatment guidelines. Novartis has also had to counter skepticism from external stakeholders that its commitment will not be long term and concern from internal colleagues regarding the potential risk of harming its core business in developing countries. Much progress has been made in this regard, and people increasingly understand that most of the Novartis social businesses have been designed to become scalable and fully self-supporting over time.

In many discussions about healthcare, the word *disruption* keeps coming up.[39] However, social business is more like the catalytic innovation that Christensen and colleagues described in 2006:

Catalytic innovations challenge organizational incumbents by offering simpler, good-enough solutions aimed at underserved groups. Unlike disruptive innovations, though, catalytic innovations are focused on creating social change. Catalytic innovators are defined by five distinct qualities. First, they create social change through scaling and replication. Second, they meet a need that is either overserved (that is, the existing solution is more complex than necessary for many people) or not served at all. Third, the products and services they offer are simpler and cheaper than alternatives, but recipients view them as good enough. Fourth, they bring in resources in ways that initially seem unattractive to incumbents. And fifth, they are often ignored, put down, or even encouraged [sic] by existing organizations, which don't see the catalytic innovators' solutions as viable.[40]

For the innovation that is social business to achieve its potential, companies must work with countries to leapfrog the current healthcare paradigm, moving from traditional transactional management approaches to more integrated solutions. All partners need to accept that they might fail as they search for solutions together. And all need to look actively for lessons from experience which may call for radical changes to the established business models.

Improvements in Access to Medicines

Progress in improving access is increasingly measured against an international benchmark. The Access to Medicine Foundation[41] was founded in 2003 with the idea of encouraging the pharmaceutical industry to do more to help the world's poorest people access the medicine they need. Since 2008, the Foundation has published the *Access to Medicine Index*, which independently ranks pharmaceutical companies' efforts to improve access to medicine in developing countries. The *Index*, funded by the Bill & Melinda Gates Foundation and the United Kingdom, the Netherlands, and other donors, is published every two years. The 2016 report found "moderate progress" in the pharmaceutical industry's efforts to improve access to medicines. All companies surveyed had improved in at least one measure. (Novartis was ranked third overall and first for general access to medicines management.) The Foundation found that the four top-ranked companies all "invest in R&D for urgently needed products, even where commercial incentives are lacking. Their access strategies support commercial objectives, with clear business rationales."[42]

The *Index* also identified four key findings:

1. Collaborative research models appear effective in engaging the industry in developing urgently needed products with low commercial potential. The top 20 pharmaceutical companies are developing 420 products, including 151 with "low commercial potential but which are urgently needed." Nearly three-quarters of these products are being developed by six companies (GSK, AbbVie, Johnson & Johnson, Sanofi, Novartis, and Merck KGaA).

2. Good practice in making products affordable and available is limited. The companies generally do not target populations with the highest needs in their registration, pricing, and licensing actions. The *Index* found that companies have tried to register their newest products in only a quarter of a list of priority countries developed by the *Index*. However, there were some notable exceptions (Novartis, Novo Nordisk, and Gilead).

3. Companies increasingly view access to medicines as a way to develop their business in emerging markets. These companies identify where access strategies support the bottom line. Half of the companies in the *Index* have set clear access-related goals linked to global health targets, such as the SDGs.

4. Six companies (AstraZeneca, GSK, Johnson & Johnson, Merck & Co., Inc., Merck KGaA, and Novartis) are using capacity-building activities to address independently prioritized gaps. These companies are doing this in R&D, manufacturing, supply chain management, and drug safety. They work with governments, NGOs, and others, often in formal partnerships, to understand where action is most needed.

These findings highlight the potential of well-designed initiatives from the pharmaceutical industry, but those initiatives cannot thrive in a vacuum. To achieve the leapfrog effect, industry initiatives must be part of integrated partnerships with fast-evolving health systems.

"Smart" Programs

In some countries, it may be necessary for governments to extensively reform health systems that were designed to deal with acute illness. Because of the massive external assistance needed to address such health issues as AIDS, malaria, and tuberculosis, many countries have developed vertical health programs that tend to deal with specific health issues in isolation. We need more horizontal and patient-centric programs that are able to treat patients with different conditions at the same time.

Appropriate technology can help build integrated and efficient systems. In many resource-constrained countries, supply chain problems make it difficult to get essential medicines and commodities to patients in a timely way, particularly in remote areas.[43] In an attempt to help address this challenge, Novartis launched SMS for Life[44] in 2009 to prevent stock-outs of antimalarial drugs in Tanzania, and it has since been rolled out in more than 10,000 public health facilities in Cameroon, Kenya, Ghana, and the Democratic Republic of Congo. To build on the success of this program, an enhanced version, SMS for Life 2.0, was launched in 2016 in Nigeria to help health workers use smartphones and tablets to track stock levels of essential antimalarials, vaccines, and treatments for HIV, TB, and leprosy. The system sends notifications to district medical officers when stock levels are low and also allows for disease monitoring for malaria, maternal and infant deaths, and seven other diseases. Furthermore, it improves training of health workers at remote locations using on-demand e-learning modules. Beyond Nigeria, SMS for Life 2.0 is planned for deployment in 500 health facilities in Zambia.

Partnerships with the Private Sector: A Critical Element in UHC

Novartis now has differentiated approaches to target different income segments of the population. These include generics; Novartis Social Business (the NMI, Healthy Family, NA, SMS for Life, and other elements); and donations and strategic philanthropy. Many other Novartis programs, within R&D and in the company's various regions, are also working on access.

C. K. Prahalad's challenge to the Novartis board of directors could have become just one more discussion of apparently intractable challenges. Instead, it sped up changes already under way at Novartis, and it has now helped lead to initiatives serving millions of people. Within the company, new ideas on access are welcomed and nurtured, in particular those that can be turned into contributors to net revenues. These profits will never be a major part of the return to investors; instead, profits mean that initiatives like

NA will not get passed by on the basis that they would be a drain on the corporate bottom line—one that would need to be justified. Just as important, successful initiatives will be able to grow quickly to their full potential because expansion will not mean higher costs to the company without an accompanying contribution to income. Indeed, NA may be a model both for future undertakings at Novartis and for efforts by other corporations.

The Novartis programs are also aligned with Prahalad's vision because all involve partnerships (with NGOs, faith-based groups, for-profit concerns, and governments) and assume that people at the base of the pyramid will embrace innovation that delivers results that these communities find worthwhile. The programs aim to link communities to health systems and to provide pathways that can be followed as families in L-LMICs become more financially secure.

The global community is still in the early stages of the journey in social business. There is no single solution to improving access to medicines. However, the NMI, Healthy Family, NA, and other programs offer compelling examples of how the pharmaceutical industry can partner with others to overcome access issues in L-LMICs. Many—perhaps most—of the new ideas will not have the impact their designers had hoped they would. Some will fail. Rigorous measurement is needed to ensure that the things that do not work are dropped and those that do work are given more resources. All of those working in global health must acknowledge the failures and learn from them. At the same time, momentum can only be built and maintained if there is generous sharing of success and clear accounts of how success was achieved. Honesty and transparency are critical. The private sector must share experiences frankly and publicly, even if its inclination is to treat the data as proprietary. If it does not, there will be redundant efforts and lost opportunities for synergy and efficiency.

If the private sector seizes the opportunities and partners effectively with the public sector and others in the private sector, it can scale up the fight against infectious disease, manage the growing incidence of NCDs in an increasingly sustainable way, and become a critical partner in achieving UHC.

NOTES

1. World Health Organization, "Health financing: What Is Universal Coverage?" http://www.who.int/health_financing/universal_coverage_definition/en/.

2. World Health Organization, "New Report Shows That 400 Million Do Not Have Access to Essential Health Services," Joint World Health Organization/World Bank news release, 12 June, 2015. http://www.who.int/mediacentre/news/releases/2015/uhc -report/en/.

3. Jenny Lei Ravelo, "Here's How Much Is Needed to Meet SDGs' Global Health Targets by 2030," Devex, https://www.devex.com/news/here-s-how-much-is-needed-to-meet -sdgs-global-health-targets-by-2030-90693.

4. Private email from Results for Development based on the most recently available data from national health accounts of 23 sub-Saharan African countries, November 2017.

5. According to data drawn from the World Health Organization Global Health Expenditures Database, last modified February 12, 2018, http://apps.who.int/nha/database.

6. Rose Calnin Kagawa, Andrew Anglemyer, and Dominic Montagu, "The Scale of Faith Based Organization Participation in Health Service Delivery in Developing Countries: Systemic Review and Meta-Analysis," *PLOS ONE* 7, no. 11 (2012): e48457.

7. Oona Campbell, Lenka Benova, D. Macleod, C. Goodman, K. Footman, A. L. Pereira, and C. A. Lynch, "Who, What, Where: An Analysis of Private Sector Family Planning Provision in 57 Low- and Middle-Income Countries," *Tropical Medicine and International Health* 20, no. 12 (December 2015): 1639–56.

8. "Exploring the Future of Access to Healthcare in Lower-Income Countries," panel discussion at the third Novartis Social Business stakeholder dialogue, November 21, 2017, Basel, Switzerland, https://www.novartis.com/news/exploring-future-access -healthcare-lower-income-countries.

9. "How Can the Private Sector Support Universal Health Coverage to Help Deliver on the Promise to Leave No One Behind?" Panel discussion during the UN High-Level Political Forum on the Sustainable Development Goals, July 13, 2016, https://sustain abledevelopment.un.org/index.php?page=view&type=20000&nr=492&menu =2993.

10. World Health Organization, "Time to Deliver: Report of the WHO Independent High-Level Commission on Noncommunicable Diseases" (Geneva: WHO, 2018).

11. Coimbatore Krishnarao Prahalad, *The Fortune at the Bottom of the Pyramid: Eradicating Poverty through Profits* (Delhi: Pearson Education India, 2004).

12. Novartis Healthy Family 2017 10-Year Report, December 2017, https://www.novartis .com/sites/www.novartis.com/files/2017-healthy-family-report.pdf.

13. Novartis, "The Novartis Malaria Initiative: Committed to Malaria Control and Elimination," 2016.

14. Deborah Spar and Brian Delacey, *The Coartem Challenge* (Boston: Harvard Business School, 2008).

15. The Global Fund, "Antimalarial Medicines," https://www.theglobalfund.org/en /sourcing-management/health-products/antimalarial-medicines.

16. Novartis, "Healthy Family: Connecting Business Success with Social Progress: 10 Years on the Ground (Preliminary Version)," November 2017, https://www.novartis.com /sites/www.novartis.com/files/2017-healthy-family-report.pdf.

17. Arogya Parivar was the subject of both a 2013 *Harvard Business Review* case study and a 2014 INSEAD case study. Michael E. Porter, Mark R. Kramer, and David Lane,

"Social Business at Novartis: Arogya Parivar," *Harvard Business School Case 715–411*, December 2014 (revised October 2017). Amitava Chattopadhyay, Anuj Pasrija, Olivier Jarry, and Jean Wee, "Arogya Parivar: Novartis' BOP Strategy for Healthcare in Rural India," https://cases.insead.edu/arogya-parivar/.

18. Pratibha Desai, "Role of Accredited Social Health Activists in the Improvement of Health Status of Villagers under NRHM in Kolhapur District, Maharashtra," *Journal of Community Medicine & Health Education* 6, no. 2 (April 2016): 416.

19. Michael E. Porter, Mark R. Kramer, and David Lane, "Social Business at Novartis: Arogya Parivar," *Harvard Business School Case 715–411*, December 2014 (revised October 2017).

20. The product portfolio addresses pain and inflammation, infectious diseases, respiratory diseases, malnutrition (iron, calcium, folic acid, and pregnancy supplementation), and pediatric health (anti-infection, deworming, and calcium supplements).

21. An Hodgson, "Top 5 Bottom of the Pyramid Markets," Euromonitor International, March 4, 2017, http://blog.euromonitor.com/2017/03/top-5-bottom-pyramid-markets-diverse-spending-patterns-future-potential.html.

22. World Health Organization, http://www.who.int/mediacentre/factsheets/fs355/en/.

23. World Health Organization, "Global Status Report on Noncommunicable Diseases 2014," 2014.

24. "New Global Study Finds Countries Saving More Lives, Despite a 'Triad of Troubles' in Obesity, Violence, and Mental Illness," Annual Global Burden of Disease Study 2016, Institute for Health Metrics and Evaluation, September 2017, http://www.healthdata.org/news-release/new-global-study-finds-countries-saving-more-lives-despite-'triad-troubles'-obesity.

25. Rachel Nugent and Andrea Feigl, *Where Have All the Donors Gone? Scarce Donor Funding for Non-Communicable Diseases* (Washington, DC: Center for Global Development, 2011): 5.

26. The initial Novartis Access portfolio includes Novartis Pharmaceuticals products Valsartan (hypertension), Vildagliptin (diabetes), and Letrozole (breast cancer), as well as 12 generic medicines from Sandoz: Amlodipine, Bisoprolol, HCT, Furosemide, and Ramipril (heart failure and hypertension); Simvastatin (dyslipidemia); Glimepiride and Metformin (diabetes); Anastrozole and Tamoxifen (breast cancer); Salbutamol (asthma and chronic obstructive pulmonary disease); and Amoxicillin 250 mg dispersible tablets (childhood pneumonia).

27. Access to Medicine Foundation, "Access to Medicine Index," 2016, https://accesstomedicineindex.org.

28. Novartis, "Novartis Access 2017, Two-Year Report" (Preliminary Version), November 2017, https://www.novartis.com/sites/www.novartis.com/files/novartis-access-report-2017.pdf.

29. D. Barakat, P. C. Rockers, T. Vian, M. A. Onyango, R. O. Laing, and V. J. Wirtz, "Access to Asthma Medicines at the Household Level in Eight Counties of Kenya," *International Journal of Tuberculosis and Lung Disease* 22, no. 5 (2018): 585–90.

30. P. C. Rockers, R. O. Laing, and V. J. Wirtz, "Equity in Access to Non-Communicable Disease Medicines: A Cross-Sectional Study in Kenya," *BMJ Global Health* 3, no. 3 (2018): e000828.

31. Harald Nusser, "How Independent Measurement of Access Programs can Help Ensure Their Success," May 16, 2017, https://www.linkedin.com/pulse/how-independent -measurement-access-programs-can-help-ensure-nusser/.

32. Peter C. Rockers, Veronika J. Wirtz, Chukwuemeka A. Umeh, Preethi M. Swamy, and Richard O. Laing, "Industry-Led Access-To-Medicines Initiatives In Low- and Middle-Income Countries: Strategies and Evidence," *Health Affairs* 36, no. 4 (April 2017), http:// sites.bu.edu/evaluatingaccess-accessaccelerated/resources/health-affairs/.

33. The authors explained in their article how they assessed the quality of the evaluations: "Three of us read the full text of each published evaluation that we included and independently determined the quality of evidence rating using the Grading of Recommendations, Assessment, Development and Evaluation (GRADE) system. This system is recommended by the Cochrane Collaboration for use in grading the quality of evidence and the strength of study recommendations. In the GRADE system, study design is a strong determinant of whether the quality of evidence is high, moderate, low, or very low. The quality of evidence from a randomized controlled trial is initially graded as high, while the quality of evidence from an observational study is initially graded as low. The initial quality grading based on study design is then raised or lowered as appropriate, based on other key aspects of the study—for example, how well a randomized controlled trial is implemented and its results reported. We assigned an overall quality rating of high, moderate, low, or very low to each article based on consensus or a majority among the three independent author ratings. Descriptive information was also extracted from each publication, including the aim of the evaluation and the study design."

34. "Evaluation of Novartis Access: An (NCD) Medicine Access Initiative," Boston University School of Public Health, http://sites.bu.edu/evaluatingaccess-novartisaccess/.

35. Peter Rockers, Veronika Wirtz, Taryn Vian, Monica Onyango, Paul Ashigbie, and Richard Laing, "Study Protocol for a Cluster-Randomised Controlled Trial of an NCD Access to Medicines Initiative: Evaluation of Novartis Access in Kenya," *BMJ Open* 6, no. 11 (2016): e013386, http://bmjopen.bmj.com/content/6/11/e013386.long.

36. Those seeking access to the full database may request it through http://sites.bu.edu /evaluatingaccess-novartisaccess/kenya/baseline-database-download/.

37. For more information, see the website of Access Accelerated, www.accessaccelerated .org.

38. Interview with Richard Laing, "Novartis Access 2017: Two-Year Report" (Preliminary Version), November 2017.

39. See, for example, Clayton M. Christensen, Michael Raynor, and Rory McDonald, "What Is Disruptive Innovation?" *Harvard Business Review* 93, no. 12 (December 2015): 44–53

40. Clayton Christensen, H. Baumann, R. Ruggles, and Thomas M. Sadtler, "Disruptive Innovation for Social Change," *Harvard Business Review* 84, no. 12 (December 2006): 94–101, 163.

41. Access to Medicine Foundation, www.accesstomedicinefoundation.org.

42. Access to Medicine Foundation, "Access to Medicine Index," 2016, https://accesstome dicineindex.org.

43. Prashant Yadav, "Health Product Supply Chains in Developing Countries: Diagnosis of the Root Causes of Underperformance and an Agenda for Reform," *Health Systems & Reform* 1, no. 2 (2015): 142–54.

44. Novartis, "SMS for Life," https://www.novartis.com/our-company/corporate-respon sibility/expanding-access-healthcare/novartis-social-business/sms-life.

The Outlook for Universal Health Coverage and the New Health Economy

Christian Franz, Louis Galambos, Ilona Kickbusch,
and Jeffrey L. Sturchio

After noting in the previous chapters what is already under way and what has been proposed in the public health movement toward universal health coverage, you have probably come to a conclusion about whether the UN's goals will be achieved by 2030. You might also have an opinion about the role the private sector is likely to play as this complex, multisectoral, multinational movement continues to evolve. Clearly, the editors of this book are convinced that UHC is a laudable and achievable goal, an objective that promises to have significant positive implications for billions of people around the world—and for their economies, their political systems, their health, and their social relations. The basis for our optimism is grounded in the history of public and private advances in healthcare in the modern era.

Before commenting on some of the salient developments, we want to acknowledge that there has long been a tension in global health between two different conceptions of what the right agenda for change should be. On the one hand was a view of what Anne-Emanuelle Birn has called "biomedical reductionism," with an emphasis on technical campaigns to address specific disease threats, rather than an integrated approach to health as the outcome of the complex interaction of myriad sociopolitical and economic factors. The World Health Organization's constitution, adopted in 1948, reflects these tensions.[1] It includes an expansive and ambitious definition of health as a human right: "Health is a state of complete physical, mental and social well-being and not merely the absence of disease or infirmity. The enjoyment of the highest attainable standard of health is one of the fundamental rights of every human being without distinction of race, religion, political belief, economic or social condition." Further, health is too important to be left to the health sector alone—and is a core responsibility of government: "Health of all peoples is fundamental to the attainment of peace and security and is dependent upon the fullest co-operation of individuals and States . . . Governments have a responsibility for the health of their peoples which can be fulfilled only by the provision of adequate health and social measures."[1]

Under Halfdan Mahler, WHO director-general from 1973 to 1988, the WHO convened a historic conference on primary healthcare in Alma-Ata, Kazakhstan (then in the USSR), which addressed this tension directly, emphasizing the importance of "health for all" as a new guiding ambition for global health.[2] That led to a new focus on equity, intersectoral action, integrated health systems, and a renewed effort to get back to the WHO's constitutional roots in helping to make a reality of health as a human right. In the intervening decades, the interactions of politics and power at the World Health Assembly, between UN organizations and an increasing number of stakeholders, have created a complex tapestry of policies and programs designed to address the most urgent global health concerns. As a consequence of these dynamics, the work of the WHO secretariat and the focus of WHO directors-general was also subject to changing priorities. Epidemiological transitions, technological innovations, new patterns of financing health (with both domestic and donor resources), new organizations, and the particular mix of public health challenges that each country has faced have created a complex mosaic of WHO cooperation with Member States. Global health—and the role of the World Health Organization—is evolving in response to these pressures, with a new emphasis on country ownership and global cooperation in the context of aspirations to achieve the goal of UHC by 2030.[3] Now considered a key component of the sustainable development agenda, UHC will require strong political commitments from governments to ensure that no one is left behind.

From the perspective of this new dynamic of global health governance, our goal has been to explore the impact of the new health economy and the different roles the private sector has played and will continue to play in helping countries navigate the transition to UHC. We realize that this history is a story of conflict and contention, which is understandable, given the importance of what is at stake. We come back to this point below after a brief consideration of the interaction of public and private sector interests in health systems innovation in the years since Alma-Ata.

Learning from the Past

Long before there was a United Nations or a World Health Organization, advances in the medical sciences opened new opportunities to prevent and treat a variety of human diseases. To take advantage of these opportunities, however, there had to be both public and private innovations in policies and performances, changes that seemed at first to be beyond society's resources and capabilities. Over time, governments and private interests found the necessary resources and developed the capabilities necessary to provide citizens with efficient sewage removal and clean water. The results included measurable increases in the elimination of diseases—especially cholera—and in life expectancy. Similar positive effects occurred after the provision of the pasteurized milk that sharply reduced infant mortality.[4] These innovations required just the same types of collective responses—at different levels in different societies in both public and private institutions—that the UHC movement now embraces at the global level. Had they not succeeded, most of us would not be alive today.

As the new science-based medicine evolved in the twentieth century, the opportunities to prevent and treat disease greatly expanded. This was a decisive turning point in world history.[5] Improved living conditions and nutrition combined with advances in medicine. For the first time, physicians could treat internal infections and look forward to the possibility that certain diseases could be eliminated entirely. The new anti-infectives and vaccines of the 1930s, 1940s, and 1950s were especially important means of treating diseases or preventing their transmission, but these innovations could not be delivered around the world without important changes in public and private institutions and their health policies.[6]

Changes came quickly in the developed nations that had the resources, the trained professionals, and the public and private institutions capable of implementing public health measures and delivering healthcare and the new medicines to their populations. Similar changes in the developing nations were slow in coming, because they needed an entirely new array of national, local, and international public and private organizations to ensure the health of their populations. Their situations were, unfortunately, even worse than the conditions in Sierra Leone discussed in chapter 8.[7]

Fortunately, in the aftermath of World War II, the interest in preventing another such devastating conflict had persuaded most of the world's countries to cooperate in new ways. This cooperation was facilitated by an entirely new array of international institutions, including the United Nations, the World Bank, and the International Monetary Fund.[8] A new World Health Organization took a leadership role in developing and maintaining programs to improve water supply and sewage removal, distribution of vaccines and other medicines, and public health and clinical facilities around the world.[9]

Were there obstacles to the new effort to improve global health? Of course there were. Lack of political commitment and shortages of funds and health professionals in many nations left some of the new programs lagging. Economic crises in the 1970s and 1980s made it difficult to continue expanding support and building new primary care facilities. Mistaken priorities set by multilateral economic organizations and national governments weakened public services in many countries. New diseases—especially HIV/AIDS—created new crises in country after country. Most recently, the Ebola outbreak in West Africa in 2014–15 brought awareness of the critical role of health systems strengthening to the fore again, after decades in which disease-specific programs had dominated much of the global health landscape.[10]

But through all of this turmoil and tension, the joint efforts to improve healthcare around the world continued to grow. New nongovernmental organizations (NGOs) emerged to bolster the national and international efforts. Even during the Cold War conflict, areas of agreement were staked out and professionals in medicine, public health, and pharmaceuticals cooperated across national, international, and ethnic/religious boundaries. They created entirely new patterns of cooperation as they promoted healthcare in a world that still blundered, from time to time, close to the outbreak of another great war.[11]

As we face present challenges we often forget what has been achieved. As Hans Rosling reminds us, "it turns out that the world, for all its imperfections, is in a much better state than we might think . . . Step-by-step, year-by-year, the world is improving. Not on every single measure every single year, but as a rule. Though the world faces huge challenges, we have made tremendous progress."[12] By 2016, average global life expectancy at birth in the world's least developed countries had improved since 1960 from 40 years to 64 years. For the nations in the Organisation for Economic Co-operation and Development, the comparable increase was from 67 to 80 years. There were nations that continued to lag greatly behind the most successful countries. The increase for Haiti (from 42 to 60 years) was distressing, as was the change in Sierra Leone. But the populations in both of these countries still had significantly better chances of living longer in 2016 than had been the case half a century before.[13]

Other more refined indicators were also positive. Of particular concern for many years had been the levels of mortality among pregnant women and infants. In recent years, however, a persistent campaign led by the UN and the WHO has logged considerable progress in combating infectious diseases, improving under-5 child mortality and lowering maternal mortality. As the chapter "Healthy Women, Healthy Economies" reminds us, women are both users and providers of healthcare. In both capacities, successful public-private partnerships have already marked a path for future global policies that will achieve faster economic growth as well as healthier lives for women and children.

Similar combinations of public and private resources and expertise have made progress in confronting the HIV/AIDS crisis in developing nations. The development of effective drugs, reporting systems, and treatment routines have transformed a life-threatening infection to a chronic disease for millions of survivors. Without that combination of publicly funded basic research, privately funded medical research and development, and public-private efforts to deliver lifesaving drugs and monitor their use, the HIV/AIDS pandemic had the potential to become the counterpart of the Black Death.[14] Ebola presents a different sort of challenge, and the lessons learned in coping with HIV/AIDS have had a visible impact on the response to this relatively new disease.[15] Lessons can and have been learned about prevention and treatment of disease, and the first and most powerful lesson is that sustained, multisectoral, public-private coalitions can provide society with powerful tools for disease prevention and treatment.[16]

Looking to the Future

The essays in this book provide a variety of perspectives on how such public-private cooperation will help countries achieve their goal of universal health coverage by 2030. We began with the conceptual framework of the "new health economy" (as proposed by Ilona Kickbusch and

Christian Franz), which looks holistically at the resources, services, and products devoted to health in national contexts and the impact these have on the overall economy—a message that is important not just to national-level health policy makers but also to those who work in economic and fiscal policy. Successive chapters explored different dimensions of the private sector role in achieving universal health coverage. Pascal Zurn, Jim Campbell, and colleagues focused in particular on the impact that creating jobs for health workers has in improving population health and social cohesion and also in increasing economic growth. Seeing the health workforce—both public and private—as an investment, rather than a cost, opens the door to a richer understanding of how countries can accelerate progress toward UHC.

The chapter by Nathan J. Blanchet, Adeel Ishtiaq, and Cicely Thomas offered a pragmatic approach to understanding how to engage the private sector successfully in advancing UHC, based on an analysis of the political, organizational, economic, and legal/regulatory challenges faced in different national contexts. The authors concluded that achieving UHC will require an ability for public officials to provide stewardship for mixed health systems that bring both public and private resources together to deliver quality health services for all. Donika Dimovska and John Campbell, Jr., provided a deeper dive into how private sector innovations are helping countries to achieve UHC, through an analysis of more than 1,300 initiatives in 130 countries that reported to the Center for Health Market Innovations (Results for Development). Their paper shows how private sector models are important sources of experimentation, learning, and potential system-level health impact. They called for continued collaboration, adaptation, and co-creation of private sector solutions that can complement what governments are already doing to improve the financing and delivery of quality health services to broader segments of their populations.

The chapters by Michael Fürst; Felicia Marie Knaul, Belén Garijo, Christine Bugos, Héctor Arreola-Ornelas, and Yasmine Rouai; Justin McCarthy and Snow Yang; and Harald Nusser explored the relationship between the private sector and UHC with case studies of innovative ways in which pharmaceutical companies are already responding to the challenges and opportunities of improving population health, through new business models that support UHC by increasing access to medicines and helping to strengthen healthcare systems. Michael Fürst provided an astute analysis that begins with the premise that pharmaceutical companies can combine an ethical approach to supporting the right to health with a portfolio approach to addressing the challenges of improving access to medicines in countries at different levels of economic development. In this way, companies can find new opportunities to help countries achieve UHC in a sustainable way. The chapters by Knaul et al. and McCarthy and Yang showed how Merck KGaA and Pfizer, respectively, have worked with a range of partners to support "healthy women, healthy economies" and to address oncology in lower- and middle-income countries and cardiovascular disease in China. Harald Nusser's review of Novartis's social business initiatives demonstrated how the private sector is supporting governments in moving toward UHC by developing sustainable businesses that deliver care to underserved populations, while also helping to build integrated and efficient systems to supply health technologies to patients in resource-constrained settings.

Finally, Sowmya Kadandale and Robert Marten and K. Srinath Reddy offered case studies of how two countries at very different levels of development are approaching UHC. In Sierra Leone, government is necessarily focused on the basics of establishing effective healthcare infrastructure while recovering from years of political instability and the added strain of an Ebola outbreak in 2014–15. With a nascent private sector, there are limits to how much the public sector in Sierra Leone can depend on their support as they rebuild their health system and plan for implementing UHC. This case suggests that the sharp constraints on both the public and private sectors in Sierra Leone call for a new order of institutions and a new approach among development partners to help the country plan with long-term sustainability in mind. Regarding India, on the other hand, K. Srinath Reddy provided a detailed and informative overview of how India's ambitious plans for UHC will build in part on a vibrant private health sector that can partner effectively with government to reach millions more Indians by 2030.

If history is a good guide to the future—as it frequently is—optimism about achieving universal health coverage is well placed. The growing role of the private sector and public-private partnerships is firmly established—with health constituting one of the largest economic sectors worldwide. The accomplishments in healthcare, in sustained economic development, and in gender equality will vary from country to country, from region to region, from locality to locality. Sustained political commitment from governments will be required to ensure that no one is left out. The path will not be entirely smooth, given the complexity of balancing the social goals of UHC and the agendas of private sector actors. Standards and regulations will be critical, as governments and their partners work together to ensure responsible stewardship of mixed health systems. Just as not all governments always act responsibly to invest in the health of their people, the private sector does not always act collectively or responsibly. We suggest that both the public and private sectors have in the recent past learned a great deal about cooperation and about the new institutions we need to foster that common effort. Still, as Richard Horton has trenchantly observed, "UHC is not a destination . . . it's a constant political struggle."[17] The results will never be definitive, as some experiments will fail and others succeed, but they will continue to be positive as the UHC movement presses forward to 2030.

As these essays demonstrate, we are confident that in the coming decades, the new health economy will provide an important supporting framework for improvements in population health. The private sector, in all its varieties, will continue to be an essential partner to governments and civil society in expanding the scope and effectiveness of the UHC movement as it pursues the bold vision of "health for all" articulated 40 years ago at Alma-Ata.

NOTES

1. "Constitution of the World Health Organization," 1948. http://www.who.int/governance/eb/who_constitution_en.pdf.
2. Declaration of Alma-Ata: International Conference on Primary Health Care, Alma-Ata, USSR, 6–12 September 1978 (Geneva: World Health Organization, 1978). http://www.who.int/publications/almaata_declaration_en.pdf. Accessed 20 July 2018.
3. Ariel Pablos-Méndez and Mario Raviglione, "A new world health era," Global Health: Science and Practice 6 (2018): 8–16.
4. Angus Deaton, The Great Escape: Health, Wealth and the Origins of Inequality (Princeton, NJ: Princeton University Press, 2013): 93, 95–97. Life expectancy (from birth) increased globally from 31 years in 1900 to 49 years by 1950: Angus Maddison, Contours of the World Economy, 1–2030 AD: Essays in Macro-Economic History (Oxford: Oxford University Press, 2007), 72.
5. Louis Galambos and Jeffrey L. Sturchio, "The pharmaceutical industry in the twentieth century: a reappraisal of the sources of innovation," History and Technology 13, no. 2 (1996): 83–100; Ralph Landau, Basil Achilladelis, and Alexander Scriabine, eds.,

Pharmaceutical Innovation: Revolutionizing Human Health (Philadelphia, PA: Chemical Heritage Press, 1999); and Walter E. Sneader, *Drug Discovery (The History)* (New York: John Wiley & Sons, Inc., 2007).

6. Stanley A. Plotkin, ed. *History of Vaccine Development* (New York: Springer Science + Business Media, 2011); Plotkin and Edward A. Mortimer, Jr., eds., *Vaccines* (Philadelphia, PA: W. B. Saunders, 1994); Maurice R. Hilleman, "Six decades of vaccine development—a personal history," *Nature medicine* 4, no. 5 (1998): 507–14; Hilleman, "Vaccines in historic evolution and perspective: a narrative of vaccine discoveries," *Vaccine* 18, no. 15 (2000): 1436–47; and Louis Galambos and Jane Eliot Sewell, *Networks of Innovation: Vaccine Development at Merck, Sharp and Dohme, and Mulford, 1895–1995* (Cambridge: Cambridge University Press, 1997).

7. See Kadandale and Marten, chapter 8 in this book. See also Paul Farmer's account of the problems in Haiti, *Pathologies of Power: Health, Human Rights, and the New War on the Poor* (Berkeley: University of California Press, 2003).

8. On the World Bank, later the World Bank Group, see Devesh Kapur, John P. Lewis, and Richard Webb, eds., *The World Bank: Its First Half Century* (Washington, DC: Brookings, 1997). On the IMF, see Margaret Garritseen deVries, *The IMF in a Changing World, 1945–85* (Washington, DC: IMF, 1986); and Harold James, *International Monetary Cooperation since Bretton Woods* (Oxford: Oxford University Press, 1996). On the United Nations and the World Health Organization see World Health Organization, *The First Ten Years of the World Health Organization* (Geneva: WHO, 1958), available at http://apps.who.int/iris/handle/10665/37089.

9. See Amy Staples, *The Birth of Development: How the World Bank, Food and Agricultural Organization and the World Health Organization Changed the World, 1945–1965* (Kent, Ohio: Kent State University Press, 2006). For additional information on the history of the WHO, see http://www.who.int/global_health_histories/en/.

10. Randall M. Packard, *A History of Global Health: Interventions into the Lives of Other Peoples* (Baltimore: Johns Hopkins University Press, 2016).

11. For personal accounts of some of the leading campaigns, see D. A. Henderson, *Smallpox: The Death of a Disease* (Amherst: Prometheus Books, 2009); William H. Foege, *House on Fire: The Fight to Eradicate Smallpox* (Berkeley: University of California Press, 2011); and Peter Piot, *No Time to Lose: A Life in Pursuit of Deadly Viruses* (New York: W. W. Norton & Co., 2012).

12. Hans Rosling with Ola Rosling and Anna Rosling Rönnlund, *Factfulness: Ten Reasons We're Wrong about the World—And Why Things Are Better Than You Think* (New York: Flatiron Books, 2018), 13.

13. World Bank, Life Expectancy at Birth. https://data.worldbank.org/indicator/SP .DYN.LEOO.IN.

14. World Health Organization, *HIV/AIDS, Treat All: Policy Adoption and Implementation Status in Countries* (November 2017). http://www.who.int/hiv/pub/arv/treat-all -uptake/en/.

15. World Health Organization, "WHO Secretariat response to the Report of the Ebola Interim Assessment Panel" (August 19, 2015). www.who.int?esr/resources/publications /ebola/who-response-to-ebola-report.pdf. See also Lawrence O. Gostin et al., "Toward

a common secure future: four global commissions in the wake of Ebola," *PLoS Medicine* (May 2016): e1002042; and Olushayo Oluseun Olu, "The Ebola Virus Disease outbreak in West Africa: a wake-up call to revitalize implementation of the International Health Regulations," *Frontiers in Public Health*, 4 (2016), 120.

16. See, for example, National Academies of Sciences, Engineering, and Medicine, *The role of public–private partnerships in health systems strengthening: workshop summary* (Washington, DC: National Academies Press, 2016); *Engaging the private sector and developing partnerships to advance health and the Sustainable Development Goals: proceedings of a workshop series* (Washington, DC: National Academies Press, 2017); *Exploring partnership governance in global health: proceedings of a workshop* (Washington, DC: National Academies Press, 2018); and Jo Ivey Boufford, Renuka Gadde, Christian Acemah, George Alleyne, Simon Bland, and Brenda Colatrella, "A proposed framework for developing health-focused public-private partnerships based on national Sustainable Development Priorities," NAM Perspectives. Discussion Paper (Washington, DC: National Academy of Medicine, 2017). https://nam.edu/wp-content/uploads/2017/07/A-Proposed-Framework-for-Developing-Health-Focused-Public-Private-Partnerships.pdf.

17. Quoted in Dana Kerecman Myers, "Fogarty's 50 years and new frontiers," *Global Health Now*, 2 May 2018. https://www.globalhealthnow.org/2018-05/fogartys-50-years-and-new-frontiers. See also Richard Horton, "Offline: UHC—one promise and two misunderstandings," *Lancet* 391 (7 April 2018): 1342.

Contributors

Jean-Louis Arcand is Professor of International Economics at the Graduate Institute of International and Development Studies in Geneva. He holds a PhD in economics from the Massachusetts Institute of Technology. His research focuses on the microeconomics of development, with a current focus on evaluating the impact of social programs in West Africa and the Maghreb.

Héctor Arreola-Ornelas is an Economics Research Coordinator at the Mexican Health Foundation (FUNSALUD), where he works on the project Universality and Competition in Health. A health economist with more than a decade of experience in government and research, Arreola-Ornelas is also an Associate Researcher and Member of the Board of Tómatelo a Pecho, a nongovernmental organization based in Mexico that focuses on reducing the lethality of breast cancer in Latin America through early detection and effective treatment.

Nathan J. Blanchet is a Program Director at Results for Development and a Visiting Scientist at the Harvard T. H. Chan School of Public Health. A health economist with more than 15 years of experience, he leads the teams focused on the design and implementation of national health insurance and other means of achieving universal health coverage, including reform of health benefits policies, strengthening primary healthcare, and integrating standalone health programs and private health services into domestic health financing systems in low- and middle-income countries. Blanchet holds a Doctor of Science (ScD) degree in global health and population from the Harvard T. H. Chan School of Public Health and an MA in international relations from the Johns Hopkins University School of Advanced International Studies.

Christine Bugos is Vice President of Global Policy and External Affairs at EMD Serono, the North America biopharma business of Merck KGaA. Bugos joined EMD Serono in February 2012 after spending over

20 years with Sanofi and its predecessor companies, where she last served as Vice President for Global Institutional Relations. Over the past 15 years, Bugos worked in international public affairs, with increasing geographical scope and a strong focus on emerging markets. Earlier in her career, Christine worked in various roles within US Medical Affairs as well as in Global Marketing and Medical. Prior to joining the biopharmaceutical industry, Christine was a clinical pharmacist. She has Doctor of Pharmacy and Master of Business Administration degrees. She is fluent in French, English, and Spanish and proficient in Hungarian.

Jim Campbell is director of the Health Workforce Department at the World Health Organization (WHO). He oversees the development and implementation of global public goods, evidence, and tools to inform national and international investments in the education, development, and retention of the health and social sector workforce in pursuit of global health security, universal health coverage, and the Sustainable Development Goals that were established at the 70th United Nations General Assembly in 2015. He coordinates the Global Health Workforce Network in engaging member states and relevant partners in the WHO's work.

John Campbell, Jr., is a scientist turned global health innovations specialist with more than eight years of experience conducting quantitative research, most recently focused on health systems strengthening and capacity building in emerging economies. Campbell is a program officer currently overseeing Results for Development's (R4D) Center for Health Market Innovations database and research portfolio. He holds an MS in international health policy from Georgetown University and a BS in biochemistry from North Carolina State University.

Ibadat Dhillon is a Technical Officer in the Department of Health Workforce at the World Health Organization, with a background in law and public health. Dhillon's current work focuses on health workforce education and migration. He has previously served as a health advisor for the Danish Government, the Irish Government, and the Centers for Disease Control and Prevention in the United States. Dhillon received his JD from Washington University in St. Louis, LLM from Georgetown University, and MPH from Emory University.

Donika Dimovska has more than 10 years of experience in health and education with a focus on promoting the uptake and scale-up of innovations and their effective integration into systems. A senior program director at Results for Development (R4D), Donika leads R4D's Scaling Innovations practice area. She holds an MA in international affairs from Syracuse University's Maxwell School of Citizenship and Public Affairs and a BA from the State University of New York.

Christian Franz is Managing Director of the data and policy analysis firm CPC Analytics, which is based in Berlin and Pune. In global health he has worked and published on the commercial determinants of health, the role of banking for health, and on Germany's role in global health. Currently, he is facilitating the Community of Practice on NCDs and commercial determinants of health for the World Health Organization GCM/NCD. At the German Institute for Economic Research (DIW Berlin), Franz worked on income inequality and an economic analysis of the German election in 2017. He has a BA in business administration and economics from Ludwig Maximilian University in Munich and an MA from Hertie School of Governance Berlin.

Michael Fürst has close to 20 years of experience in corporate responsibility (CR) and business ethics and is currently responsible for CR strategy and innovation at Novartis AG. He works primarily on CR strategy, access to medicines, inclusive business model innovation, measurement and evaluation, innovative finance in healthcare, and human rights and stakeholder engagement. Fürst helped Novartis to develop and implement innovative business models such as Novartis Access and Healthy Family (e.g., Arogya Parivar) and other programs. He is an author and editor of articles and books in the areas of CR, social entrepreneurship, access to medicines, integrity management, and risk and good governance, and he is a Social Entrepreneur in Residence at INSEAD. Fürst has a PhD with honors (summa cum laude) and was awarded the German Max Weber Prize for Business Ethics (2006) for his scholarly work.

Louis Galambos is Research Professor of History and Co-director of the Institute for Applied Economics, Global Health, and the Study of Business Enterprise at Johns Hopkins University. He has written extensively on modern institutional development in America, the rise of the bureaucratic state, and the evolution of the professions. Among other publications, his books include *Networks of Innovation; Medicine, Science, and Merck*; and (with Jeffrey L. Sturchio) *Noncommunicable Diseases in the Developing World: Addressing Gaps in Global Policy and Research*. In 2018, he published *Eisenhower: Becoming the Leader of the Free World*. His major current interest is American innovation and the role professionals have played in enabling the United States to address problems at home and abroad in the twentieth and twenty-first centuries. He has received grants from the NEH and NHPRC, and he currently has a grant from the Kauffman Foundation (to study American capitalism) and the IFPMA (to study universal healthcare).

Belén Garijo is a member of the Executive Board of Merck KGaA, Darmstadt, Germany, and CEO of the Healthcare business. She assumed Executive Board responsibility for Group Human Resources in September 2017 and is an advocate for diversity and women's health. Before joining Merck KGaA, Garijo served as Senior Vice President, Global Operations Europe, at Sanofi-Aventis in France, where she was also a member of the Management Committee of the Sanofi-Aventis Group and of the Management Board of the Sanofi-Pasteur vaccines joint venture with Merck Sharp & Dohme (MSD). Prior to that, she worked in research and development for eight years, initially as Medical Director of the Abbott Laboratories Spanish affiliate, before moving to lead International Medical Affairs at Abbott headquarters in Illinois. Garijo is a medical doctor specializing in clinical pharmacology.

Adeel Ishtiaq is a Senior Program Officer at Results for Development (R4D) in Washington, DC. He focuses on reform in healthcare financing, service delivery, and governance mechanisms in countries pursuing universal health coverage and seeking to sustainably finance pressing health needs in priority disease areas. Currently, in Nigeria, Tanzania, Uganda, Cambodia, and Kenya, Ishtiaq's work on primary healthcare services in the private sector centers on mitigating financial barriers for users at the point of care and considering "health system intermediaries" to connect private providers with public sector mechanisms for financing and oversight. Ishtiaq holds an MA in international relations from Yale University and a BSc in economics from the Lahore University of Management Sciences.

Sowmya Kadandale has extensive experience working in international and nonprofit settings. She is currently Chief of Health at UNICEF Indonesia, prior to which she was with the World Health Organization (WHO) for a decade, advising countries on strengthening their health systems. Kadandale has been actively engaged in a variety of programs across Africa, Asia, and Europe; her most recent WHO posting was in Sierra Leone in support of the government's Ebola response and recovery efforts.

Ilona Kickbusch is Director of the Global Health Centre at the Graduate Institute of International and Development Studies in Geneva. She chairs the International Advisory Board on Global Health of the German Ministry of Health. She is co-chair of UHC2030 and is a member of the Global Preparedness Monitoring Board and the World Health Organization's High-Level Independent Commission on Noncommunicable Diseases. In 2016 she was awarded the Cross of the Order of Merit of the Federal Republic of Germany (*Bundesverdienstkreuz*) in recognition of her invaluable contributions to innovation in governance for global health and global health diplomacy.

Felicia Marie Knaul has a PhD from Harvard University in economics and is an international health economist and expert in Latin American health systems and social sectors. She is Director of the Institute for Advanced Study of the Americas and Professor at the Miller School of Medicine at the University of Miami. She has produced more than 200 academic and policy publications; chaired the *Lancet* Commission on Global Access to Palliative Care and Pain Relief; was a leading member of the *Lancet* Commission on Women and Health; and led the *Lancet* series on health system reform in Mexico. Knaul maintains a strong program of research and advocacy focused on the Latin American and Caribbean region, especially in Mexico, where she is Senior Economist at the Mexican Health Foundation (FUNSALUD), member of the National Academy of Medicine of Mexico, and Level III of the Mexican National System of Researchers. She is the Founding President of Tómatelo a Pecho, a Mexican nongovernmental organization that undertakes and promotes research, advocacy, awareness, and early detection initiatives for breast cancer in Latin America.

Jeremy Lauer is an economist in the Department of Health Systems Governance and Financing at the World Health Organization. He has an AB in mathematics and philosophy from St. John's College in Annapolis, Maryland, an MSc and MA in economics and in agricultural and applied economics from the University of Wisconsin, Madison, and a PhD from Erasmus University Rotterdam on the use of population models in cost-effectiveness analysis. Recently, Lauer studied the economics of fiscal space for workforce expansion, as well as interactions between the health system and the broader economy, for the UN Secretary-General's High-Level Commission on Health Employment and Economic Growth. He is currently working on the economics of taxes in health policy.

Robert Marten is a Council on Foreign Affairs Hitachi Fellow based in Tokyo at the Japan Center for International Exchange, studying Japan's role in global health. He previously worked for the World Health Organization in Sierra Leone on health systems strengthening in the post-Ebola phase. Prior to this position, he worked at the Rockefeller Foundation in New York. He managed a $20 million grant portfolio focused on global health policy, including research and advocacy efforts to embed health systems and universal health coverage within the post-2015 development agenda as well as the foundation's response to the Ebola crisis.

Justin McCarthy is Senior Vice President, Patient and Health Impact group, part of the Strategy and Commercial Operations division at Pfizer. Prior to this role, he was Senior Vice President, Global Policy and International Public Affairs, responsible for defining Pfizer's public policy positions and advancing government and public affairs strategies internationally. McCarthy has been with Pfizer for 25 years and was formerly Chief Counsel for Pfizer's Worldwide Research and Development division, advising on regulatory, licensing, and clinical trial issues and overseeing global intellectual property activities. He serves on the boards of the National Pharmaceutical Council, Business Council for International Understanding, the Global Intellectual Property Center, Vivli Inc., the US Council for International Business, and the harmonization subcommittee of the Health and Human Services Secretary's Advisory Committee on Human Research Protections. Before joining Pfizer, McCarthy was an associate in the law firm of Keller and Heckman. He holds a BA in pharmacy from the University of Rhode Island and a law degree from the Catholic University of America.

Harald Nusser, PhD, MBA, has been leading Novartis Access since June 2015. Since October 2016, he has also taken on responsibility for the Novartis Malaria Initiative, the Novartis Healthy Family programs, SMS for Life, and NGO supply, which have been combined with Novartis Access into a newly formed unit called Novartis Social Business. Nusser started his career at Schering AG in 2000 as a mathematician in global research and development. Having worked in both exploratory research as well as clinical research, he held positions of increasing responsibility between 2004 and 2010 in corporate strategy and strategic planning at Schering AG and, as of 2006, at Bayer. As Head of Portfolio Management, he managed the Holistic R&D Portfolio Review for Bayer Pharma and the annual strategic planning process for Bayer HealthCare, led restructuring activities, and became Managing Director for Bayer spol. s r.o. in Slovakia in 2010. Starting in 2012, Dr. Nusser led the Bayer HealthCare business (comprising Animal Health, Radiology, Diabetes Care, OTC and Pharmaceuticals) in sub-Saharan Africa, Uruguay, Paraguay, Bolivia, Peru, Laos, Myanmar, and Cambodia before joining Sandoz International, the Novartis generics and biosimilars division, in June 2015 as Global Head, Novartis Access. Nusser is a member of the Novartis Access to Medicines Committee. He graduated with a PhD in mathematics from the Free University of Berlin in 1998 and with an MBA from the University of Bradford, United Kingdom, in 2003.

K. Srinath Reddy is President, Public Health Foundation of India (PHFI), and formerly headed the Department of Cardiology at All India Institute of Medical Sciences. He served as the First Bernard Lown Visiting Professor of Cardiovascular Health at the Harvard School of Public Health (2009–13) and is an Adjunct Professor at Harvard and Emory Universities and an Honorary Professor of Medicine at the University of Sydney. He has served on many expert panels for the World Health Organization and has been President of the World Heart Federation (2013–14). He chaired the High-Level Expert Group on Universal Health Coverage for the Planning Commission of India. Reddy is a member of the Leadership Council of the Sustainable Development Solutions Network (SDSN), established to assist the United Nations in developing the post-2015 goals, and he chairs the Thematic Group on Health in the SDSN. He is a member of the Global Panel on Agriculture and Food Systems for Nutrition. He has published more than 500 scientific papers and is the author of multiple books and book chapters. Reddy's several honors include the WHO Director-General's Award and the Luther Terry Medal of the American Cancer Society for Outstanding Contributions to Global Tobacco Control and the Queen Elizabeth Medal for health promotion. He was conferred Padma Bhushan by the President of India in 2005.

Yasmine Rouai is Associate Director, Global Health Policy, of Government and Public Affairs at EMD Serono. In her current role, she works on increasing internal capabilities for public-private partnerships as well as on Healthy Women, Healthy Economies, an initiative that originated in the Asia-Pacific Economic Cooperation Forum and tackles women's health barriers through policy interventions to increase their labor force participation. Prior to joining EMD Serono in 2015, Rouai started her career at the World Bank, where she worked on economic development issues affecting the Middle East and North Africa region. She also served as Global Trade Specialist at Sandler Trade LLC, where she focused on trade policy and advocacy for US trade preference programs. Rouai holds both an MA in international commerce and policy from George Mason University and an MS in finance from Johns Hopkins University. She received her BA from George Washington University in international affairs, with a concentration in Middle Eastern studies.

Jeffrey L. Sturchio is President and CEO at Rabin Martin, a global health strategy consulting firm; a visiting scholar at the Institute for Applied Economics, Global Health, and the Study of Business Enterprise at Johns Hopkins University; and former President and CEO of the Global Health Council. Before joining the council in 2009, Sturchio was Vice President of Corporate Responsibility at Merck & Co., Inc., and president of The Merck Company Foundation. He currently serves as chairman of the Corporate Council on Africa, chairman of the BroadReach Institute for Training and Education, and as a member of the boards of ACHAP, the Science History Institute, and Friends of the Global Fight Against AIDS, Tuberculosis and Malaria. Sturchio is a senior associate at the Center for Strategic and International Studies; a principal of the Modernizing Foreign Assistance Network; Fellow of the American Association for the Advancement of Science; a member of the Council on Foreign Relations and the Arthur W. Page Society; and an advisor to amfAR, Intrahealth International, and the Partnership for Quality Medical Donations. He received an AB in history from Princeton University and a PhD in the history and sociology of science from the University of Pennsylvania. His publications include *Noncommunicable Diseases in the Developing World: Addressing Gaps in Global Policy and Research* (edited with L. Galambos, Johns Hopkins University Press, 2013).

Cicely Thomas is a Program Director at Results for Development (R4D), where her work focuses broadly on health system strengthening and financing, with a focus on mixed health systems, health benefit package reform, and subnational health system capacity building. She leads the Private Sector Engagement Collaborative of the Joint Learning Network's Primary Health Care Initiative, providing technical assistance to individual country partners aiming to achieve universal health coverage. She also leads work in sustainable health financing in Ghana and Guinea, including work on costing and resource mobilization. Thomas holds an MSc in health, population, and society and an MA in geography and art history.

Tana Wuliji is a senior health workforce specialist, policy advisor, and researcher. As a Technical Officer in the Health Workforce Department at the World Health Organization, she is responsible for coordinating the Working for Health program—a five-year ILO, OECD, WHO action plan for health employment and inclusive economic growth to expand and transform the health and social workforce. She has advised on health workforce planning, supported workforce strategy implementation, and led research on health workforce education, training, regulation, performance, and productivity in 15 countries in Africa, Asia, and the Middle East. She received her PhD from the University College London and a BPharm from the University of Otago.

Snow Yang is Director (Asia Pacific and China), Global Policy and International Public Affairs, at Pfizer's Corporate Affairs division in New York. She currently leads health policy development for all 15 markets across the Asia-Pacific region, including Japan, China, and Korea. Her responsibilities mainly focus on establishing Pfizer's public policy positions and building partnerships with a wide range of cross-sectoral stakeholders to promote pro-innovation healthcare policies and improve patient access to quality medicines. Prior to this role, she was Global Market Access Lead for Inflammation at Pfizer's Specialty Care Business Unit (SCBU) Market Access, driving and implementing payer and access strategy for Pfizer's Inflammation Portfolio outside the United States. Through her various jobs at Pfizer headquarters and China, Merck & Co., Inc., and IMS Consulting, she has gained extensive experience that spans clinical development, commercialization, market access, and public affairs. She holds an MBA from Wharton at the University of Pennsylvania.

Pascal Zurn is Health Labour Market Unit Coordinator in the Health Workforce Department at the World Health Organization. This unit is responsible for providing policy advice and technical support for the development of health workforce policies, plans, and capacity-building initiatives, with a particular focus on health labor market analysis, health workforce planning, forecasting, and modeling. Zurn is a health economist with an MA in health economics from the University of York and a PhD in economics from the University of Lausanne. He joined the World Health Organization in August 2001.

Index